# Toxoplasmosis: A Comprehensive Clinical Guide

# Toxoplasmosis: A Comprehensive Clinical Guide

Editor: Lawson Williams

MURPHY & MOORE
www.murphy-moorepublishing.com

www.murphy-moorepublishing.com

MURPHY & MOORE

**Cataloging-in-Publication Data**

Toxoplasmosis : a comprehensive clinical guide / edited by Lawson Williams.
p. cm.
Includes bibliographical references and index.
ISBN 978-1-63987-536-8
1. Toxoplasmosis. 2. Toxoplasmosis--Diagnosis. 3. Toxoplasmosis--Treatment.
4. Coccidiosis. I. Williams, Lawson.
RC186.T75 T69 2022
616.936--dc23



Murphy & Moore Publishing,
1 Rockefeller Plaza,
New York City, NY 10020, USA

ISBN 978-1-63987-536-8 (Hardback)

# Contents

# Preface

The disease caused by the Toxoplasma gondii parasite is termed as toxoplasmosis. A few of its symptoms are body aches, headache, fever and fatigue. Transmission of this parasite can occur through exposure to infected cat feces, consumption of contaminated meat which has not been cooked adequately, and from a mother to her child during pregnancy. The risk factors for toxoplasmosis are taking immunosuppressant medications, chemotherapy and HIV/AIDS. Most healthy people do not require serious medical help, but people with a weakened immune system are at risk of suffering from severe complications such as seizures and encephalitis. This book elucidates the concepts and innovative models around prospective developments with respect to the research on toxoplasmosis. It presents studies on this disease in the most comprehensible and easy to understand language. This book includes contributions of experts and scientists which will provide innovative insights into this field.

The information contained in this book is the result of intensive hard work done by researchers in this field. All due efforts have been made to make this book serve as a complete guiding source for students and researchers. The topics in this book have been comprehensively explained to help readers understand the growing trends in the field.

I would like to thank the entire group of writers who made sincere efforts in this book and my family who supported me in my efforts of working on this book. I take this opportunity to thank all those who have been a guiding force throughout my life.

**Editor**

# 1

# *Toxoplasma gondii* and Schizophrenia: A Relationship that is not Ruled Out

Antonio Sorlozano-Puerto and
Jose Gutierrez-Fernandez

**Abstract**

Over recent years, it has been proposed that some diseases of unknown origin, such as schizophrenia, may be caused by persistent chronic infections coupled with a genetic component and may be perpetuated by the immune system. This hypothesis is supported by epidemiological and biological evidence on the exposure of schizophrenics to infectious diseases during prenatal or postnatal periods, including *Toxoplasma gondii*, chlamydia, human herpes virus, human endogenous retroviruses, parvovirus B19, mumps, and flu viruses. This growing list of microbes will undoubtedly continue to increase in the future. Linking infection to schizophrenia is a complex challenge that requires further experimental and epidemiological research. *T. gondii* is the infectious agent that has most frequently been related to neuropsychiatric disorders, including schizophrenia, and it is considered to represent a highly useful model to analyze the influence of a microorganism on human behavior and the development of psychiatric disease. It may also help to detect patient subpopulations susceptible to treatment with specific antimicrobials by improving definition of the differential phenotype of the disease, and it offers the possibility of a preventive approach.

**Keywords:** schizophrenia, *Toxoplasma gondii*, antibodies, behavior, cytokine, neurotransmitter, gene-infection interaction

## 1. Introduction

Over the past few years, it has been proposed by some authors that schizophrenia may be caused by central nervous system (CNS) disorders during neurodevelopment (i.e., congenital) or during the postnatal period, at least in some patient subgroups [1]. These disorders may be related to environmental exposure to toxic products, radiation, stress, fetal hypoxia, nutritional problems, infections (especially when chronic and persistent), and/or, according to more recent data, gut microbiota [2, 3]. Any of these exposures could possibly affect cognitive functions and behavior patterns with important neuropsychiatric consequences, including irreversible neurological lesions leading to neuronal dysfunction, behavior problems, mental retardation, learning difficulties, or mood disorders [4–9]. Participation by microbial agents in the development of schizophrenia is suggested by medical evidence, with prenatal or perinatal infection being the most frequent cause of severe congenital malformations and mental impairment [10]. Their involvement is also supported by epidemiological evidence on the exposure of schizophrenic patients to *T. gondii*, chlamydia, human herpes virus, human endogenous retroviruses, parvovirus B19, and rubella, mumps, or influenza viruses, among other microorganisms [11].

According to current pathogenic models, microorganisms may produce various inflammatory and/or immunological disorders in the infected brain, giving rise to neurotransmitter synthesis disorders with important clinical repercussions [7]. Schizophrenia has been related to the production of inflammatory cytokines that alter the synthesis of dopamine and other neurotransmitters [12] and to fetal neuronal tissue damage due to the transplacental transfer of maternal antibodies, which might underlie development of the disease decades later [13]. This association with inflammatory and immunologic disorders has been observed in studies of animal models and human cells. Thus, maternal infection of mice and rats during pregnancy was associated with behavioral disorders in the offspring that were very similar to those reported in schizophrenic patients. Various studies in murine models revealed an association between prenatal infection and marked deficits in sensory information processing, in the expression of certain neurotransmitters (e.g., dopamine) and of cytokines, and in the immune function, all of which emerged in the offspring. Their onset is at an age equivalent to human adolescence and is earlier, with more severe effects, in male *versus* female rats, and these alterations can be reverted by the administration of antipsychotic drugs. In short, the fetus can be damaged by numerous infectious agents, whether or not they are primarily neurotropic, which may favor in a direct or immune-mediated manner the development of neurological damage, disorders in neurotransmitter expression, and modifications in sensory information processing [14].

There is intense and increasing research interest in the relationship between schizophrenia and infectious agents. Irreversible mild or severe neurophysiologic alterations may result from fetal infection, maternal infection with secondary fetal involvement *via* inflammatory and/or immunological mechanisms, or postnatal infection and may lead to the emergence of schizophrenia over the years. The full elucidation of these associations may allow specific antimicrobial treatments to be added to current symptomatic (or antipsychotic) treatments for these patients [5], potentially offering a preventive and curative approach to the disease, given that they would act on known and treatable etiologic factors.

*T. gondii* is the infectious agent that has most frequently been related to neuropsychiatric disorders, including schizophrenia, and it is considered to represent a useful model to analyze the influence of a microorganism on human behavior and the development of psychiatric disease [15]. It is an obligate intracellular protozoa belonging to the *Coccidia* subclass of the phylum *Apicomplexa* and causes toxoplasmosis. Its definitive hosts are cats and other felines, which are the only animals in which the sexual stage of their life cycle takes place (in intestines), forming oocysts that are eliminated through the feces. Hot-blooded vertebrates such as birds and other mammals, including humans, are intermediate hosts. Humans can become infected by various pathways, such as: the intake of undercooked meat containing latent forms of the parasite (bradyzoites in tissue cysts), fresh food (e.g., fruit and vegetables), or water contaminated with oocysts from cat feces; blood transfusions; transplantation of solid organ or stem cells, or transplacental transmission. Upon reaching tissues, *T. gondii* rapidly replicates in the form of tachyzoites until tissue proliferation and expansion of the parasite are impeded by the immune response, after which its replication slows and it remains in tissue cysts in latent or bradyzoite form. Cysts are most frequently found in skeletal muscle, myocardium, CNS, and eyes and are responsible for persistent infection [16, 17].

Primary infection usually takes place during childhood, when only a small percentage of people show symptoms, which are mild and include general discomfort, lethargy, cervical lymphadenopathy, and/or eye disease, among others. Most parasitized individuals remain asymptomatic for a long time period, even throughout their life, and host the latent form of *T. gondii*. However, chronic infection can be reactivated in immunocompromised individuals (AIDS, transplanted, and oncology patients, etc.), giving rise to various symptoms and even, in death. This reactivation is often associated with nervous system symptoms, such as Guillain-Barré syndrome, diffuse encephalopathy, meningoencephalitis, or brain abscesses [17, 18]. Human parasitizations, although generally considered asymptomatic, may cause behavioral disorders and the development of a psychiatric disease such as schizophrenia due to damage resulting from the initial infection, from the host immune response to the parasite, or from the persistence of cysts in the CNS [19]. Accordingly, the concept of asymptomatic chronic parasitization is currently under debate [20].

*T. gondii* is a plausible candidate as an infectious origin of schizophrenia and has attracted considerable research attention for the following reasons: the possibility of its transplacental transmission; its marked neurotropism; its capacity for persistent infection, remaining in latent form but with the possibility of reactivation; its association with brain development disorders and anomalies; its relationship with behavior disorders in animal and human models; and *in vitro* evidence of the inhibition of its growth in cell culture by antipsychotic drugs.

## 2. Epidemiologic data on the association between toxoplasmosis and schizophrenia

One of the first approaches adopted to explore a possible relationship between *T. gondii* infection and schizophrenia was to analyze epidemiological data on the two diseases. Initial conclusions were as follows:

- Both have a familial incidence. This is explained in the case of schizophrenia by the possible participation of certain genes in its pathogeny [21], and in the case of toxoplasmosis by the possible common exposure of family members to the parasite, although a genetic influence has also been proposed [22].

- There is a relatively high frequency of stillborns among both schizophrenic [23] and parasitized [24] mothers.
- Both diseases typically show a decreased prevalence in geographic areas with small populations of felines [25, 26].
- Initial symptoms in both diseases commonly manifest between the second and third decade of life [27, 28].
- The prevalence of both diseases is higher among populations with lower socioeconomic level and living in overcrowded conditions [29, 30].

These and other published findings indicate that the two diseases have some similar features and may even be epidemiologically related. However, they are inadequate to establish etiological relationships, and a pathophysiological approach is required to explore causality.

## 3. Studies based on the detection of anti-*Toxoplasma gondii* antibodies

For more than six decades, the relationship between schizophrenia and toxoplasmosis has been explored by studying a specific immune response [31]. Various meta-analyses have demonstrated a significantly higher prevalence of anti-*T. gondii* antibodies in schizophrenic patients than in controls, with odds ratios ranging between 2.7 [11, 32–34] and 1.8 [35].

In the natural time course of toxoplasmosis, IgM antibodies against *T. gondii* are the first to be detected in serum, a few days after infection. These are usually negativized between weeks 4 and 12 but can remain detectable for months or even years in a large number of patients. IgG antibodies are detected at around 2 weeks later than IgM antibodies, reaching a maximum level in the 2nd to 3rd month and persisting throughout life in residual titers. The presence of IgM antibodies in the absence of IgG indicates recent infection, while the presence of IgG indicates chronic infection, especially in the absence of IgM. The reactivation of a persistent infection can be accompanied by increased IgG and/or IgM values, although these antibodies can be undetectable in immunocompromised patients [36].

Most studies have centered on the humoral immune response, comparing anti-*T. gondii* IgG and IgM antibodies between schizophrenic patients (in different clinical/therapeutic situations) and controls. This method is widely employed because of the ease with which samples (usually serum, occasionally cerebrospinal fluid) can be gathered and the high degree of reproducibility, specificity, and sensitivity obtained. Many of these studies reported higher levels of antibodies (IgG and, in some studies, IgM) against *T. gondii* in patients with schizophrenia than in other populations, including patients with a different psychiatric disorder [32, 37–51]. However, findings have been inconsistent [52, 53], and account should be taken of the publication bias against studies without significant results [11].

Clinical manifestations differ between seropositive and seronegative schizophrenic patients, with a predominance in the former of positive symptoms (delirium, hallucinations, disorganized thinking), cognitive disorders (abstract thinking difficulties, disorientation, attention deficit), and agitation [50, 54]. Some researchers also observed that patients with schizophrenia and anti-*T. gondii* antibodies had a significantly higher risk of dying from natural causes [55] and were more likely to attempt suicide [56] in comparison with seronegative patients.

The above studies suggest a strong association between these diseases, with a significantly higher frequency of chronic parasitization in schizophrenic patients than in other population groups. However, if schizophrenia is a consequence of chronic CNS infection, which usually takes place at an early age, the question arises as to why it typically appears between the second and third decades of life. According to Yolken et al. [51], a significant increase in IgG titers observed in patients with a first schizophrenia episode may be compatible with a reactivation of the infection (previously in latent phase) that becomes clinically manifest in the onset of the disease *via* an immune-mediated mechanism. Some authors proposed that the immunoglobulins may cross the blood-brain barrier in this situation and react with brain tissue antigens due to their molecular mimicry with *T. gondii* antigens. This is similar to observations in such autoimmune diseases as systemic lupus erythematosus or in paraneoplastic syndromes [57]. Associations with the presence of anti-*Toxoplasma* IgM are less well documented [35], although Monroe et al. [58] reported in their meta-analysis a significant 1.7-fold greater likelihood of *T. gondii* IgM antibodies in patients with acute psychosis than in controls. It was concluded that *T. gondii* IgM antibodies may indicate either an acute/recent infection or a reinfection, possibly with a different genotype.

However, although a strong association has been described between schizophrenia and parasitization, these studies do not provide evidence to confirm the hypothesis on the infectious etiology of schizophrenia, and a causal relationship has not been demonstrated. Contact with *T. gondii* may be favored by the anomalous behavior, disorganized lifestyle, and/or weaker socioeconomic situation of schizophrenics, with infection being the consequence rather than the cause of their disease, which may explain the positive serological results [50].

## 4. Seroprevalence studies in mothers and newborns

The possible transplacental transmission of *T. gondii* has attracted considerable attention in seroprevalence studies. Maternal infection during the first or second trimester of pregnancy can lead to severe problems in the offspring, including intracranial calcifications, chorioretinitis, blindness, deafness, hydrocephaly, microcephaly, mental retardation, psychomotor retardation, pancytopenia, or epilepsy. The timing of the transmission is an influential factor: early maternal infection less frequently affects the fetus but is associated with a more severe congenital toxoplasmosis that may result in intrauterine death and miscarriages, while later maternal infection (third trimester) increases the risk of affecting the fetus but is associated with offspring who are asymptomatic [17]. Complications, possibly including schizophrenia, can appear decades later in patients with initially undetected infection due to its reactivation [59].

This type of study can be classified into two groups: those on the presence of antibodies in pregnant women and the development of schizophrenia in their offspring; those on the presence of antibodies in newborns and their later development of schizophrenia. Among the former, Brown et al. [60] and Blomström et al. [61] demonstrated associations between increased anti-*Toxoplasma* IgG levels in pregnant mothers and risk of schizophrenia in their offspring, although other researchers published discrepant results [62]. Xiao et al. [63] observed a significant association between the presence of maternal antibodies against type I *T. gondii* (but not against types II or III) and the onset of psychotic disorders in the offspring. Among the latter group of studies, Mortensen et al. [59] demonstrated that newborn levels of anti-*T. gondii* IgG levels (from the mother) were significantly higher in individuals who developed schizophrenia in adulthood.

Published data suggest that schizophrenia risk in offspring is associated with persistent maternal infection by *T. gondii* but is not directly related to acute maternal infection [64]. If this were the case, a significant association could be expected between the presence of IgM in the serum of mothers and/or newborns and the presence of the disease, which has not been demonstrated [60]. However, this relationship may be masked by the low frequency of anti-*Toxoplasma* IgM detection in pregnant women [24, 65].

As noted above, increased maternal IgG levels can cross the placenta (unlike IgM antibodies) and may damage fetal brain development by molecular mimicry [60, 64]. However, the presence of maternal IgG may indicate a reactivation of latent infection due to the impact of immune system disorders on protozoan replication control during pregnancy [66]; hence, brain development could also be impaired by transplacental transmission and/or the passage of inflammatory cytokines to the fetus [67, 68].

The majority of schizophrenic patients do not have anti-*Toxoplasma* antibodies, and the majority of seropositive patients are not schizophrenic. Therefore, *T. gondii* would only explain a minority of cases. Other factors under investigation that may explain why only some parasitized individuals develop schizophrenia include genetic susceptibility, the infective genotype of the parasite, the existence of different infection pathways, and the timing of toxoplasmosis onset [20, 33, 63].

## 5. Studies based on *Toxoplasma gondii* nucleic acid detection

Studies of animal brain biopsies have shown *T. gondii* to have high neurotropism, with the capacity to infect glial cells (especially microglia and astrocytes) and neurons, forming persistent cysts in brain tissue [69]. Although no tropism for specific brain regions has been observed, with cysts being detected in many areas, the most frequently parasitized regions are the hippocampus, thalamus, cerebral cortex, cerebellum, olfactory bulb, and, especially, the amygdala [70–73].

However, the presence of brain cysts can only be detected in *postmortem* biopsies, explaining the few studies of this type and the predominance of serological techniques for the detection of chronic infection by *T. gondii* in humans. The presence of glial anomalies, including a reduced amount of astrocytes, has been reported in the brains of schizophrenic patients [74], and it has been speculated that these may possibly result from infection by *T. gondii* [31].

Imaging techniques have revealed a lower density of gray matter in certain brain regions of schizophrenic patients [75], which may be directly related to the infection, given that non-parasitized schizophrenic patients were found to have the same brain morphology as healthy controls [76].

One of the few studies of *postmortem* brain biopsies found no parasite DNA in any subject (14 schizophrenic patients and 26 healthy controls) [77]. There appear to be three possible explanations: first, there was truly no association with the infection; second, the biopsies missed infected brain areas; and finally, the sensitivity of the nucleic acid detection technique might be inadequate. In addition, the detection of parasite DNA only demonstrates the presence of the parasite not its possible effect on the parasitized individual and would not establish an etiological relationship with schizophrenia. Thus, the detection of parasite DNA in brain tissues does not distinguish between asymptomatic patients with latent parasitization and those with encephalitis [17].

A study of blood samples detected parasite DNA in 33 out of 101 samples from schizophrenic patients *versus* 2 out of 55 samples from controls, a significant difference [46]. In contrast, Gutiérrez-Fernández et al. [32] detected parasite DNA in only 1 out of 128 blood samples from schizophrenic patients and in none of 143 samples from controls (nonsignificant difference). However, although the presence of parasite DNA in blood indicates acute infection [17], it does not necessarily signify infection of the brain, and no relationship was found between anti-*Toxoplasma* IgM and schizophrenia in the aforementioned study [46].

## 6. Studies on behavioral disorders in animals and humans

Research on this issue has included experimental animal studies, mainly in rats and mice. Parasitized animals have shown various behavioral changes, becoming more active, expressing less fear when examining new stimuli, reducing their natural aversion to cat odor or even becoming attracted to it, and demonstrating reduced learning ability and attention or memory deficits [78–83]. According to the "behavioral manipulation hypothesis," these disorders in their intermediate hosts (rodents) represent an evolutionary adaptation of the parasite, facilitating their capture by their definitive host (felines) and completing their life cycle [84, 85]. Although the mechanism by which *T. gondii* induces these behavioral changes is poorly understood, various possibilities have been proposed. It may be due to a direct effect on tissue cysts in specific brain areas such as the amygdala or hippocampus, given that the host response to predator odors was changed by the parasite in male rats infected with *T. gondii* by inducing hypomethylation of the neuropeptide arginine vasopressin in the posterodorsal part of the medial amygdala, an important node of the extrahypothalamic vasopressin system that contains a large number of arginine vasopressin neurons. This epigenetic manipulation produced a greater activation of vasopressinergic neurons after exposure to cat odor, leading to the reversion of fear into attraction [86]. It may also result from the effect of a more diffuse and wider involvement of brain tissues, with no apparent changes, that nevertheless give rise to a series of neurophysiological disorders. Changes may also result from inflammation (encephalitis) caused by the immune activation induced by parasitization, which would increase inflammatory cytokines in the rodent brain, such as tumor necrosis factor alpha (TNF-$\alpha$), interleukin-1$\beta$ (IL-1$\beta$), IL-10, interferon gamma (IFN$\gamma$), C-reactive protein, tissue inhibitor of metalloproteinases 1 (TIMP-1), or vascular cell adhesion molecule 1 (VCAM-1), similar to observations in *postmortem* biopsies of schizophrenic patients. Finally, the behavioral changes have also been related to neurochemical mechanisms, with an increase in dopamine and homovanillic acid and a decrease in norepinephrine levels [73, 84, 85, 87–90].

Any of the above mechanisms in rodents could also produce behavioral changes in the brains of other intermediate hosts, including humans. Thus, research in humans also suggests that toxoplasmosis may alter behavior, psychomotor abilities, or personality, with the corresponding clinical consequences [84]. These disorders would be more related to latent rather than acute toxoplasmosis, given that its emergence, frequently several years after primary infection and not during the acute phase, would indicate that it results from slow and possibly accumulative changes induced by parasite activity [91–93]. The study by Horacek et al. [76] demonstrates that, in seropositive schizophrenic patients, latent parasitization is associated with a significant reduction in gray matter volume in specific brain areas (cortical regions, hippocampus, and caudate nucleus), which is not observed in seronegative patients.

Reinforcing the relationship between the parasite and the psychiatric disease, it has been demonstrated that haloperidol, an antipsychotic drug that blocks D2 dopaminergic receptors in the mesolimbic system and often used in the symptomatic treatment of schizophrenia, inhibits the replication of tachyzoites in cell cultures *in vitro*. This effect may at least partly be due to the capacity of this drug to inhibit calcium transport, blocking cell ion channels [94]. The interaction between tachyzoites and host cells is calcium-dependent; hence, cell invasion capacity can be inhibited by the presence of drugs that block calcium channels, such as haloperidol [95]. Experimental studies with rodents have also demonstrated that some behavioral changes caused by the infection are reverted by using the antipsychotic, and that there are fewer parasitized neurons and glial cells after the treatment; this is observed using immunohistochemical techniques [96]. It is therefore possible that its therapeutic effect can be explained in patients with schizophrenia by various mechanisms, given that on the one hand, it blocks dopamine, whose levels are often elevated in schizophrenia patients parasitized with *T. gondii* [89, 97], and on the other hand, it can inhibit parasite replication in brain cells [96]. Other antipsychotic drugs such as fluphenazine, thioridazine, trifluoperazine, or zuclopenthixol, and mood stabilizers, e.g., valproic acid, were also found to inhibit *T. gondii* proliferation in cell cultures [94, 98, 99].

Antipsychotics are especially indicated in patients with a predominance of positive symptoms and agitation (as in the acute phase of schizophrenia), which are significantly more frequent in those parasitized with *T. gondii*, as noted above. The greater effectiveness of these drugs in these situations may be due not only to their dopamine blocking effect but also to their anti-*Toxoplasma* activity. Thus, these treatments were found to reduce anti-*Toxoplasma* antibody levels in seropositive schizophrenic patients, indicating their antiparasitic effect [44]. These findings suggest that these drugs may possibly have a beneficial effect on schizophrenic patients parasitized with *T. gondii*.

Studies to date on the possible effect in these patients of drugs with anti-*Toxoplasma* activity (e.g., pyrimethamine, sulfadiazine, azithromycin, or trimethoprim-sulfamethoxazole) have not demonstrated significant improvements in psychotic symptoms [100, 101]. In fact, drugs used to treat toxoplasmosis are largely active during the tachyzoite replication phase, and their effectiveness against bradyzoites in tissue cysts is drastically reduced once chronic infection by *T. gondii* is established [102].

The etiological relationship between parasitization and schizophrenia has not yet been established, despite the above data on behavioral changes in animals or humans and on the effects of antipsychotic drugs on symptoms. In addition, differences in behavioral disorders between humans and rodents may mean that results in animal models cannot be extrapolated to humans. It should also be borne in mind that the mild behavioral modifications associated with the infection cannot necessarily be considered symptoms of a psychotic disease.

## 7. The role of proinflammatory cytokines

The host response to the parasitization of glial cells and neurons involves the activation of immune system cells, including T lymphocytes (CD4+ and CD8+), B lymphocytes, NK cells, macrophages, and dendritic and glial cells. These produce a wide variety of inflammatory cytokines such as IFN$\gamma$, interleukins (IL-1, IL-1$\beta$, IL-2, IL-4, IL-6, IL-10, IL-12, IL-15, IL-17, IL-18, IL-23), granulocyte macrophage colony-stimulating factor (GM-CSF), and/or TNF$\alpha$ [69, 103]. These cytokines halt protozoan proliferation and limit their replication, playing a key role in regulating the infection of host cells, thereby favoring the formation of tissue cysts and the development of the chronic latent form [20]. These and other inflammatory responses have also been reported in schizophrenia [104] and are therefore involved in brain disorders both in this disease and in *T. gondii* infection [105].

Thus, infection of brain tissue by *T. gondii* produces activation of the Jak/STAT pathway, which is recognized as an important regulatory mechanism in CNS development, function, and disease progression [106, 107]. This pathway comprises three elements: a ligand receptor, the majority are receptors of cytokines such as IFN$\gamma$; Janus kinase (Jak) proteins associated with the receptor within the cell, which possess tyrosine-kinase activity; and signal transducer and activator of transcription (STAT) proteins, which act as transcription factors that move toward the cell nucleus after their phosphorylation, where they bind with regulatory sequences of genes designated gamma interferon activation sites (GAS) [108]. In mammals, the Jak/STAT pathway induces the transcription of genes that participate in multiple processes, including antimicrobial activity and the production of proinflammatory cytokines [109]. Among other effects, an increase is produced in the expression of NADPH oxidase enzyme (NOX2) and inducible nitric oxide synthase (iNOS). These enzymes are responsible for the production of reactive oxygen species (ROS) and reactive nitrogen species (RNS), which assist the destruction of foreign pathogens [110, 111] but have been linked to seizures, stroke, neurodegenerative diseases, and schizophrenia [111, 112] as a consequence of their toxic effect on neurons [113]. Scientific evidence points to ROS-mediated oxidative damage as a key pathogenic pathway involved in infection-mediated neuropathy. According to these findings, it can be expected that a high degree of degenerated neuron degeneration and cognitive impairment is associated with the presence of *T. gondii* in the brain [111].

## 8. The importance of dopamine and other neurotransmitters

As already noted, some experimental animal and human studies concluded that behavioral changes may be explained by increased dopamine levels in the parasitized brain, and that these disorders could largely be resolved by administration of a dopaminergic receptor antagonist (e.g., haloperidol) or dopamine reuptake inhibitor (e.g., GBR-12909) [96, 114, 115]. It is therefore possible that dopamine represents the link between toxoplasmosis and schizophrenia [97]. This neurotransmitter is synthesized in the cytosol of neurons from L-tyrosine amino acid by the action of the tyrosine hydroxylase enzyme, which converts it to L-3,4-dihydroxyphenylalanine (L-DOPA). L-DOPA is in turn converted by the action of DOPA-decarboxylase (DDC) to dopamine, a precursor of norepinephrine (noradrenalin) and epinephrine (adrenalin) in the synthesis pathway of these catecholamines. It is subsequently packaged in vesicles and transported through the axon to the synapse, where it is released by exocytosis in response to an electrical stimulus. Dopamine is one of the main neurotransmitters in the prefrontal cortex and the mesolimbic system (mainly formed by the nucleus accumbens, amygdala, and hippocampus), where the presence of *T. gondii* tissue cysts is especially frequent [73].

The definitive mechanism by which *T. gondii* induces changes in the dopaminergic pathway has not been fully elucidated. However, an increase in dopamine with no modification of cellular tyrosine hydroxylase was demonstrated *in vitro* after parasitization of a rat pheochromocytoma cell line (PC12) and *in vivo* after the parasitization of mouse brains. This dopamine synthesis is attributable to the additional activity of the aromatic amino acid hydroxylase, which is encoded by two *T. gondii* genes [116] and has homologous activities to those of mammalian tyrosine hydroxylase, associated with the entry of cellular DDC enzymes into parasitophorous vacuoles (compartments formed by the parasite to invade the cell) and into tissue cysts (the protozoan encodes no enzyme with DDC activity) [114, 117]. Experiments in cell cultures have demonstrated that dopamine increases the replication of *T. gondii* tachyzoites [118]. This biochemical mechanism may play a role in the behavioral changes observed, which would result from the involvement of catecholaminergic neurons and consequent dopaminergic hyperactivity [19].

Parasitization in the fetal period may also impair the development of mesolimbic dopaminergic or prefrontal cortex neurons (inappropriate migration, altered position, reduced synapses, etc.) leading to neurodevelopmental disorders. Disease symptoms would not be induced immediately by these early anomalies but would rather manifest after a latency period of one to three decades. This is because the proliferation, migration, differentiation, and maturation of glial progenitor cells continue throughout childhood [119] and the volume of gray matter increases to a peak in puberty before beginning to diminish [120].

However, the hypothesis that increased dopamine levels or dopaminergic hyperactivity is the underlying cause of schizophrenia does not account for the negative symptoms in these patients, which are more likely to result from dopaminergic hypoactivity. Therefore, neurotransmitters other than dopamine may play an important role in the development of this disease. Thus, it has been proposed that deficits in glutamatergic brain systems also participate in the physiopathology of schizophrenia based on findings of higher kynurenic acid levels in patients with psychotic symptoms than in healthy controls [121]. Kynurenic acid is a metabolite of tryptophan with important biological effects on the nervous system, related to its antagonism for the glutamate receptor in the human brain (it is a glutamatergic NMDA receptor antagonist). Increased kynurenic acid levels due to blockade of NMDA receptors in glutamatergic neurons have been related to changes in dopamine level in different brain areas. These modifications include cortical dopaminergic hypoactivity and mesolimbic dopaminergic hyperactivity, which would explain the negative and positive symptoms in patients. This relationship between glutamate pathway disorders and dopamine level changes may explain the presence of different symptoms in the psychosis [122].

Indoleamine-2,3-dioxygenase and therefore the metabolism of tryptophan, a precursor metabolite in serotonin (and melatonin) synthesis, are induced by the proinflammatory cytokines released in response to *T. gondii* infection, especially IFNγ [123]. Tryptophan is an essential amino acid for the parasite, and decreased levels inhibit its growth and replication capacity [124]. However, induction of this metabolite in turn increases kynurenic acid levels and therefore alters dopamine levels through the glutamatergic receptor antagonist effect of this acid [114]. Tryptophan degradation also reduces serotonin levels, which has been related to a higher incidence of depression and suicide [125, 126], as also observed in patients with high anti-*T. gondii* antibody levels [56].

Patients with schizophrenia also show anomalous levels of gamma-aminobutyric acid (GABA), another important neurotransmitter [20], which is synthesized from glutamate by the action of glutamic acid decarboxylase (GAD) [127]. GABA activates $GABA_A$ receptors, which are ion channels, and $GABA_B$ receptors, which are G-protein-coupled receptors [128]. It is the main neurotransmitter with inhibiting effect in the CNS, regulating dopaminergic activity and playing a key role in the reduction of neuronal excitability throughout the nervous system. Dopaminergic neurons in basal ganglia would be directly inhibited by GABAergic neurons, so that any GABAergic hypofunction would be accompanied by an increase in subcortical dopaminergic activity, as observed in schizophrenia.

More direct evidence of the involvement of this neurotransmitter in the etiology of schizophrenia derives from data on the reduction in neurons in the GABAergic system or in brain regions such as the hippocampus, temporal lobe, and prefrontal cortex of schizophrenic patients [129–131]. *Postmortem* molecular studies have demonstrated: a reduction in messenger RNA (mRNA) levels of isoform 67 of glutamic acid decarboxylase (GAD67) and of type 1 GABA transporter (GAT-1) in the prefrontal cortex of schizophrenics [132, 133]; an increase in subunit $\alpha 2$ of the $GABA_A$ receptor in the initial segment of the axon of pyramidal neurons [134]; and a reduced expression of the receptor $GABA_{B,}$ which regulates GABA release as a possible compensatory mechanism for GABAergic dysfunction [135]. As noted above, these findings may be the consequence of alterations during neurodevelopment in the differentiation and migration of these neurons toward their definitive localizations in the brain. This would give rise to structural alterations and neurochemical dysregulation that would have a global effect on all of these neurotransmitters (dopamine, glutamate, serotonin, GABA) and would become manifest from adolescence onward, inducing the appearance of the disease. Once more, infection by *T. gondii* may play an important role in this process.

Outside the nervous system, GABAergic mechanisms have been observed in different tissues and peripheral organs, and GABA has also been found to exert a major role in the immune system, with important inter-regulatory functions between this and the CNS [136]. It has been reported that *T. gondii* infection is followed by an increase in the motility and migratory capacity of infected dendritic cells, permitting propagation of the parasite to different tissues, including the brain [128]. Although dendritic cells are considered guardians of the immune system, they can also, paradoxically, mediate in the spread of the parasite. This mechanism is produced by the induction in these cells of the GAD enzyme and therefore of GABA production and secretion, which in turn activate GABA receptors expressed by these same cells, stimulating their motility [137]. In experimental mouse models, inhibition of the GABAergic pathway by blockade of GABAA receptors or inhibition of the GAD enzyme markedly reduced the hypermotility and spread of *T. gondii*-infected dendritic cells and therefore of the parasite itself [137, 138]. Finally, it has also been reported that brain infection by *T. gondii* can interfere with the GABAergic system by inducing changes in the distribution of the GAD67 enzyme, although this event has been related more to possible neurological complications of toxoplasmic encephalitis, such as seizures [139], than to possible complications of latent toxoplasmosis, such as schizophrenia.

Accordingly, the inflammatory response of the host to parasitization, which aims to control parasite replication and alterations in differentiation and migration processes, can change levels of dopamine, tryptophan, kynurenic acid, serotonin, and GABA, leading to behavioral changes and giving rise to different psychotic symptoms.

In order to establish dopamine and other related neurotransmitters as a causal link between toxoplasmosis and schizophrenia development, it is necessary to confirm that this neurotransmitter is also involved in the disease genesis when there is infection by other pathogens [140], and this mechanism should also explain the possible contribution of *T. gondii* parasitization in other dopaminergic pathway diseases, e.g., Parkinson's disease [114].

## 9. The *N*-methyl-D-aspartate receptor hypofunction theory: anti-NMDAr antibodies

Encephalitis due to antibodies against the glutamatergic NMDA receptor (anti-NMDAr antibodies) is an autoimmune disease caused when antibodies produced by the host immune system identify NMDA receptors as foreign antigens. This receptor forms a heterotetramer between two GluN1 and two GluN2 subunits and participates in essential functions for reality perception, memory, and the control of unconscious activities. The disease is characterized by the hypofunction of NMDA receptors, which would account for the psychotic symptoms, personality changes, memory impairment, and psychomotor agitation

[141, 142]. It usually arises during the course of a paraneoplastic process and is frequently associated with the development of ovarian teratomas, explaining its higher incidence among females [143, 144]. Likewise, 14–75% of patients with systemic erythematous lupus, another autoimmune disease, have been reported to manifest psychiatric symptoms related to the presence of the same antibodies [145, 146]. This involvement of anti-NMDAr antibodies (and other neurotransmission receptors) indicates an important link between immune abnormalities and altered neurotransmission in schizophrenia, major depression, or bipolar disorder [147, 148].

The presence of anti-NMDAr antibodies has been documented in schizophrenic patients in the absence of seizures, movement disorders, or other neurological signs or symptoms [149–151], although other researchers were unable to replicate these findings [152, 153]. For various reasons, the production of anti-NMDAr antibodies is a plausible mechanism to explain at least a percentage of schizophrenic cases [149]: several studies reported that 5–10% of cases are associated with the presence of these antibodies in serum and cerebrospinal fluid [150, 151, 154]; kynurenic acid is an antagonist of glutamate *via* blockade of NMDA receptors, as commented in the previous section, suggesting that it contributes to the pathogenesis of schizophrenia [122]; persistent blockade of NMDA receptors in experimental animals recreates clinical characteristics of schizophrenia [155]; selective elimination of subunit GluN1 of the NMDA receptor in neurons of the cortex and hippocampus in early postnatal development contributes to the pathophysiology of schizophrenia-related disorders in mice [156]; some of the genes associated with schizophrenia are related to the NMDA receptor [157]; NMDA receptors are reduced in medication-free schizophrenic patients [158]; blockade of the receptor with ketamine or phencyclidine produces psychotic symptoms [159, 160]; and *de novo* mutations (large chromosomal copy number changes) affect genes that encode one or more nucleotides among the glutamatergic postsynaptic proteins that form part of the receptor, providing insight into possible etiological mechanisms underlying schizophrenia [161].

Maternal infection during brain development or infection during childhood may produce anti-NMDAr antibodies, while other environmental or genetic factors may influence the age of disease onset [149]. Certain pathogens have been associated with elevated anti-NMDAr antibodies [162, 163]. Thus, a *T. gondii*-infected mouse model showed a significantly higher increase in serum GluN2A autoantibodies among juvenile- *versus* adult-infected mice. Adolescence is a critical window in neurodevelopment, and the authors hypothesized that early infection would have greater effects on behavior and the brain in comparison with adult infection. It is possible that chronic infection with *T. gondii* affects pre- or postnatal brain development by altering synaptic maturation. An increase in NMDAr autoantibodies due to *T. gondii* exposure might underlie behavioral alterations in symptomatic individuals [164].

## 10. Studies on gene-infection interaction

Various studies have demonstrated the participation of numerous genes in schizophrenia, providing firm evidence on the involvement of genetics in the etiology of the disease

[165]. Some authors have described inheritability in >80% of cases, and schizophrenia has been associated with polymorphic variability in certain genes [21, 166–168]. However, the genetic hypothesis alone cannot explain the familial association of schizophrenia with other diseases, the seasonal peaks of schizophrenia births, the different prevalences among residents of urban and rural areas, discordant results between monozygotic and dizygotic twins or between dizygotic twins and full siblings, or correlations in adopted children, which are, however, consistent with an infectious etiology [1]. Schizophrenia is likely a genetically complex disease that does not follow a Mendelian transmission pattern but rather involves multiple genes, each with a small effect, which act in combination with epigenetic and environmental factors [169]. Accordingly, epidemiological findings suggest that a combination of intrinsic (genetic) and extrinsic or environmental factors, including infections, may participate in the origin of this disease, operating during the development of the individual at some time between conception and adolescence [7]. Tomonaga [170] proposed that persistent chronic infections or the expression of microbial proteins may directly and/or indirectly affect CNS functions in infected individuals, changing the expressions of genes related to schizophrenia and increasing the risk of suffering this disease or at least some of its varied clinical phenotypes.

Genes whose variants or polymorphisms have been associated with the risk of schizophrenia include some that encode proteins with important functions in neurodevelopment or neurodegeneration and in neuronal neurotransmission circuits. This is the case of the gene that encodes neuregulin 1 (NRG1), a key molecule in maintaining brain synaptic plasticity in adults, which has been related to schizophrenia etiology [171, 172], and the genes that encode catechol-O-methyltransferase (COMT) [173], proline dehydrogenase (PRODH) [174], dysbindin protein (DTNBP1) [175], a regulator of G4 protein (RGS4) [176], a regulator of potassium calcium channels (KCNN3) [177], and D-amino-oxidase complex (G72, DAAO) [178], among others [179]. The genes that encode these proteins are located in chromosomal regions that have been described as relevant for the study of schizophrenia, and many of these proteins participate in glutamatergic, dopaminergic, or serotonergic neurotransmission circuits.

Genetic polymorphisms that increase susceptibility to schizophrenia, including some of the above, have also been related to resistance or susceptibility to certain infections through their important role in the life cycle of some pathogens, including *T. gondii* [169, 179, 180]. Schizophrenia may possibly correspond to a model in which various genes may interact with microbial agents in a process that is probably mediated by the inflammatory and immune response of the individual, increasing the risk of developing psychiatric disease [169, 179–182]. It appears reasonable to assume that infections may interact, thereby changing the expressions of schizophrenia-related genes and increasing the risk of suffering this condition.

Various rodent [79, 183, 184] and human [185, 186] studies have supported the existence of genetic susceptibility to *T. gondii* parasitization, suggesting that if the parasite were one of the possible causes underlying schizophrenia development, this genetic susceptibility might also explain familial cases of schizophrenia [1]. As commented above, some *T. gondii* genes encode proteins with a similar activity to that of enzymes (e.g., tyrosine hydroxylase) in the cells of their intermediate hosts. Therefore, this parasite has genes that allow it to "manipulate" the behavior of the host and facilitate its capture by the cat, its definitive host, thereby favoring parasite survival. The presence of these genes is consequently an evolutionary advantage of *T. gondii* [19].

Genetic studies (in animals and humans) currently center on the possible presence of genes or specific allelic variants that interact with the genes of microorganisms that can infect the patient (gene-infection interaction hypothesis), increasing the risk of schizophrenia [187–189]. Thus, it has been demonstrated that a critical role in human congenital *T. gondii* infection is played by the *ALOX12* gene, which encodes arachidonate 5-lipoxygenase enzyme, which is involved in fatty acid metabolism and has been related to schizophrenia, at least in a Korean population [190, 191]. HLA-related genes such as *SGK1* on chromosome 6, which plays a role in regulating different brain functions [192] and mediates the effects of cortisol on hippocampal neurogenesis [193], have a modulating effect on some infectious agents, including *T. gondii*, consistent with the proposition that parasitization may modify the risk of schizophrenia [187]. In a study of mice parasitized with *T. gondii*, heterozygous deletion of the *Nurr1* gene (Nurr1 ± genotype), an orphan nuclear receptor essential for the development of mesencephalic dopamine neurons [194], predisposed the animals to behavioral disorders that involve dopamine neurotransmission associated with schizophrenia symptoms [195].

A further example in support of this hypothesis is the Akt cell signaling system. The *Akt* gene encodes a serine-threonine kinase with three isoforms (Akt1, 2, and 3), whose activation mediates cell survival processes and whose inhibition favors apoptosis. As commented above, the innate immune system induces a range of processes after infection of brain cells by *T. gondii*, including antimicrobial activity and the generation of ROS to assist in the destruction of foreign pathogens. However, increases in ROS concentrations activate the Akt system, which guarantees cell survival and allows the pathogen to persist and replicate within the infected cell. Akt is above all activated in pathophysiological situations in which ROS increase as the result of ischemia-reperfusion, playing an important role in the protection of the different cells and tissues involved, including nerve tissue [196]. On the other hand, Akt is known to affect dopaminergic signaling, and polymorphisms of the *Akt1* gene have been found to increase the risk of developing schizophrenia through its relationship with dopaminergic pathways of the prefrontal cortex [197].

Other researchers reported similar associations between schizophrenia risk and other human pathogens, supporting the gene-infection interaction hypothesis [198–201]. This research line on the effects of interaction between genes or genetic variants on the risk of schizophrenia related to *T. gondii* parasitization is highly likely to establish the true causes of the disease, at least in some types of patient.

## 11. Is there an etiological association between *Toxoplasma gondii* infection and schizophrenia development?

Numerous studies have contributed evidence on the involvement of toxoplasmosis in the pathogenesis of numerous CNS diseases, including bipolar disorder, depression, Alzheimer's disease, Parkinson's disease, and epilepsy [49, 202–204]. However, the main advances over the past few years have been achieved by research on deciphering the molecular mechanisms underlying the physiopathology of schizophrenia.

This chapter analyzes data from *in vitro* and animal and human *in vivo* studies in order elucidate points of connection between *T. gondii* and schizophrenia. It can be concluded that infection by *T. gondii* is highly likely to be a cause of the disease for the following reasons: it is a neurotropic microorganism that persistently invades glial cells and neurons; it generates brain development anomalies; it reduces brain gray matter density; it elicits an inflammatory and immune response that alters neurotransmission systems; it affects cognitive function and behavior; and its replication is inhibited by some antipsychotics. All disorders reported for the parasite are associated with the development of psychotic symptoms. Furthermore, specific genetic polymorphisms linked to an increased risk of schizophrenia have also been associated with a higher likelihood of infection by this parasite. Nevertheless, despite all of the above evidence on this possible pathogenic association, one important

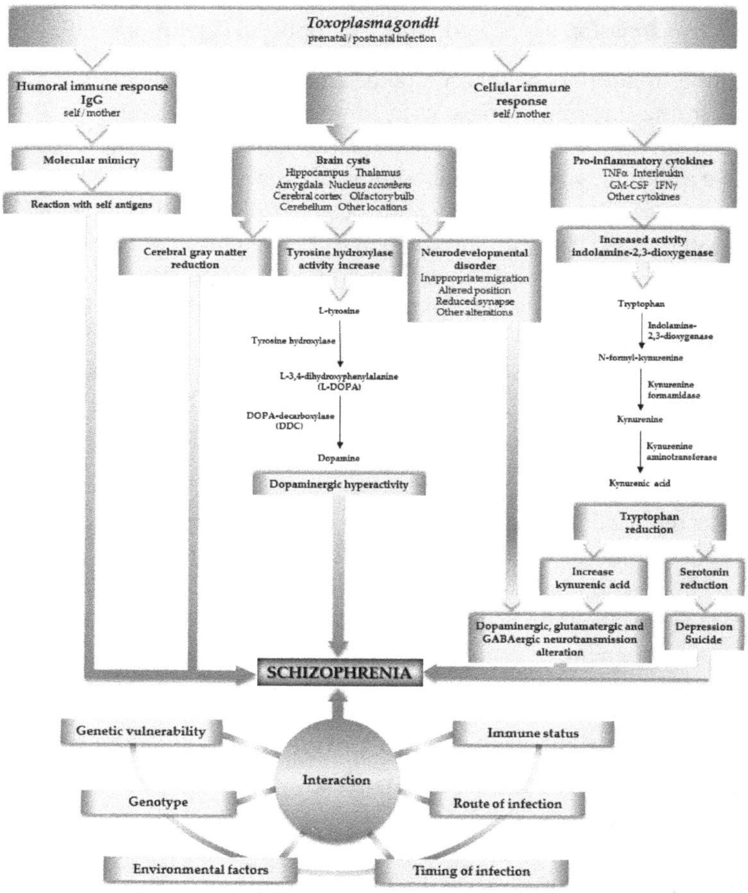


**Figure 1.** Likely involvement of infection by *Toxoplasma gondii* in the development of schizophrenia.

question remains to be resolved, which is why most individuals with signs of infection by *T. gondii* are asymptomatic and only a few develop psychiatric disorders.

Schizophrenia is a complex disease with innumerable symptoms, and its presentation and severity vary among patients. According to the infectious hypothesis of this disease (**Figure 1**), differences among patients would be influenced by their genetic predisposition or vulnerability, their immune status, the timing of parasitization (congenital, neonatal, or adult), the time interval since their first contact, and/or the particular brain area(s) affected. Characteristics of the infection also play a role, including its source (oocysts or tissue cysts), possible interactions with other infectious agents, and the genotype; thus, genotypes II and III more frequently establish chronic infections and show a greater expression of tyrosine hydroxylase genes in comparison with genotype I, and they may be more strongly related to behavioral changes [205].

Finally, the biology of schizophrenia must be fully elucidated to support the appropriate design of disease-modifying therapies or novel antipsychotic drugs. There appears to be sufficient evidence to suggest that schizophrenic patients with *T. gondii* infection could clinically benefit from a combined therapeutic approach based on the prescription of current or future antipsychotic drugs with antitoxoplasmic activity. However, published results have not been conclusive [206], and randomized controlled prospective trials are required in wider samples, stratifying schizophrenic patients into subgroups (e.g., by clinical phenotype, pathophysiological mechanism, or response to treatment) and in relation to specific types of *T. gondii* parasitization. Translational research must play a key role, with the involvement of psychiatric, neurologic, immunologic, biochemical, genetic, pharmacological, and microbiological investigators, among others, offering the possibility of using new and more effective methodologies. It appears highly likely that different causal agents are responsible for schizophrenia and that the pathogenic action of a particular microorganism such as *T. gondii* would only be relevant in certain patient subgroups, endorsing the need for personalized medicine.

## Author details

Antonio Sorlozano-Puerto[1] and Jose Gutierrez-Fernandez[1,2*]

*Address all correspondence to: josegf@ugr.es

1 Department of Microbiology, School of Medicine, University of Granada and Biosanitary Research Institute ibs, Granada, Spain

2 Area of Microbiology, Granada University Hospital Complex, Spain

## References

[1] Ledgerwood LG, Ewald PW, Cochran GM. Genes, germs, and schizophrenia: an evolutionary perspective. Perspect Biol Med. 2003;**46**(3):317–348. doi:10.1353/pbm.2003.0038

[2] Tsuang M. Schizophrenia: genes and environment. Biol Psychiatry. 2000;**47**(3):210–220. doi:10.1016/S0006-3223(99)00289-9

[3] Dinan TG, Borre YE, Cryan JF. Genomics of schizophrenia: time to consider the gut microbiome? Mol Psychiatry. 2014;**19**(12):1252–1257. doi:10.1038/mp.2014.93

[4] Arseneault L, Cannon M, Witton J, Murray RM. Causal association between cannabis and psychosis: examination of the evidence. Br J Psychiatry. 2004;**184**:110–117. doi:10.1192/bjp.184.2.110

[5] Brown AS. The risk for schizophrenia from childhood and adult infections. Am J Psychiatry. 2008;**165**(1):7–10. doi:10.1176/appi.ajp.2007.07101637

[6] Fatemi SH, Folsom TD. The neurodevelopmental hypothesis of schizophrenia, revisited. Schizophr Bull. 2009;**35**(3):528–548. doi:10.1093/schbul/sbn187

[7] Matheson SL, Shepherd AM, Carr VJ. How much do we know about schizophrenia and how well do we know it? Evidence from the Schizophrenia Library. Psychol Med. 2014;**44**(16):3387–3405. doi:10.1017/S0033291714000166

[8] Moore TH, Zammit S, Lingford-Hughes A, Barnes TR, Jones PB, Burke M, Lewis G. Cannabis use and risk of psychotic or affective mental health outcomes: a systematic review. Lancet. 2007;**370**(9584):319–328. doi:10.1016/S0140-6736(07)61162-3

[9] Sullivan PF, Kendler KS, Neale MC. Schizophrenia as a complex trait: evidence from a meta-analysis of twin studies. Arch Gen Psychiatry. 2003;**60**(12):1187–1192. doi:10.1001/archpsyc.60.12.1187

[10] Rawlins S. Nonviral sexually transmitted infections. J Obstet Gynecol Neonatal Nurs. 2001;**30**(3):324–331. doi:10.1111/j.1552-6909.2001.tb01551.x

[11] Arias I, Sorlozano A, Villegas E, de Dios Luna J, McKenney K, Cervilla J, Gutierrez B, Gutierrez J. Infectious agents associated with schizophrenia: a meta-analysis. Schizophr Res. 2012;**136**(1–3):128–136. doi:10.1016/j.schres.2011.10.026

[12] Müller N, Riedel M, Ackenheil M, Schwarz MJ. The role of immune function in schizophrenia: an overview. Eur Arch Psychiatry Clin Neurosci. 1999;**249**(Suppl 4):62–68. doi:10.1007/PL00014187

[13] Nahmias AJ, Nahmias SB, Danielsson D. The possible role of transplacentally acquired antibodies to infectious agents, with molecular mimicry to nervous system sialic acid epitopes, as causes of neuromental disorders: prevention and vaccine implications. Clin Dev Immunol. 2006;**13**(2–4):167–183. doi:10.1080/17402520600801745

[14] Gomez-Sintes R, Bortolozzi A, Artigas F, Lucas JJ. Reduced striatal dopamine DA D2 receptor function in dominant-negative GSK-3 transgenic mice. Eur Neuropsychopharmacol. 2014;**24**(9):1524–1533. doi:10.1016/j.euroneuro.2014.07.004

[15] Flegr J. Influence of latent *Toxoplasma* infection on human personality, physiology and morphology: pros and cons of the *Toxoplasma*-human model in studying the manipulation hypothesis. J Exp Biol. 2013;**216**(Pt 1):127–133. doi:10.1242/jeb.073635

[16] Gagne SS. Toxoplasmosis. Prim Care Update Ob Gyns. 2001;**8**(3):122–126. doi:10.1016/S1068-607X(00)00083-4

[17] Montoya JG, Liesenfeld O. Toxoplasmosis. Lancet. 2004;**363**(9425):1965–1976. doi:10.1016/S0140-6736(04)16412-X

[18] Bossi P, Caumes E, Paris L, Dardé ML, Bricaire F. *Toxoplasma gondii*-associated Guillain-Barré syndrome in an immunocompetent patient. J Clin Microbiol. 1998;**36**(12):3724–3725.

[19] McConkey GA, Martin HL, Bristow GC, Webster JP. *Toxoplasma gondii* infection and behaviour—location, location, location? J Exp Biol. 2013;**216**(Pt 1):113–119. doi:10.1242/jeb.074153.

[20] Fabiani S, Pinto B, Bruschi F. Toxoplasmosis and neuropsychiatric diseases: can serological studies establish a clear relationship? Neurol Sci. 2013;**34**(4):417–425. doi:10.1007/s10072-012-1197-4

[21] Jablensky AV, Kalaydjieva LV. Genetic epidemiology of schizophrenia: phenotypes, risk factors, and reproductive behavior. Am J Psychiatry. 2003;**160**(3):425–429. doi:10.1176/appi.ajp.160.3.425

[22] Johnson J, Suzuki Y, Mack D, Mui E, Estes R, David C, Skamene E, Forman J, McLeod R. Genetic analysis of influences on survival following *Toxoplasma gondii* infection. Int J Parasitol. 2002;**32**(2):179–185. doi:10.1016/S0020-7519(01)00321-6

[23] Bennedsen BE, Mortensen PB, Olesen AV, Henriksen TB. Congenital malformations, stillbirths, and infant deaths among children of women with schizophrenia. Arch Gen Psychiatry. 2001;**58**(7):674–679. doi:10.1001/archpsyc.58.7.674

[24] Sever JL, Ellenberg JH, Ley AC, Madden DL, Fuccillo DA, Tzan NR, Edmonds DM. Toxoplasmosis: maternal and pediatric findings in 23,000 pregnancies. Pediatrics. 1988;**82**(2):181–192.

[25] Torrey EF, Torrey BB, Burton-Bradley BG. The epidemiology of schizophrenia in Papua New Guinea. Am J Psychiatry. 1974;**131**(5):567–573.

[26] Wallace GD, Zigas V, Gajdusek DC. Toxoplasmosis and cats in New Guinea. Am J Trop Med Hyg. 1974;**23**(1):8–14.

[27] Ryan M, Hall SM, Barrett NJ, Balfour AH, Holliman RE, Joynson DH. Toxoplasmosis in England and Wales 1981 to 1992. Commun Dis Rep CDR Rev. 1995;**5**(2):R13–R21.

[28] Watt DC, Szulecka TK. The effect of sex, marriage and age at first admission on the hospitalization of schizophrenics during 2 years following discharge. Psychol Med. 1979;**9**(3):529–539. doi:10.1017/S0033291700032098

[29] Kruszon-Moran D, McQuillan GM. Seroprevalence of six infectious diseases among adults in the United States by race/ethnicity: data from the third national health and nutrition examination survey, 1988–94. Adv Data. 2005;**352**:1–9.

[30] Regier DA, Farmer ME, Rae DS, Myers JK, Kramer M, Robins LN, George LK, Karno M, Locke BZ. One-month prevalence of mental disorders in the United States and sociode-

mographic characteristics: the Epidemiologic Catchment Area study. Acta Psychiatr Scand. 1993;**88**(1):35–47. doi:10.1111/j.1600-0447.1993.tb03411.x

[31] Torrey EF, Yolken RH. *Toxoplasma gondii* and schizophrenia. Emerg Infect Dis. 2003;**9**(11):1375–1380.

[32] Gutiérrez-Fernández J, Luna Del Castillo J de D, Mañanes-González S, Carrillo-Ávila JA, Gutiérrez B, Cervilla JA, Sorlózano-Puerto A. Different presence of *Chlamydia pneumoniae*, herpes simplex virus type 1, human herpes virus 6, and *Toxoplasma gondii* in schizophrenia: meta-analysis and analytical study. Neuropsychiatr Dis Treat. 2015;**11**:843–852. doi:10.2147/NDT.S79285

[33] Torrey EF, Bartko JJ, Lun ZR, Yolken RH. Antibodies to *Toxoplasma gondii* in patients with schizophrenia: a meta-analysis. Schizophr Bull. 2007;**33**(3):729–736. doi:10.1093/schbul/sbl050

[34] Torrey EF, Bartko JJ, Yolken RH. *Toxoplasma gondii* and other risk factors for schizophrenia: an update. Schizophr Bull. 2012;**38**(3):642–647. doi:10.1093/schbul/sbs043

[35] Sutterland AL, Fond G, Kuin A, Koeter MW, Lutter R, van Gool T, Yolken R, Szoke A, Leboyer M, de Haan L. Beyond the association. *Toxoplasma gondii* in schizophrenia, bipolar disorder, and addiction: systematic review and meta-analysis. Acta Psychiatr Scand. 2015;**132**(3):161–179. doi:10.1111/acps.12423

[36] Dard C, Fricker-Hidalgo H, Brenier-Pinchart MP, Pelloux H. Relevance of and new developments in serology for toxoplasmosis. Trends Parasitol. 2016;**32**(6):492–506. doi:10.1016/j.pt.2016.04.001.

[37] Ahmad D, Mehdi S, Sayed HH, Sayed AK, Shirzad G. Serological survey of *Toxoplasma gondii* in schizophrenia patients referred to Psychiatric Hospital, Sari City, Iran. Trop Biomed. 2010;**27**(3):476–482.

[38] Alvarado-Esquivel C, Alanis-Quiñones OP, Arreola-Valenzuela MA, Rodríguez-Briones A, Piedra-Nevarez LJ, Duran-Morales E, Estrada-Martínez S, Martínez-García SA, Liesenfeld O. Seroepidemiology of *Toxoplasma gondii* infection in psychiatric inpatients in a northern Mexican city. BMC Infect Dis. 2006;**6**:178. doi:10.1186/1471-2334-6-178

[39] Alvarado-Esquivel C, Urbina-Álvarez JD, Estrada-Martínez S, Torres-Castorena A, Molotla-de-León G, Liesenfeld O, Dubey JP. *Toxoplasma gondii* infection and schizophrenia: a case control study in a low *Toxoplasma* seroprevalence Mexican population. Parasitol Int. 2011;**60**(2):151–155. doi:10.1016/j.parint.2010.12.003

[40] Amminger GP, McGorry PD, Berger GE, Wade D, Yung AR, Phillips LJ, Harrigan SM, Francey SM, Yolken RH. Antibodies to infectious agents in individuals at ultra-high risk for psychosis. Biol Psychiatry. 2007;**61**(10):1215–1217. doi:10.1016/j.biopsych.2006.09.034

[41] Cetinkaya Z, Yazar S, Gecici O, Namli MN. Anti-*Toxoplasma gondii* antibodies in patients with schizophrenia—preliminary findings in a Turkish sample. Schizophr Bull. 2007;**33**(3):789–791. doi:10.1093/schbul/sbm021

[42] El-Sahn AA, Shatat HZ, Ghitany EM. Seropositivity of toxoplasmosis in patients with schizophrenia. J Egypt Public Health Assoc. 2005;**80**(5–6):509–524.

[43] Hamidinejat H, Ghorbanpoor M, Hosseini H, Alavi SM, Nabavi L, Jalali MH, Borojeni MP, Jafari H, Mohammadaligol S. *Toxoplasma gondii* infection in first-episode and inpatient individuals with schizophrenia. Int J Infect Dis. 2010;**14**(11):e978–e981. doi:10.1016/j.ijid.2010.05.018

[44] Leweke FM, Gerth CW, Koethe D, Klosterkötter J, Ruslanova I, Krivogorsky B, Torrey EF, Yolken RH. Antibodies to infectious agents in individuals with recent onset schizophrenia. Eur Arch Psychiatry Clin Neurosci. 2004;**254**(1):4–8. doi:10.1007/s00406-004-0481-6

[45] Niebuhr DW, Millikan AM, Cowan DN, Yolken R, Li Y, Weber NS. Selected infectious agents and risk of schizophrenia among US military personnel. Am J Psychiatry. 2008;**165**(1):99–106. doi:10.1176/appi.ajp.2007.06081254

[46] Omar A, Bakar OC, Adam NF, Osman H, Osman A, Suleiman AH, Manaf MR, Selamat MI. Seropositivity and serointensity of *Toxoplasma gondii* antibodies and DNA among patients with schizophrenia. Korean J Parasitol. 2015;**53**(1):29–34. doi:10.3347/kjp.2015.53.1.29

[47] Pedersen MG, Stevens H, Pedersen CB, Nørgaard-Pedersen B, Mortensen PB. *Toxoplasma* infection and later development of schizophrenia in mothers. Am J Psychiatry. 2011;**168**(8):814–821. doi:10.1176/appi.ajp.2011.10091351

[48] Tamer GS, Dundar D, Yalug I, Caliskan S, Yazar S, Aker A. The schizophrenia and *Toxoplasma gondii* connection: infectious, immune or both? Adv Ther. 2008;**25**(7):703–709. doi:10.1007/s12325-008-0063-5

[49] Tedla Y, Shibre T, Ali O, Tadele G, Woldeamanuel Y, Asrat D, Aseffa A, Mihret W, Abebe M, Alem A, Medhin G, Habte A. Serum antibodies to *Toxoplasma gondii* and *Herpesvidae* family viruses in individuals with schizophrenia and bipolar disorder: a case-control study. Ethiop Med J. 2011;**49**(3):211–220.

[50] Wang HL, Wang GH, Li QY, Shu C, Jiang MS, Guo Y. Prevalence of *Toxoplasma* infection in first-episode schizophrenia and comparison between *Toxoplasma*-seropositive and *Toxoplasma*-seronegative schizophrenia. Acta Psychiatr Scand. 2006;**114**(1):40–48. doi:10.1111/j.1600-0447.2006.00780.x

[51] Yolken RH, Bachmann S, Ruslanova I, Lillehoj E, Ford G, Torrey EF, Schroeder J. Antibodies to *Toxoplasma gondii* in individuals with first-episode schizophrenia. Clin Infect Dis. 2001;**32**(5):842–844. doi:10.1086/319221

[52] Xiao Y, Yin J, Jiang N, Xiang M, Hao L, Lu H, Sang H, Liu X, Xu H, Ankarklev J, Lindh J, Chen Q. Seroepidemiology of human *Toxoplasma gondii* infection in China. BMC Infect Dis. 2010;**10**:4. doi:10.1186/1471-2334-10-4.

[53] Nascimento FS, de Rosalmeida Dantas C, Netto MP, Mella LF, Suzuki LA, Banzato CE, Rossi CL. Prevalence of antibodies to *Toxoplasma gondii* in patients with schizophrenia and mood disorders. Schizophr Res. 2012;**142**(1–3):244–245. doi:10.1016/j.schres.2012.08.036

[54] Holub D, Flegr J, Dragomirecká E, Rodriguez M, Preiss M, Novák T, Čermák J, Horáček J, Kodym P, Libiger J, Höschl C, Motlová LB. Differences in onset of disease and severity of psychopathology between toxoplasmosis-related and toxoplasmosis-unrelated schizophrenia. Acta Psychiatr Scand. 2013;**127**(3):227–238. doi:10.1111/acps.12031

[55] Dickerson F, Boronow J, Stallings C, Origoni A, Yolken R. *Toxoplasma gondii* in individuals with schizophrenia: association with clinical and demographic factors and with mortality. Schizophr Bull. 2007;**33**(3):737–740. doi:10.1093/schbul/sbm005

[56] Okusaga O, Langenberg P, Sleemi A, Vaswani D, Giegling I, Hartmann AM, Konte B, Friedl M, Groer MW, Yolken RH, Rujescu D, Postolache TT. *Toxoplasma gondii* antibody titers and history of suicide attempts in patients with schizophrenia. Schizophr Res. 2011;**133**(1–3):150–155. doi:10.1016/j.schres.2011.08.006

[57] Rice JS, Kowal C, Volpe BT, DeGiorgio LA, Diamond B. Molecular mimicry: anti-DNA antibodies bind microbial and nonnucleic acid self-antigens. Curr Top Microbiol Immunol. 2005;**296**:137–151. doi:10.1007/3-540-30791-5_8

[58] Monroe JM, Buckley PF, Miller BJ. Meta-Analysis of anti-*Toxoplasma gondii* IgM antibodies in acute psychosis. Schizophr Bull. 2015;**41**(4):989–998. doi:10.1093/schbul/sbu159

[59] Mortensen PB, Nørgaard-Pedersen B, Waltoft BL, Sørensen TL, Hougaard D, Torrey EF, Yolken RH. *Toxoplasma gondii* as a risk factor for early-onset schizophrenia: analysis of filter paper blood samples obtained at birth. Biol Psychiatry. 2007;**61**(5):688–693. doi:10.1016/j.biopsych.2006.05.024

[60] Brown AS, Schaefer CA, Quesenberry CP Jr, Liu L, Babulas VP, Susser ES. Maternal exposure to toxoplasmosis and risk of schizophrenia in adult offspring. Am J Psychiatry. 2005;**162**(4):767–773. doi:10.1176/appi.ajp.162.4.767

[61] Blomström A, Karlsson H, Wicks S, Yang S, Yolken RH, Dalman C. Maternal antibodies to infectious agents and risk for non-affective psychoses in the offspring-a matched case-control study. Schizophr Res. 2012;**140**(1–3):25–30. doi:10.1016/j.schres.2012.06.035

[62] Buka SL, Tsuang MT, Torrey EF, Klebanoff MA, Wagner RL, Yolken RH. Maternal cytokine levels during pregnancy and adult psychosis. Brain Behav Immun. 2001;**15**(4):411–420. doi:10.1006/brbi.2001.0644

[63] Xiao J, Buka SL, Cannon TD, Suzuki Y, Viscidi RP, Torrey EF, Yolken RH. Serological pattern consistent with infection with type I *Toxoplasma gondii* in mothers and risk of psychosis among adult offspring. Microbes Infect. 2009;**11**(13):1011–1018. doi:10.1016/j.micinf.2009.07.007

[64] Mortensen PB, Nørgaard-Pedersen B, Waltoft BL, Sørensen TL, Hougaard D, Yolken RH. Early infections of *Toxoplasma gondii* and the later development of schizophrenia. Schizophr Bull. 2007;**33**(3):741–744. doi:10.1093/schbul/sbm009

[65] Lebech M, Andersen O, Christensen NC, Hertel J, Nielsen HE, Peitersen B, Rechnitzer C, Larsen SO, Nørgaard-Pedersen B, Petersen E. Feasibility of neonatal screening for toxoplasma infection in the absence of prenatal treatment. Danish Congenital Toxoplasmosis Study Group. Lancet. 1999;**353**(9167):1834–1837.

[66] Pope RM. Immunoregulatory mechanisms present in the maternal circulation during pregnancy. Baillieres Clin Rheumatol. 1990;**4**(1):33–52. doi:10.1016/S0950-3579(05)80242-0

[67] Brown AS, Hooton J, Schaefer CA, Zhang H, Petkova E, Babulas V, Perrin M, Gorman JM, Susser ES. Elevated maternal interleukin-8 levels and risk of schizophrenia in adult offspring. Am J Psychiatry. 2004;**161**(5):889–895. doi:10.1176/appi.ajp.161.5.889

[68] Buka SL, Tsuang MT, Torrey EF, Klebanoff MA, Bernstein D, Yolken RH. Maternal infections and subsequent psychosis among offspring. Arch Gen Psychiatry. 2001;**58**(11):1032–1037. doi:10.1001/archpsyc.58.11.1032

[69] Carruthers VB, Suzuki Y. Effects of *Toxoplasma gondii* infection on the brain. Schizophr Bull. 2007;**33**(3):745–751. doi:10.1093/schbul/sbm008

[70] Berenreiterová M, Flegr J, Kuběna AA, Němec P. The distribution of *Toxoplasma gondii* cysts in the brain of a mouse with latent toxoplasmosis: implications for the behavioral manipulation hypothesis. PLoS One. 2011;**6**(12):e28925. doi:10.1371/journal.pone.0028925

[71] Di Cristina M, Marocco D, Galizi R, Proietti C, Spaccapelo R, Crisanti A. Temporal and spatial distribution of *Toxoplasma gondii* differentiation into bradyzoites and tissue cyst formation *in vivo*. Infect Immun. 2008;**76**(8):3491–3501. doi:10.1128/IAI.00254-08

[72] Hermes G, Ajioka JW, Kelly KA, Mui E, Roberts F, Kasza K, Mayr T, Kirisits MJ, Wollmann R, Ferguson DJ, Roberts CW, Hwang JH, Trendler T, Kennan RP, Suzuki Y, Reardon C, Hickey WF, Chen L, McLeod R. Neurological and behavioral abnormalities, ventricular dilatation, altered cellular functions, inflammation, and neuronal injury in brains of mice due to common, persistent, parasitic infection. J Neuroinflamm. 2008;**5**:48. doi:10.1186/1742-2094-5-48

[73] Vyas A, Kim SK, Giacomini N, Boothroyd JC, Sapolsky RM. Behavioral changes induced by *Toxoplasma* infection of rodents are highly specific to aversion of cat odors. Proc Natl Acad Sci U S A. 2007;**104**(15):6442–6447. doi:10.1073/pnas.0608310104

[74] Cotter DR, Pariante CM, Everall IP. Glial cell abnormalities in major psychiatric disorders: the evidence and implications. Brain Res Bull. 2001;**55**(5):585–595. doi:10.1016/S0361-9230(01)00527-5

[75] Shenton ME, Dickey CC, Frumin M, McCarley RW. A review of MRI findings in schizophrenia. Schizophr Res. 2001;**49**(1–2):1–52. doi:10.1016/S0920-9964(01)00163-3

[76] Horacek J, Flegr J, Tintera J, Verebova K, Spaniel F, Novak T, Brunovsky M, Bubenikova-Valesova V, Holub D, Palenicek T, Höschl C. Latent toxoplasmosis reduces gray matter density in schizophrenia but not in controls: voxel-based-morphometry (VBM) study. World J Biol Psychiatry. 2012;**13**(7):501–509. doi:10.3109/15622975.2011.573809

[77] Conejero-Goldberg C, Torrey EF, Yolken RH. Herpesviruses and *Toxoplasma gondii* in orbital frontal cortex of psychiatric patients. Schizophr Res. 2003;**60**(1):65–69. doi:10.1016/S0920-9964(02)00160-3

[78] Berdoy M, Webster JP, Macdonald DW. Parasite-altered behaviour: is the effect of *Toxoplasma gondii* on *Rattus norvegicus* specific? Parasitology. 1995;**111**(Pt 4):403–409. doi:10.1017/S0031182000065902

[79] Berdoy M, Webster JP, Macdonald DW. Fatal attraction in rats infected with *Toxoplasma gondii*. Proc Biol Sci. 2000;**267**(1452):1591–1594. doi:10.1098/rspb.2000.1182

[80] Hay J, Aitken PP, Graham DI. Toxoplasma infection and response to novelty in mice. Z Parasitenkd. 1984;**70**(5):575–588. doi:10.1007/BF00926588

[81] Webster JP. The effect of *Toxoplasma gondii* and other parasites on activity levels in wild and hybrid *Rattus norvegicus*. Parasitology. 1994;**109**(Pt 5):583–589. doi:10.1017/S0031182000076460

[82] Webster JP, Brunton CF, MacDonald DW. Effect of *Toxoplasma gondii* upon neophobic behaviour in wild brown rats, *Rattus norvegicus*. Parasitology. 1994;**109**(Pt 1):37–43. doi:10.1017/S003118200007774X

[83] Witting PA. Learning capacity and memory of normal and *Toxoplasma*-infected laboratory rats and mice. Z Parasitenkd. 1979;**61**(1):29–51.

[84] Webster JP. Rats, cats, people and parasites: the impact of latent toxoplasmosis on behaviour. Microbes Infect. 2001;**3**(12):1037–1045. doi:10.1016/S1286-4579(01)01459-9

[85] Webster JP. The effect of *Toxoplasma gondii* on animal behavior: playing cat and mouse. Schizophr Bull. 2007;**33**(3):752–756. doi:10.1093/schbul/sbl073

[86] Hari Dass SA, Vyas A. *Toxoplasma gondii* infection reduces predator aversion in rats through epigenetic modulation in the host medial amygdala. Mol Ecol. 2014;**23**(24):6114–6122. doi:10.1111/mec.12888

[87] Daniels BP, Sestito SR, Rouse ST. An expanded task battery in the Morris water maze reveals effects of *Toxoplasma gondii* infection on learning and memory in rats. Parasitol Int. 2015;**64**(1):5–12. doi:10.1016/j.parint.2014.09.002

[88] Holliman RE. Toxoplasmosis, behaviour and personality. J Infect. 1997;**35**(2):105–110. doi:10.1016/S0163-4453(97)91380-3

[89] Stibbs HH. Changes in brain concentrations of catecholamines and indoleamines in *Toxoplasma gondii* infected mice. Ann Trop Med Parasitol. 1985;**79**(2):153–157.

[90] Tomasik J, Schultz TL, Kluge W, Yolken RH, Bahn S, Carruthers VB. Shared immune and repair markers during experimental *Toxoplasma* chronic brain infection and schizophrenia. Schizophr Bull. 2016;**42**(2):386–395. doi:10.1093/schbul/sbv134

[91] Flegr J, Zitková S, Kodym P, Frynta D. Induction of changes in human behaviour by the parasitic protozoan *Toxoplasma gondii*. Parasitology. 1996;**113**(Pt 1):49–54. doi:10.1017/S0031182000066269

[92] Flegr J, Kodym P, Tolarová V. Correlation of duration of latent *Toxoplasma gondii* infection with personality changes in women. Biol Psychol. 2000;**53**(1):57–68. doi:10.1016/S0301-0511(00)00034-X

[93] Havlícek J, Gasová ZG, Smith AP, Zvára K, Flegr J. Decrease of psychomotor performance in subjects with latent 'asymptomatic' toxoplasmosis. Parasitology. 2001;**122**(Pt 5):515–520. doi:10.1017/S0031182001007624

[94] Jones-Brando L, Torrey EF, Yolken R. Drugs used in the treatment of schizophrenia and bipolar disorder inhibit the replication of *Toxoplasma gondii*. Schizophr Res. 2003;**62**(3):237–244. doi:10.1016/S0920-9964(02)00357-2

[95] Pezzella N, Bouchot A, Bonhomme A, Pingret L, Klein C, Burlet H, Balossier G, Bonhomme P, Pinon JM. Involvement of calcium and calmodulin in *Toxoplasma gondii* tachyzoite invasion. Eur J Cell Biol. 1997;**74**(1):92–101.

[96] Webster JP, Lamberton PH, Donnelly CA, Torrey EF. Parasites as causative agents of human affective disorders? The impact of anti-psychotic, mood-stabilizer and anti-parasite medication on *Toxoplasma gondii*'s ability to alter host behaviour. Proc Biol Sci. 2006;**273**(1589):1023–1030. doi:10.1098/rspb.2005.3413

[97] Flegr J, Preiss M, Klose J, Havlícek J, Vitáková M, Kodym P. Decreased level of psychobiological factor novelty seeking and lower intelligence in men latently infected with the protozoan parasite *Toxoplasma gondii*. Dopamine, a missing link between schizophrenia and toxoplasmosis? Biol Psychol. 2003;**63**(3):253–268. doi:10.1016/S0301-0511(03)00075-9

[98] Fond G, Macgregor A, Tamouza R, Hamdani N, Meary A, Leboyer M, Dubremetz JF. Comparative analysis of anti-toxoplasmic activity of antipsychotic drugs and valproate. Eur Arch Psychiatry Clin Neurosci. 2014;**264**(2):179–183. doi:10.1007/s00406-013-0413-4

[99] Goodwin DG, Strobl JS, Lindsay DS. Evaluation of five antischizophrenic agents against *Toxoplasma gondii* in human cell cultures. J Parasitol. 2011;**97**(1):148–151. doi:10.1645/GE-2536.1

[100] Dickerson FB, Stallings CR, Boronow JJ, Origoni AE, Yolken RH. A double-blind trial of adjunctive azithromycin in individuals with schizophrenia who are seropositive for *Toxoplasma gondii*. Schizophr Res. 2009;**112**(1–3):198–199. doi:10.1016/j.schres.2009.05.005

[101] Shibre T, Alem A, Abdulahi A, Araya M, Beyero T, Medhin G, Deyassa N, Negash A, Nigatu A, Kebede D, Fekadu A. Trimethoprim as adjuvant treatment in schizophrenia: a double-blind, randomized, placebo-controlled clinical trial. Schizophr Bull. 2010;**36**(4):846–851. doi:10.1093/schbul/sbn191

[102] Wei HX, Wei SS, Lindsay DS, Peng HJ. A systematic review and meta-analysis of the efficacy of anti-*Toxoplasma gondii* medicines in humans. PLoS One. 2015;**10**(9):e0138204. doi:10.1371/journal.pone.0138204

[103] da Silva RC, Langoni H. *Toxoplasma gondii*: host-parasite interaction and behavior manipulation. Parasitol Res. 2009;**105**(4):893–898. doi:10.1007/s00436-009-1526-6

[104] Khandaker GM, Cousins L, Deakin J, Lennox BR, Yolken R, Jones PB. Inflammation and immunity in schizophrenia: implications for pathophysiology and treatment. Lancet Psychiatry. 2015;**2**(3):258–270. doi:10.1016/S2215-0366(14)00122-9

[105] Doorduin J, de Vries EF, Willemsen AT, de Groot JC, Dierckx RA, Klein HC. Neuroinflammation in schizophrenia-related psychosis: a PET study. J Nucl Med. 2009;**50**(11):1801–1807. doi:10.2967/jnumed.109.066647

[106] Lin G, Zhang H, Sun F, Lu Z, Reed-Maldonado A, Lee YC, Wang G, Banie L, Lue TF. Brain-derived neurotrophic factor promotes nerve regeneration by activating the JAK/STAT pathway in Schwann cells. Transl Androl Urol. 2016;**5**(2):167–175. doi:10.21037/tau.2016.02.03

[107] Qin H, Buckley JA, Li X, Liu Y, Fox TH 3rd, Meares GP, Yu H, Yan Z, Harms AS, Li Y, Standaert DG, Benveniste EN. Inhibition of the JAK/STAT pathway protects against $\alpha$-synuclein-induced neuroinflammation and dopaminergic neurodegeneration. J Neurosci. 2016;**36**(18):5144–5159. doi:10.1523/JNEUROSCI.4658-15.2016

[108] Gavrilescu LC, Butcher BA, Del Rio L, Taylor GA, Denkers EY. STAT1 is essential for antimicrobial effector function but dispensable for gamma interferon production during *Toxoplasma gondii* infection. Infect Immun. 2004;**72**(3):1257–1264. doi:10.1128/IAI.72.3.1257-1264.2004

[109] Kim SK, Fouts AE, Boothroyd JC. *Toxoplasma gondii* dysregulates IFN-gamma-inducible gene expression in human fibroblasts: insights from a genome-wide transcriptional profiling. J Immunol. 2007;**178**(8):5154–5165.

[110] Sun GY, Horrocks LA, Farooqui AA. The roles of NADPH oxidase and phospholipases A2 in oxidative and inflammatory responses in neurodegenerative diseases. J Neurochem. 2007;**103**(1):1–16.

[111] Elsheikha HM, Büsselberg D, Zhu XQ. The known and missing links between *Toxoplasma gondii* and schizophrenia. Metab Brain Dis. 2016;**31**(4):749–759. doi:10.1007/s11011-016-9822-1

[112] Vasconcelos AR, Yshii LM, Viel TA, Buck HS, Mattson MP, Scavone C, Kawamoto EM. Intermittent fasting attenuates lipopolysaccharide-induced neuroinflammation and memory impairment. J Neuroinflamm. 2014;**11**:85. doi:10.1186/1742-2094-11-85

[113] Zindler E, Zipp F. Neuronal injury in chronic CNS inflammation. Best Pract Res Clin Anaesthesiol. 2010;**24**(4):551–562. doi:10.1016/j.bpa.2010.11.001

[114] Prandovszky E, Gaskell E, Martin H, Dubey JP, Webster JP, McConkey GA. The neurotropic parasite *Toxoplasma gondii* increases dopamine metabolism. PLoS One. 2011;**6**(9):e232866. doi:10.1371/journal.pone.0023866

[115] Skallová A, Kodym P, Frynta D, Flegr J. The role of dopamine in *Toxoplasma*-induced behavioural alterations in mice: an ethological and ethopharmacological study. Parasitology. 2006;**133**(Pt 5):525–535. doi:10.1017/S0031182006000886

[116] Gaskell EA, Smith JE, Pinney JW, Westhead DR, McConkey GA. A unique dual activity amino acid hydroxylase in *Toxoplasma gondii*. PLoS One. 2009;**4**(3):e4801. doi:10.1371/journal.pone.0004801

[117] Martin HL, Alsaady I, Howell G, Prandovszky E, Peers C, Robinson P, McConkey GA. Effect of parasitic infection on dopamine biosynthesis in dopaminergic cells. Neuroscience. 2015;**306**:50–62. doi:10.1016/j.neuroscience.2015.08.005

[118] Strobl JS, Goodwin DG, Rzigalinski BA, Lindsay DS. Dopamine stimulates propagation of *Toxoplasma gondii* tachyzoites in human fibroblast and primary neonatal rat astrocyte cell cultures. J Parasitol. 2012;**98**(6):1296–1299. doi:10.1645/GE-2760.1

[119] Stiles J, Jernigan TL. The basics of brain development. Neuropsychol Rev. 2010;**20**(4):327–348. doi:10.1007/s11065-010-9148-4

[120] Paus T. Mapping brain maturation and cognitive development during adolescence. Trends Cogn Sci. 2005;**9**(2):60–88. doi:10.1016/j.tics.2004.12.008

[121] Nilsson LK, Linderholm KR, Engberg G, Paulson L, Blennow K, Lindström LH, Nordin C, Karanti A, Persson P, Erhardt S. Elevated levels of kynurenic acid in the cerebrospinal fluid of male patients with schizophrenia. Schizophr Res. 2005;**80**(2–3):315–322. doi:10.1016/j.schres.2005.07.013

[122] Erhardt S, Schwieler L, Nilsson L, Linderholm K, Engberg G. The kynurenic acid hypothesis of schizophrenia. Physiol Behav. 2007;**92**(1–2):203–209. doi:10.1016/j.physbeh.2007.05.025

[123] Silva NM, Rodrigues CV, Santoro MM, Reis LF, Alvarez-Leite JI, Gazzinelli RT. Expression of indoleamine 2,3-dioxygenase, tryptophan degradation, and kynurenine formation during *in vivo* infection with *Toxoplasma gondii*: induction by endogenous gamma interferon and requirement of interferon regulatory factor 1. Infect Immun. 2002;**70**(2):859–868. doi:10.1128/IAI.70.2.859-868.2002

[124] Miller CM, Boulter NR, Ikin RJ, Smith NC. The immunobiology of the innate response to *Toxoplasma gondii*. Int J Parasitol. 2009;**39**(1):23–39. doi:10.1016/j.ijpara.2008.08.002

[125] Lidberg L, Belfrage H, Bertilsson L, Evenden MM, Asberg M. Suicide attempts and impulse control disorder are related to low cerebrospinal fluid 5-HIAA in mentally disordered violent offenders. Acta Psychiatr Scand. 2000;**101**(5):395–402.

[126] Widner B, Laich A, Sperner-Unterweger B, Ledochowski M, Fuchs D. Neopterin production, tryptophan degradation, and mental depression—what is the link? Brain Behav Immun. 2002;**16**(5):590–595. doi:10.1016/S0889-1591(02)00006-5

[127] Buddhala C, Hsu CC, Wu JY. A novel mechanism for GABA synthesis and packaging into synaptic vesicles. Neurochem Int. 2009;**55**(1–3):9–12. doi:10.1016/j.neuint.2009.01.020

[128] Barragan A, Weidner JM, Jin Z, Korpi ER, Birnir B. GABAergic signalling in the immune system. Acta Physiol (Oxf). 2015;**213**(4):819–827. doi:10.1111/apha.12467

[129] Simpson MD, Slater P, Deakin JF, Royston MC, Skan WJ. Reduced GABA uptake sites in the temporal lobe in schizophrenia. Neurosci Lett. 1989;**107**(1–3):211–215. doi:10.1016/0304-3940(89)90819-7

[130] Reynolds GP, Czudek C, Andrews HB. Deficit and hemispheric asymmetry of GABA uptake sites in the hippocampus in schizophrenia. Biol Psychiatry 1990;**27**(9):1038–1044. doi:10.1016/0006-3223(90)90039-5

[131] Lewis DA, Pierri JN, Volk DW, Melchitzky DS, Woo TU. Altered GABA neurotransmission and prefrontal cortical dysfunction in schizophrenia. Biol Psychiatry. 1999;**46**(5):616–626. doi:10.1016/S0006-3223(99)00061-X

[132] Volk D, Austin M, Pierri J, Sampson A, Lewis D. GABA transporter-1 mRNA in the prefrontal cortex in schizophrenia: decreased expression in a subset of neurons. Am J Psychiatry. 2001;**158**(2):256–265. doi:10.1176/appi.ajp.158.2.256

[133] Woo TU, Walsh JP, Benes FM. Density of glutamic acid decarboxylase 67 messenger RNA-containing neurons that express the *N*-methyl-D-aspartate receptor subunit NR2A in the anterior cingulate cortex in schizophrenia and bipolar disorder. Arch Gen Psychiatry. 2004;61(7):649–657.

[134] Volk DW, Pierri JN, Fritschy JM, Auh S, Sampson AR, Lewis DA. Reciprocal alterations in pre- and postsynaptic inhibitory markers at chandelier cell inputs to pyramidal neurons in schizophrenia. Cereb Cortex. 2002;**12**(10):1063–1070. doi:10.1093/cercor/12.10.1063

[135] Fatemi SH, Folsom TD, Thuras PD. Deficits in GABA(B) receptor system in schizophrenia and mood disorders: a postmortem study. Schizophr Res. 2011;**128**(1–3):37–43. doi:10.1016/j.schres.2010.12.025

[136] Olofsson PS, Rosas-Ballina M, Levine YA, Tracey KJ. Rethinking inflammation: neural circuits in the regulation of immunity. Immunol Rev. 2012;**248**(1):188–204. doi:10.1111/j.1600-065X.2012.01138.x

[137] Fuks JM, Arrighi RB, Weidner JM, Kumar Mendu S, Jin Z, Wallin RP, Rethi B, Birnir B, Barragan A. GABAergic signaling is linked to a hypermigratory phenotype in dendritic cells infected by *Toxoplasma gondii*. PLoS Pathog. 2012;**8**(12):e1003051. doi:10.1371/journal.ppat.1003051

[138] Weidner JM, Kanatani S, Hernandez-Castaneda MA, Fuks JM, Rethi B, Wallin RP, Barragan A. Rapid cytoskeleton remodelling in dendritic cells following invasion by *Toxoplasma gondii* coincides with the onset of a hypermigratory phenotype. Cell Microbiol. 2013;**15**(10):1735–1752. doi:10.1111/cmi.12145

[139] Brooks JM, Carrillo GL, Su J, Lindsay DS, Fox MA, Blader IJ. *Toxoplasma gondii* infections alter GABAergic synapses and signaling in the central nervous system. MBio. 2015;**6**(6):e01428–15. doi:10.1128/mBio.01428-15

[140] Xiao J, Li Y, Prandovszky E, Karuppagounder SS, Talbot CC Jr, Dawson VL, Dawson TM, Yolken RH. MicroRNA-132 dysregulation in *Toxoplasma gondii* infection has implications for dopamine signaling pathway. Neuroscience. 2014;**268**:128–138. doi:10.1016/j.neuroscience.2014.03.015

[141] Dalmau J, Gleichman AJ, Hughes EG, Rossi JE, Peng X, Lai M, Dessain SK, Rosenfeld MR, Balice-Gordon R, Lynch DR. Anti-NMDA-receptor encephalitis: case series and analysis of the effects of antibodies. Lancet Neurol. 2008;**7**(12):1091–1098. doi:10.1016/S1474-4422(08)70224-2

[142] Irani SR, Bera K, Waters P, Zuliani L, Maxwell S, Zandi MS, Friese MA, Galea I, Kullmann DM, Beeson D, Lang B, Bien CG, Vincent A. *N*-methyl-D-aspartate antibody encephalitis: temporal progression of clinical and paraclinical observations in a predominantly non-paraneoplastic disorder of both sexes. Brain. 2010;**133**(Pt 6):1655–1667. doi:10.1093/brain/awq113

[143] Dalmau J, Tüzün E, Wu HY, Masjuan J, Rossi JE, Voloschin A, Baehring JM, Shimazaki H, Koide R, King D, Mason W, Sansing LH, Dichter MA, Rosenfeld MR, Lynch DR. Paraneoplastic anti-*N*-methyl-D-aspartate receptor encephalitis associated with ovarian teratoma. Ann Neurol. 2007;**61**(1):25–36. doi:10.1002/ana.21050

[144] Fawcett RG. Acute psychosis associated with anti-NMDA-receptor antibodies and bilateral ovarian teratomas: a case report. J Clin Psychiatry. 2010;**71**(4):504. doi:10.4088/JCP.09l05609yel

[145] Benros ME, Mortensen PB, Eaton WW. Autoimmune diseases and infections as risk factors for schizophrenia. Ann N Y Acad Sci. 2012;**1262**:56–66. doi:10.1111/j.1749-6632.2012.06638.x

[146] DeGiorgio LA, Konstantinov KN, Lee SC, Hardin JA, Volpe BT, Diamond B. A subset of lupus anti-DNA antibodies cross-reacts with the NR2 glutamate receptor in systemic lupus erythematosus. Nat Med. 2001;**7**(11):1189–1193.

[147] Pearlman DM, Najjar S. Meta-analysis of the association between *N*-methyl-D-aspartate receptor antibodies and schizophrenia, schizoaffective disorder, bipolar disorder, and major depressive disorder. Schizophr Res. 2014;**157**(1–3):249–258. doi:10.1016/j.schres.2014.05.001

[148] Smyth AM, Lawrie SM. The neuroimmunology of schizophrenia. Clin Psychopharmacol Neurosci. 2013;**11**(3):107–117. doi:10.9758/cpn.2013.11.3.107

[149] Deakin J, Lennox BR, Zandi MS. Antibodies to the *N*-methyl-D-aspartate receptor and other synaptic proteins in psychosis. Biol Psychiatry. 2014;**75**(4):284–291. doi:10.1016/j.biopsych.2013.07.018

[150] Steiner J, Walter M, Glanz W, Sarnyai Z, Bernstein HG, Vielhaber S, Kästner A, Skalej M, Jordan W, Schiltz K, Klingbeil C, Wandinger KP, Bogerts B, Stoecker W. Increased prevalence of diverse *N*-methyl-D-aspartate glutamate receptor antibodies in patients with an initial diagnosis of schizophrenia: specific relevance of IgG NR1a antibodies for distinction from *N*-methyl-D-aspartate glutamate receptor encephalitis. JAMA Psychiatry. 2013;**70**(3):271–278. doi:10.1001/2013.jamapsychiatry.86

[151] Zandi MS, Irani SR, Lang B, Waters P, Jones PB, McKenna P, Coles AJ, Vincent A, Lennox BR. Disease-relevant autoantibodies in first episode schizophrenia. J Neurol. 2011;**258**(4):686–688. doi:10.1007/s00415-010-5788-9

[152] Masdeu JC, González-Pinto A, Matute C, Ruiz De Azúa S, Palomino A, De Leon J, Berman KF, Dalmau J. Serum IgG antibodies against the NR1 subunit of the NMDA receptor not detected in schizophrenia. Am J Psychiatry. 2012;**169**(10):1120–1121. doi:10.1176/appi.ajp.2012.12050646

[153] Rhoads J, Guirgis H, McKnight C, Duchemin AM. Lack of anti-NMDA receptor autoantibodies in the serum of subjects with schizophrenia. Schizophr Res. 2011;**129**(2–3):213–214. doi:10.1016/j.schres.2010.12.018

[154] Tsutsui K, Kanbayashi T, Tanaka K, Boku S, Ito W, Tokunaga J, Mori A, Hishikawa Y, Shimizu T, Nishino S. Anti-NMDA-receptor antibody detected in encephalitis, schizophrenia, and narcolepsy with psychotic features. BMC Psychiatry. 2012;**12**:37. doi:10.1186/1471-244X-12-37

[155] Coyle JT. NMDA receptor and schizophrenia: a brief history. Schizophr Bull. 2012;**38**(5):920–926. doi:10.1093/schbul/sbs076

[156] Belforte JE, Zsiros V, Sklar ER, Jiang Z, Yu G, Li Y, Quinlan EM, Nakazawa K. Postnatal NMDA receptor ablation in corticolimbic interneurons confers schizophrenia-like phenotypes. Nat Neurosci. 2010;**13**(1):76–83. doi:10.1038/nn.2447

[157] Timms AE, Dorschner MO, Wechsler J, Choi KY, Kirkwood R, Girirajan S, Baker C, Eichler EE, Korvatska O, Roche KW, Horwitz MS, Tsuang DW. Support for the *N*-methyl-D-aspartate receptor hypofunction hypothesis of schizophrenia from exome sequencing in multiplex families. JAMA Psychiatry. 2013;**70**(6):582–590. doi:10.1001/jamapsychiatry.2013.1195

[158] Pilowsky LS, Bressan RA, Stone JM, Erlandsson K, Mulligan RS, Krystal JH, Ell PJ. First *in vivo* evidence of an NMDA receptor deficit in medication-free schizophrenic patients. Mol Psychiatry. 2006;**11**(2):118–119. doi:10.1038/sj.mp.4001751

[159] Pomarol-Clotet E, Honey GD, Murray GK, Corlett PR, Absalom AR, Lee M, McKenna PJ, Bullmore ET, Fletcher PC. Psychological effects of ketamine in healthy volunteers. Phenomenological study. Br J Psychiatry. 2006;**189**:173–179. doi:10.1192/bjp.bp.105.015263

[160] Javitt DC. Glutamate and schizophrenia: phencyclidine, *N*-methyl-D-aspartate receptors, and dopamine-glutamate interactions. Int Rev Neurobiol. 2007;**78**:69–108.

[161] Fromer M, Pocklington AJ, Kavanagh DH, Williams HJ, Dwyer S, Gormley P, Georgieva L, Rees E, Palta P, Ruderfer DM, Carrera N, Humphreys I, Johnson JS, Roussos P, Barker DD, Banks E, Milanova V, Grant SG, Hannon E, Rose SA, Chambert K, Mahajan M, Scolnick EM, Moran JL, Kirov G, Palotie A, McCarroll SA, Holmans P, Sklar P, Owen MJ, Purcell SM, O'Donovan MC. *De novo* mutations in schizophrenia implicate synaptic networks. Nature. 2014;**506**(7487):179–184. doi:10.1038/nature12929

[162] Prüss H, Finke C, Höltje M, Hofmann J, Klingbeil C, Probst C, Borowski K, Ahnert-Hilger G, Harms L, Schwab JM, Ploner CJ, Komorowski L, Stoecker W, Dalmau J, Wandinger KP. *N*-methyl-D-aspartate receptor antibodies in herpes simplex encephalitis. Ann Neurol. 2012;**72**(6):902–911. doi:10.1002/ana.23689

[163] Hammer C, Stepniak B, Schneider A, Papiol S, Tantra M, Begemann M, Sirén AL, Pardo LA, Sperling S, Mohd Jofrry S, Gurvich A, Jensen N, Ostmeier K, Lühder F, Probst C, Martens H, Gillis M, Saher G, Assogna F, Spalletta G, Stöcker W, Schulz TF, Nave KA, Ehrenreich H. Neuropsychiatric disease relevance of circulating anti-NMDA receptor autoantibodies depends on blood-brain barrier integrity. Mol Psychiatry. 2014;**19**(10):1143–1149. doi:10.1038/mp.2013.110

[164] Kannan G, Crawford JA, Yang C, Gressitt KL, Ihenatu C, Krasnova IN, Cadet JL, Yolken RH, Severance EG, Pletnikov MV. Anti-NMDA receptor autoantibodies and associated neurobehavioral pathology in mice are dependent on age of first exposure to *Toxoplasma gondii*. Neurobiol Dis. 2016;**91**:307–314. doi:10.1016/j.nbd.2016.03.005

[165] Freedman R. Schizophrenia. N Engl J Med. 2003;**349**(18):1738–1749.

[166] Cardno AG, Marshall EJ, Coid B, Macdonald AM, Ribchester TR, Davies NJ, Venturi P, Jones LA, Lewis SW, Sham PC, Gottesman II, Farmer AE, McGuffin P, Reveley AM, Murray RM. Heritability estimates for psychotic disorders: the Maudsley twin psychosis series. Arch Gen Psychiatry. 1999;**56**(2):162–168. doi:10.1001/archpsyc.56.2.162

[167] Fatemi SH, Pearce DA, Brooks AI, Sidwell RW. Prenatal viral infection in mouse causes differential expression of genes in brains of mouse progeny: a potential animal model for schizophrenia and autism. Synapse. 2005;**57**(2):91–99. doi:10.1002/syn.20162

[168] Harrison PJ, Owen MJ. Genes for schizophrenia? Recent findings and their pathophysiological implications. Lancet. 2003;**361**(9355):417–419. doi:10.1016/S0140-6736(03)12379-3

[169] Carter CJ. Schizophrenia: a pathogenetic autoimmune disease caused by viruses and pathogens and dependent on genes. J Pathog. 2011;**2011**:128318. doi:10.4061/2011/128318

[170] Tomonaga K. Virus-induced neurobehavioral disorders: mechanisms and implications. Trends Mol Med. 2004;**10**(2):71–77. doi:10.1016/j.molmed.2003.12.001

[171] Harrison PJ, Law AJ. Neuregulin 1 and schizophrenia: Genetics, gene expression, and neurobiology. Biol Psychiatry. 2006;**60**(2):132–140. doi:10.1016/j.biopsych.2005.11.002

[172] Rico B, Marín O. Neuregulin signaling, cortical circuitry development and schizophrenia. Curr Opin Genet Dev. 201;**21**(3):262–270. doi:10.1016/j.gde.2010.12.010

[173] Chen CY, Lu RB, Yeh YW, Shih MC, Huang SY. Association study of catechol-O-methyltransferase gene polymorphisms with schizophrenia and psychopathological symptoms in Han Chinese. Genes Brain Behav. 2011;**10**(3):316–324. doi:10.1111/j.1601-183X.2010.00670.x

[174] Willis A, Bender HU, Steel G, Valle D. PRODH variants and risk for schizophrenia. Amino Acids. 2008;**35**(4):673–679. doi:10.1007/s00726-008-0111-0

[175] Voisey J, Swagell CD, Hughes IP, Connor JP, Lawford BR, Young RM, Morris CP. A polymorphism in the dysbindin gene (DTNBP1) associated with multiple psychiatric disorders including schizophrenia. Behav Brain Funct. 2010;**6**(1):41. doi:10.1186/1744-9081-6-41

[176] Ding L, Hegde AN. Expression of RGS4 splice variants in dorsolateral prefrontal cortex of schizophrenic and bipolar disorder patients. Biol Psychiatry. 2009;**65**(6):541–545. doi:10.1016/j.biopsych.2008.10.026

[177] Ritsner M, Modai I, Ziv H, Amir S, Halperin T, Weizman A, Navon R. An association of CAG repeats at the KCNN3 locus with symptom dimensions of schizophrenia. Biol Psychiatry. 2002;**51**(10):788–794. doi:10.1016/S0006-3223(01)01348-8

[178] Madeira C, Freitas ME, Vargas-Lopes C, Wolosker H, Panizzutti R. Increased brain D-amino acid oxidase (DAAO) activity in schizophrenia. Schizophr Res. 2008; **101**(1–3):76–83. doi:10.1016/j.schres.2008.02.002

[179] Carter CJ. Schizophrenia susceptibility genes directly implicated in the life cycles of pathogens: cytomegalovirus, influenza, herpes simplex, rubella, and *Toxoplasma gondii*. Schizophr Bull. 2009;**35**(6):1163–1182. doi:10.1093/schbul/sbn054

[180] Carter CJ. Toxoplasmosis and polygenic disease susceptibility genes: extensive *Toxoplasma gondii* host/pathogen interactome enrichment in nine psychiatric or neurological disorders. J Pathog. 2013;**2013**:965046. doi:10.1155/2013/965046

[181] Pearce BD. Schizophrenia and viral infection during neurodevelopment: a focus on mechanisms. Mol Psychiatry. 2001;**6**(6):634–646. doi:10.1038/sj.mp.4000956

[182] Tsuang MT, Stone WS, Faraone SV. Genes, environment and schizophrenia. Br J Psychiatry Suppl. 2001;**178**(40):s18–s24. doi:10.1192/bjp.178.40.s18

[183] Khan IA, Murphy PM, Casciotti L, Schwartzman JD, Collins J, Gao JL, Yeaman GR. Mice lacking the chemokine receptor CCR1 show increased susceptibility to *Toxoplasma gondii* infection. J Immunol. 2001;**166**(3):1930–1937. doi:10.4049/jimmunol.166.3.1930

[184] Yap GS, Ortmann R, Shevach E, Sher A. A heritable defect in IL-12 signaling in B10.Q/J mice. II. Effect on acute resistance to *Toxoplasma gondii* and rescue by IL-18 treatment. J Immunol. 2001;**166**(9):5720–5725. doi:10.4049/jimmunol.166.9.5720

[185] Mack DG, Johnson JJ, Roberts F, Roberts CW, Estes RG, David C, Grumet FC, McLeod R. HLA-class II genes modify outcome of *Toxoplasma gondii* infection. Int J Parasitol. 1999;**29**(9):1351–1358. doi:10.1016/S0020-7519(99)00152-6

[186] Suzuki Y, Wong SY, Grumet FC, Fessel J, Montoya JG, Zolopa AR, Portmore A, Schumacher-Perdreau F, Schrappe M, Köppen S, Ruf B, Brown BW, Remington JS. Evidence for genetic regulation of susceptibility to toxoplasmic encephalitis in AIDS patients. J Infect Dis. 1996;**173**(1):265–268. doi:10.1093/infdis/173.1.265

[187] Avramopoulos D, Pearce BD, McGrath J, Wolyniec P, Wang R, Eckart N, Hatzimanolis A, Goes FS, Nestadt G, Mulle J, Coneely K, Hopkins M, Ruczinski I, Yolken R, Pulver AE. Infection and inflammation in schizophrenia and bipolar disorder: a genome wide study for interactions with genetic variation. PLoS One. 2015;**10**(3):e0116696. doi:10.1371/journal.pone.0116696

[188] Børglum AD, Demontis D, Grove J, Pallesen J, Hollegaard MV, Pedersen CB, Hedemand A, Mattheisen M, Uitterlinden A, Nyegaard M, Ørntoft T, Wiuf C, Didriksen M, Nordentoft M, Nöthen MM, Rietschel M, Ophoff RA, Cichon S, Yolken RH, Hougaard DM, Mortensen PB, Mors O. Genome-wide study of association and interaction with maternal cytomegalovirus infection suggests new schizophrenia loci. Mol Psychiatry. 2014;**19**(3):325–333. doi:10.1038/mp.2013.2

[189] Kannan G, Sawa A, Pletnikov MV. Mouse models of gene-environment interactions in schizophrenia. Neurobiol Dis. 2013;**57**:5–11. doi:10.1016/j.nbd.2013.05.012

[190] Kim T, Kim HJ, Park JK, Kim JW, Chung JH. Association between polymorphisms of arachidonate 12-lipoxygenase (ALOX12) and schizophrenia in a Korean population. Behav Brain Funct. 2010;**6**:44. doi:10.1186/1744-9081-6-44

[191] Witola WH, Liu SR, Montpetit A, Welti R, Hypolite M, Roth M, Zhou Y, Mui E, Cesbron-Delauw MF, Fournie GJ, Cavailles P, Bisanz C, Boyer K, Withers S, Noble AG, Swisher CN, Heydemann PT, Rabiah P, Muench SP, McLeod R. ALOX12 in human toxoplasmosis. Infect Immun. 2014;**82**(7):2670–2679. doi:10.1128/IAI.01505-13

[192] Lang F, Strutz-Seebohm N, Seebohm G, Lang UE. Significance of SGK1 in the regulation of neuronal function. J Physiol. 2010;**588**(Pt 18):3349–3354. doi:10.1113/jphysiol.2010.190926

[193] Anacker C, Cattaneo A, Musaelyan K, Zunszain PA, Horowitz M, Molteni R, Luoni A, Calabrese F, Tansey K, Gennarelli M, Thuret S, Price J, Uher R, Riva MA, Pariante CM. Role for the kinase SGK1 in stress, depression, and glucocorticoid effects on hippocampal neurogenesis. Proc Natl Acad Sci U S A. 2013;**110**(21):8708–8713. doi:10.1073/pnas.1300886110

[194] Kadkhodaei B, Ito T, Joodmardi E, Mattsson B, Rouillard C, Carta M, Muramatsu S, Sumi-Ichinose C, Nomura T, Metzger D, Chambon P, Lindqvist E, Larsson NG, Olson L, Björklund A, Ichinose H, Perlmann T. Nurr1 is required for maintenance of matur-

ing and adult midbrain dopamine neurons. J Neurosci. 2009;**29**(50):15923–15932. doi:10.1523/JNEUROSCI.3910-09.2009

[195] Eells JB, Varela-Stokes A, Guo-Ross SX, Kummari E, Smith HM, Cox E, Lindsay DS. Chronic *Toxoplasma gondii* in Nurr1-null heterozygous mice exacerbates elevated open field activity. PLoS One. 2015;**10**(4):e0119280. doi:10.1371/journal.pone.0119280

[196] Mullonkal CJ, Toledo-Pereyra LH. Akt in ischemia and reperfusion. J Invest Surg. 2007;**20**(3):195–203. doi:10.1080/08941930701366471

[197] Tan HY, Nicodemus KK, Chen Q, Li Z, Brooke JK, Honea R, Kolachana BS, Straub RE, Meyer-Lindenberg A, Sei Y, Mattay VS, Callicott JH, Weinberger DR. Genetic variation in AKT1 is linked to dopamine-associated prefrontal cortical structure and function in humans. J Clin Invest. 2008;**118**(6):2200–2208. doi:10.1172/JCI34725

[198] Fellerhoff B, Laumbacher B, Mueller N, Gu S, Wank R. Associations between *Chlamydophila* infections, schizophrenia and risk of HLA-A10. Mol Psychiatry. 2007;**12**(3):264–272. doi:10.1038/sj.mp.4001925

[199] Kim JJ, Shirts BH, Dayal M, Bacanu SA, Wood J, Xie W, Zhang X, Chowdari KV, Yolken R, Devlin B, Nimgaonkar VL. Are exposure to cytomegalovirus and genetic variation on chromosome 6p joint risk factors for schizophrenia? Ann Med. 2007;**39**(2):145–153. doi:10.1080/07853890601083808

[200] Prasad KM, Bamne MN, Shirts BH, Goradia D, Mannali V, Pancholi KM, Xue B, McClain L, Yolken RH, Keshavan MS, Nimgaonkar VL. Grey matter changes associated with host genetic variation and exposure to herpes simplex virus 1 (HSV1) in first episode schizophrenia. Schizophr Res. 2010;**118**(1–3):232–239. doi:10.1016/j.schres.2010.01.007

[201] Shirts BH, Kim JJ, Reich S, Dickerson FB, Yolken RH, Devlin B, Nimgaonkar VL. Polymorphisms in MICB are associated with human herpes virus seropositivity and schizophrenia risk. Schizophr Res. 2007;**94**(1–3):342–353. doi:10.1016/j.schres.2007.04.021

[202] Kusbeci OY, Miman O, Yaman M, Aktepe OC, Yazar S. Could *Toxoplasma gondii* have any role in Alzheimer disease? Alzheimer Dis Assoc Disord. 2011;**25**(1):1–3. doi:10.1097/WAD.0b013e3181f73bc2

[203] Miman O, Kusbeci OY, Aktepe OC, Cetinkaya Z. The probable relation between *Toxoplasma gondii* and Parkinson's disease. Neurosci Lett. 2010;**475**(3):129–131. doi:10.1016/j.neulet.2010.03.057

[204] Yazar S, Arman F, Yalçin S, Demirtas F, Yaman O, Sahin I. Investigation of probable relationship between *Toxoplasma gondii* and cryptogenic epilepsy. Seizure. 2003;**12**(2):107–109. doi:10.1016/S1059-1311(02)00256-X

[205] Webster JP, Kaushik M, Bristow GC, McConkey GA. *Toxoplasma gondii* infection, from predation to schizophrenia: can animal behaviour help us understand human behaviour? J Exp Biol. 2013;**216**(Pt 1):99–112. doi:10.1242/jeb.074716.

[206] Fond G, Boyer L, Gaman A, Laouamri H, Attiba D, Richard JR, Delavest M, Houenou J, Le Corvoisier P, Charron D, Krishnamoorthy R, Oliveira J, Tamouza R, Yolken R, Dickerson F, Leboyer M, Hamdani N. Treatment with anti-toxoplasmic activity (TATA) for toxoplasma positive patients with bipolar disorders or schizophrenia: a cross-sectional study. J Psychiatr Res. 2015;**63**:58–64. doi:10.1016/j.jpsychires.2015.02.011

2

# The Laboratory Diagnosis in *Toxoplasma* Infection

María de la Luz Galván Ramírez,
Laura Verónica Sánchez Orozco and
Cynthia Guadalupe Temores Ramírez

**Abstract**

The diagnosis of toxoplasmosis is of great importance due to the damage caused by this parasite in immunosuppressed people or in pregnant women, the diagnosis of an active toxoplasmosis represents a sign to initiate a pharmacological treatment immediately. The diagnosis of *Toxoplasma* can be performed with direct methods through intraperitoneal inoculation of serum or cerebrospinal fluid, in susceptible mice evaluating the survival and detection of tachyzoites of biological samples. Indirect methods detecting the IgM and IgG isotypes against *Toxoplasma* have been the tools mostly used and had leaded to discriminate between an active and acute, from a chronic toxoplasmosis. Molecular methods actually *Toxoplasma*-DNA identification by molecular biology tests like the polymerase chain reaction (PCR) allow the direct detection of the parasite. Polymerase chain reaction-restriction fragment length polymorphisms (PCR-RFLPs) have been used to identify three strain linages (type I, II and III). Recently, a high-resolution melting method was described to determine the genotype of the infection by *Toxoplasma gondii* directly from biological samples.

**Keywords:** *Toxoplasma* infection, diagnosis, toxoplasmosis, methods

## 1. Introduction

The diagnosis of toxoplasmosis represents a very important decision to whether to initiate or not an anti-parasitic treatment. The immunological methods that detect the IgM and IgG isotypes against *Toxoplasma* have been the tools mostly used and had leaded to discriminate between acute and chronic toxoplasmosis. In immunosuppressed people or in pregnant women, the diagnosis of an active toxoplasmosis represents a sign to initiate a pharmacological treatment immediately.

Several methodologies have been applied historically, including the isolation of the parasite in biological specimens and the xenodiagnostic evaluation through intraperitoneal inoculation of serum or cerebrospinal fluid, in susceptible mice evaluating the survival and detection of tachyzoites in cerebrospinal fluid. Serologic diagnosis is frequently performed for the detection in serum of IgM and IgG anti-*Toxoplasma* antibodies, and recently *Toxoplasma*-DNA identification by molecular biology tests is the polymerase chain reaction (PCR) that allows the detection of just 10 or less parasites in the reaction volume.

## 2. Direct methods

### 2.1. Isolation of the parasite or bioassay

The diagnosis of toxoplasmosis could be performed by the inoculation of suspicious blood samples, cerebrospinal fluid, lymph node or other corporal fluids or tissues, in the peritoneal cavity of the immunosuppressed mice or in a susceptible strain like BALB/c. The presence of tachyzoites in the peritoneal fluid of the mice is analysed by phase contrast microscopy from 6 to 10 days after inoculation. The parasite is observed in its characteristic half-moon fixing the specimen with methanol and stain with Wright, Giemsa or May-Grunwald and observed by a microscope. The parasites present sometimes a granular membrane, dyed blue cytoplasm and a red nucleus at the center of the cytoplasm.

In cases of new-borns with toxoplasmosis, inoculation of mice with blood of the child obtained during the first week of birth reaches 75% of positive results; however, if the sampling is delayed by 1 month, the positive results are reduced to 52%. A drawback of this method is the need of specialized personal because of the risk of contamination by the handling of *Toxoplasma*, as well as the lapse of time to get the results [1–5].

### 2.2. Cellular culture

Cellular culture is more utilized nowadays for the diagnosis and isolation of parasite *in vitro* [5, 6], the parasite has been isolated from lung [5, 6] and cerebrospinal fluid from patients with acquired immunodeficiency syndrome (AIDS) [7]. Diagnosis by cellular cultures has also been utilized in ocular toxoplasmosis [8, 9]. Cellular cultures are also used for research purposes, like the study of host-parasite interaction, identification of factors involved on innate resistance, molecular and genetic characterization of *Toxoplasma* strains [10] and for the evaluation of candidate molecules on vaccine and treatment development [11].

The cell culture to identify tachyzoites from biopsy or corporal fluid of infected patients, leads to the destruction of the cellular monolayer and is related with the initial amount of tachyzoites in the biological sample. The sensitivity of parasite detection by cell culture from intraocular liquid (aqueous and vitreous humor) is 91%, compared with antibodies detection by ELISA with 67%.

### 2.3. Histology

The detection of tachyzoites in histological sections from suspicious biopsies indicates an acute infection; on the contrary, the detection of tissue cysts that contain bradyzoites in histological samples only confirms a chronic toxoplasmosis infection. The presence of cysts in the placenta, foetus or new-born indicates a congenital infection, according to the number of cysts in histological sections, can be suggested as an active infection and needs immediate treatment. In biopsy or autopsy material, the encysted tachyzoites and bradyzoites are usually demonstrable with wright, hematoxylin and eosin dyes, where the bradyzoites contain glycogen vacuoles. The size of the cyst is important in histological sections of the brain (**Figure 1**). There are other stain techniques like Schiff-periodic acid, specific immunohistochemistry stained with inmunoperoxidase that are equally efficient. These procedures have great diagnosis value but are limited due to the difficulty to grow parasites *in vivo* as well as the identification of tachyzoites by histochemistry methods [3, 5, 8].

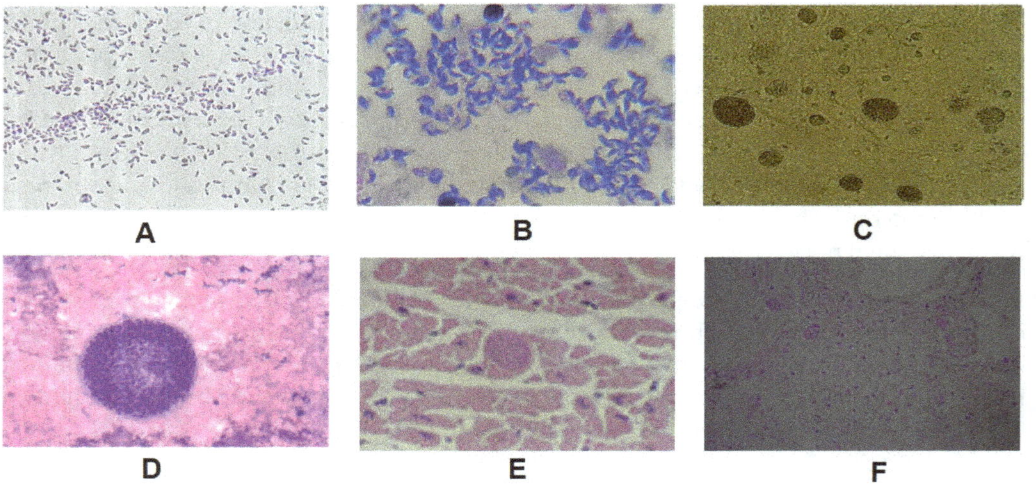


**Figure 1.** (A) Tachyzoites from mice peritoneal exudate, Diff-Quick stain, 100×. (B) Tachyzoites from mice peritoneal exudate, alkaline metilen blue, 10×. (C) Multiply tisular cysts en mouse brain, without stain, 20×. (D) Tisular cyst in mouse brain, Diff-Quick stain, 40×. (E) Histological section of the necropsy from patient (400×) cyst of *Toxoplasma gondii* in the sarcoplasm of a cardiac muscle fiber. (F) Histological section of the necropsy from patient (400×) H&E stain, in which some cysts of *Toxoplasma* are observed in the alveolar epithelium, necrosis in the adjacent cells, detritus, some inflammatory cells and proteinaceous material H&E stain. (A–D) Courtesy of Gustavo Salas Lais. Student of Doctoral Science in Biomedicine and Molecular Biotechnology, ENCB-IPN.Mexico. (E and F) Courtesy of Dr. Ramón Franco Topete: Medical Pathologist, Department of Microbiology and Pathology CUCS and the New Civil Hospital of Guadalajara, Mexico.

## 3. Immunodiagnostics'

### 3.1. Sabin and Feldman test

The Sabin and Feldman reaction, also known as the dye test [12], is considered as golden standard by detection of *Toxoplasma*-specific antibodies. The patient's serum is mixed with a suspension of live tachyzoites, and then methylene blue dye is added. If the patient's serum has anti-*Toxoplasma* antibodies, by the effect of complement factors, the parasites are lysed losing the property of capturing the dye, and as a result they are observed without colour under the microscope (positive result for toxoplasmosis). When there are no anti-*Toxoplasma* antibodies in the assayed serum, the parasites remain with their cellular layer intact and thereby capture the dye showing a blue colour under the microscope (negative result to toxoplasmosis). The problem with this test is the use of live tachyzoites, a potential risk to laboratory staff conducting the test. Also, it requires specialized infrastructure for the maintenance of the parasites, so only research and reference centres perform this diagnostic tool [12]. Interpretation of results shows that the parasites dyed blue (negative) and more than 50% non-dyed (positive) parasites are reported with the highest serum dilution with the positive result, and the values that reflect infection with the parasite are >1:16 IU.

### 3.2. Hemagglutination

The hemagglutination assay was first described by Jacobs L. in 1957. This test is based on the capacity of anti-*Toxoplasma gondii* antibodies to agglutinate sensitive erythrocytes masked with cytoplasmic *Toxoplasma* antigens [13, 14]. This test is useful, rapid and highly sensitive ideal to be used in association with indirect immunofluorescence [15]. Also, it could interfere in the diagnosis of congenital toxoplasmosis, as the identified antibodies are IgG and so on. Interpretation of the test: positive if agglutination is present and negative if the agglutination is inhibited. The result is considered the lecture at the higher dilution. Afterwards Yamamoto in 1991, standardized a test for the determination of IgM antibodies, with a sensibility of 98% and specificity of 95% [16].

### 3.3. Modified agglutination test (MAT)

For this assay, the tachyzoites are fixed with formaldehyde in microtiter plates in the form of U plates with diluted serum added. In positive serum samples, a thin layer of agglutination is produced, while in negative samples compact sediment is formed due to precipitated tachyzoites at the bottom of the well. This assay was first described by Fulton and Turk [17], with low specificity and sensitivity, due to the union of normal IgM at the surface of the parasite and improved by the preparation of the antigen using a buffer with 2-mercaptoethanol, that eliminates the non-specific IgM. This assay detects IgG antibodies, without limitation of host species, but false negative results could occur during early stages of acute infection [17]. The specificity and sensitivity of MAT are similar to the Sabin and Feldman assay in most species. Also, MAT can be used in corporal fluids, being of much used in field work.

### 3.4. Indirect immunofluorescence (IFI)

This assay was described by Garin in 1967 [18], consists of fixation of tachyzoites on microscope slides. Upon contact with the antibodies present in the patient's serum, the antibody antigen reaction is carried out, which is visible with a second antibody labelled with fluorescein. The antigen-antibody reaction is evidenced by fluorescence microscope. In positive cases, a bright yellow greenish fluorescence is evident and a red colour without fluorescence is observed in negative cases. The colour of the fluorescence depends on the fluorochrome conjugated to the antibodies. The immunofluorescence is a test that shows high precision when it is adapted for specific antibodies. It is known that when the human is infected, it responds first with the production of IgM that disappears later. The detection of specific

IgM in the new-born shows difference in the antibodies transmitted from the mother to the product (IgG goes through placental barrier and IgM is not capable to do it). The detection of specific IgG contributes to the diagnosis most of the times; however, considerable titles of antibodies may persist for months or years [18].

### 3.5. Enzyme linked immunosorbent assay (ELISA)

The enzyme linked immunosorbent assay (ELISA) was described initially in 1971 by Engvall and Perlman, uses antibodies conjugated to an enzyme [19]. The antibody conserves its capacity of specific union to the antigen, while the enzyme is capable of a redox reaction, in which the substrate precipitates in a coloured product. In this system, the antigen or the antibody is absorbed to an insoluble solid phase (micro polystyrene plates). There are several variants of ELISA: direct, indirect, capture and competitive. All of them allow the determination of antigens in biological fluids except the indirect method that only detects antibodies.

The direct ELISA methods involve attachment of the antigen to the solid phase, followed by an enzyme-labelled antibody. This type of assay generally makes measurement of crude samples difficult, since contaminating antigens compete for plastic binding sites. Whereas, indirect ELISAs also involve attachment of the antigen to a solid phase, but in this case, the primary antibody is not marked. An enzyme-conjugated secondary antibody, directed at the first antibody, is then added. This format is used most often to detect specific antibodies in serum.

The captured ELISA assay involves attachment of a captured antibody to a solid phase support. Samples containing known or unknown antigens are then added in a matrix or buffer that will minimize attachment to the solid phase. An enzyme-labelled antibody is then added for detection.

The most used enzymes are horse radish peroxidase (HRP), alkaline phosphatase (FA) and the β-ᴅ-galactosidase (BG), the substrates for the HRP enzyme are hydrogen or urea peroxide, which on reducing make certain chromogens oxidized in the enzymatic reaction, developing a coloured product. The oxidized ortho-phenylene diamine remains soluble after the oxidation reaction and is the most used. The FA substrate p-nitrophenyl phosphate that produces colour when degraded by the enzyme at temperatures over 30°C, the 5 bromo-4cloro-3-indoilphosfate can be employed in ELISA in tube or in dot-ELISA. The ELISA method detects from 70 to 80% of cases in congenital infections, a rise in the titles of IgM that extends more over the first week is indicative of acute infection, since the average of duration of maternal IgM is from 3 to 5 days. Also, antibodies can be determined in serum and aqueous humour.

Interpretation of the test: If ELISA is qualitative, a development of colour is observed in seropositive samples. If the test is quantitative, the intensity of the developed colour is measured at a determined wavelength (nanometres) and the lecture of absorbance is proportional to the magnitude of the reaction antigen-antibody [20–22].

### 3.6. Recombinant antigens

At the final of the nineteenth century, several recombinant antigens of different sites of the parasites were analysed [23, 24]. The dense granule antigen—GRA1, GRA2, GRA4, GRA6,

GRA7 and GRA8, rhoptries protein—ROP1 and ROP2, the matrix protein—MAG1, protein micronemes—MIC2, MIC3, MIC4 and MIC5 or the surface antigen—SAG1 and SAG226, were evaluated as diagnostic markers in human beings or animals by ELISA to detect IgG and IgM specific antibodies [25]. The combinations of recombinant antigens have showed more sensibility and specificity for the use of only one antigen. For example, the combinations of SAG2A, GRA2, GRA4, ROP2, GRA8 and GRA7 are potentially useful to detect antibodies IgG in human beings with the infection recently acquired [26], ROP1, SAG1, GRA7, GRA8 and GRA6 are promising to detect specific IgM antibodies while GRA7 and GRA8 are used to detect IgA specific antibodies. A specific protein of sporozoites related with embryogenesis (TgERP) was identified in a study, it can react with specific antibodies of oocysts and can be used to detect an early infection by sporozoites implying the oocysts as infection source [27, 28].

### 3.7. Avidity test

The IgG avidity test was described by Hedman et al. [24]. This assay measures the avidity of the binding of specific antibodies to *T. gondii* antigen. The proteins present in the serum are denatured with a solution of urea. The avidity can be variable during the course of infection [29, 30]. In early stages of infection, the values of avidity are low and are increasing with the course of infection [24]. Therefore, the avidity test can distinguish between acute and chronic infection. The assay is performed by different serological procedures, such as ELISA. However, there are limitations for the IgG test in pregnant women, since these antibodies can persist for several months and the treatment of *T. gondii* can affect the results [31].

### 3.8. Western blot

Western blot is an immunoenzymatic technique, based on the binding of *Toxoplasma* antigens fixed on nitrocellulose paper with specific antibodies present in the serum of infected patients. First, the protein antigens must be separated by electrophoresis in polyacrylamide gel (PAGE-SDS), then transferred and immobilized in a solid phase (nitrocellulose layer). Nitrocellulose paper must be blocked or saturated with non-antigenic protein (bovine serum albumin) to prevent the unspecific binding of the antibodies. Then a second antibody conjugated with an enzyme (horseradish peroxidase or alkaline phosphatase) is added, this antibody binds to the Fc of the first antibody, when the substrate of the enzyme is added. The substrate is transformed to a product and visible specific bands in situ indicate the antigens of *T. gondii* recognized by specific antibodies [32].

Western blot has the advantage to identify specific antigens recognized by IgG, IgM and IgA antibodies from serum and cerebrospinal fluid of patients with chronic and acute toxoplasmosis, specially in immunocompromised patients with low titers of antibodies. In immunocompetent patients this method has been used to identify parasite proteins as markers for toxoplasmosis diagnosis (**Figure 2**) [33]. Also, diagnosis of congenital toxoplasmosis from colostrum samples by Western blot is very useful, since IgA antibodies recognize a greater

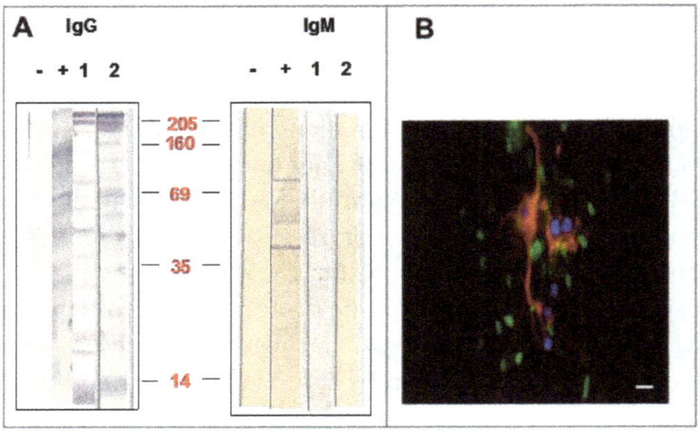


**Figure 2.** Recognition pattern of antibodies IgG and IgM by Western blot. The antibodies IgG and IgM were detected in samples of serum from a patient with acute infection. Negative control (–), positive control (+), samples 1 and 2 correspond to the bands of antigen *T. gondii* revealed by specific antibodies type IgG and IgM.

number of antigens [34]. This method has also been used with other corporal fluids such as saliva [35].

### 3.9. Immunocytochemistry and immunohistochemistry

The immunocytochemistry involves detection of epitopes expressed by the antigens of *Toxoplasma* within a tissue sample using a 'primary antibody' capable of binding those epitopes with high specificity. After the epitope-antibody binding event, a 'secondary antibody' capable of binding the primary antibody with high specificity is added. The secondary antibody is coupled to a reporter molecule and after the antibody-antibody binding event, a chemical substrate is added which reacts with the reporter molecule to produce a coloured precipitate at the site of the whole epitope-antibody complex (**Figure 2B**). The immunohistochemistry has the same base as that of the immunocytochemistry, the difference is that this one is realized on tissue slides. Studies have been done for a neuropathological test of cerebral tissue in patients with infection by the virus of human immunodeficiency VHI/AIDS, to evaluate the diffuse and spread brain multifocal lesions [36]. With immunohistochemistry there have been realized studies in different tissues to demonstrate *T. gondii*, such as ocular toxoplasmosis [37–39].

## 4. Molecular techniques

### 4.1. Generalities of the genome of *T. gondii*

Molecular biology has permitted the advance in molecular knowledge of *T. gondii*. Its genome contains approximately 65 megabases (MB), distributed in 14 chromosomes which varies from 1.9 to 7.4 MB. It contains 52.3% of GC and codifies for almost 7988 proteins and contains

296 small non-coding genes (Ensemble protists): *T. gondii:* [40, 41]. The complete genome sequence of GT1, ME49 and VEG strains classifies the *Toxoplasma* in three types I, II and III, respectively. Till date, the analysis of the restriction fragment length polymorphisms (RFLPs) with more than 900 strains of the parasite permits its classification in 140 genotypes grouped in 12 main groups. Similar results were obtained by the sequencing of introns of a smaller number of samples and also using microsatellite markers. In spite of these results, it is necessary to sequence more complete genomes for a better precision in the clarification of the linages (information taken in the page of Institute J, Craig Venter) [42].

### 4.2. Molecular diagnosis by the polymerase chain reaction (PCR)

The polymerase chain reaction (PCR) consists in making a repetitive replication *in vitro* of specific DNA sequences. Amplifying or copying several times a fragment of DNA, the analytical sensibility of the test increases proportionally. The amplified product is analysed by electrophoresis in agarose or polyacrylamide gel. This technique is useful in the detection of the parasite in serum samples, peripheral blood mono-nuclear cells (PBMC), urine, placenta, amniotic and spinal brain liquid. The sensibility and specificity of PCR depends on the technique used in the extraction of DNA, the primers and the parameters of the amplification reaction [43, 44]. The most conserved genes of *Toxoplasma* are B1 with 35 copies in the genome of the parasite, followed by the repetitive region REP of 529 base pairs (bp) with an approach of 300 copies in the genome; these genes are the most selected for the PCR test as diagnostic tool. Other sequences of unique copy, which are used in investigation laboratories mainly for genotyping purposes are SAG1, SAG2, SAG3, SAG4 and GRA4 genes [45]. The polymerase chain reaction (PCR) is a very valuable diagnosis method in acute infections, when the parasite crosses placental barrier and infects the foetus or on infected patients with AIDS and other immunosuppression or reactivation of the parasite [46–48]. Unfortunately, it is difficult to have a confidentially valor in the PCR assays. For a pre-natal diagnosis, the reported sensibility goes from 64 to 97.4% with a predictive negative value of 87.7–99.7%, respectively; in case of patients with AIDS and toxoplasmosis, the reported sensibility goes from 13 to 87.5% [49]. With the detection of the sequence REP 529-bp, a sensibility of 100% has been reported in amniotic fluids [48]. The sequence REP 529-bp is having an increase in the utility for the diagnosis of *T. gondii* by PCR since it demonstrates greater sensibility, possibly the high number of repetitions in the parasites sequence increases the possibilities of detection. The variations in the results are due to different time of infection in the patients, type of sample, storage conditions that affect sensibility. Also, actually there is no agreement in the primers that should be used in the PCR, one of the regions which is more conserved is gen B1 [47], still there exists some polymorphisms and the strains of *Toxoplasma* in clinical samples are not the same genotype, these factors can affect the parasite detection. It requires large number of studies which compare gen B1 and the sequence REP 529-bp to meet and agreement in the selection of primers. Another factor that can affect the results is the variability reported in the techniques used for DNA extraction.

In patients with AIDS, the detection of *T. gondii* by PCR in cerebrospinal liquid has shown different sensibilities, reaching to 87% of sensibility when the sample is taken soon enough preferably during the first 3 days and a maximum of 7 days after starting the specific treatment [48].

The polymerase chain reaction (PCR) can be in the future, undoubtedly a successful tool in the diagnosis of toxoplasmosis, when a satisfactory correlation exists between the patient's clinical profile and the presence of *T. gondii* DNA aspects which still have to be studied and standardized. Also, in countries with low development and still in many with high development, it has not been implemented for daily use due to its high cost.

### 4.3. PCR in real time

Unlike the conventional PCR, the real-time PCR using fluorescence probes measures the product of amplification in each cycle and can be quantified with the use of known concentration standards. Real-time PCR has been successfully used to detect the *T. gondii* DNA in human blood, cerebrospinal fluid, aqueous humour, amniotic liquid and other samples [49–51]. Also, it is used to evaluate the progression of the toxoplasmosis and the efficiency of the treatment, since it can estimate the intensity of the infection by *T. gondii.* The PCR assay in real time with REP 529-bp sequence is considered as the technique with greater efficiency for the diagnosis of toxoplasmosis in comparison with the detection of gen B1.

### 4.4. Loop mediated isothermal amplification (LAMP)

Loop mediated isothermal amplification (LAMP) is a technique of DNA amplification under isothermal conditions, which combines speed, efficiency and high specificity. The amplification of DNA proceeds from the repetition of two reactions of elongation in a structure that has loop form. It uses DNA polymerase with strand displacement activity and two inner primers and two outer primers. The inner primers contain sense and antisense sequences of DNA and initiate the LAMP reaction. The outer primers hybridize a few bases of the inner and initiate the DNA synthesis with strand displacement, forming a loop structure, which initiates a DNA synthesis by auto recognition. In this technique, 10 copies of DNA can be produced in less than one hour [52]. The final products are multiple loop DNA formed by alignment between inverted repeated sequences present in the same chain [53]. It only requires a water bath or thermo block to realize the amplification of DNA and the amplified products can be analysed by real time PCR equipment or by electrophoresis [54]. This technique is more sensitive than conventional PCR but low sensitive than real time PCR [53]. The LAMP assay has been evaluated identifying REP 529-bp, SAG1, SAG2 and B1 *T. gondii* sequences from PBMC [54]. The reported sensitivity was 0.1 tachyzoites and crossed reactivity with other parasites was not found. The detection of SAG2 showed the higher sensitivity (87.5%) followed by SAG-1 (80%) and B1 (80%). The specificity was 100% in all of them [55]. However, all techniques of nucleic acid amplification have a high sensitivity, for that reason a rigorous quality control is necessary to discard false positives.

### 4.5. Polymerase chain reaction-restriction fragment length polymorphisms (PCR-RFLPs)

The PCR-RFLP is based on the capacity of restriction endonucleases that recognize polymorphisms of only one nucleotide (SNPs). Polymerase chain reaction (PCR) products treated with restriction enzymes to generate polymorphic DNA fragments of variable length, that are visualized after electrophoresis in agarose or polyacrylamide gels with a band pattern [55]. In 1995, Howe and Sibley identified three main linages (type I, II and III) from 106 strains of *T. gondii* isolated from humans and animals by PCR-RFLP using six markers [56].

Since then, in different laboratories, several groups of different multi-locus markers have been selected, to characterize by PCR-RFLP *T. gondii* isolates from persons and animals [57, 58]. Currently, there has been developed a method for *T. gondii* classification into genotypes known as multiplex nested PCR-RFLPs (Mn-PCR-RFLPs). This method uses 10 genetic markers including the gens SAG1, SAG2, SAG3, Btub, GRA6, C22-8, c29-2, L358, PK1 and apico [59]. The Mn-PCR-RFLP has been applied broadly in the typing of positive clinically samples and has generated a big amount of data about the genetic diversity of the parasite [60, 61]. As in all techniques, where DNA amplification is performed, several negative controls must be included to have a strict quality control.

The microsatellites (MS) are short tandem repeats (STR) sequences of DNA (2 to 6 pb), that are widely distributed throughout the nuclear genomes of eukaryotes. They are highly polymorphic, the MS length varies depending the numbers of STR. The tandem repetitions in *T. gondii* are often simple, with only repetitions of two nucleotides, which occur from 2 to 20 times [62, 63]. Around 15 markers of MS have been used, including (tub2, W35, TgM-A, B18, B17; M33, IV.1, XI.1, M48, M102, N60, N82, AA, N61, N83) to determine the genotype of *T. gondii* in different laboratories [61, 62]. Ajzenberg et al. developed an easy method to genotype *T. gondii* in one multiplex PCR using 15 MS markers, in which eight MS markers (tub2, W35, TgM-A, B18, B17, M33, IV.1 and XI.1) could differentiate the types I, II and III from all the atypical genotypes, and the other seven markers (M48, M102, N60, N82, AA, N61, N83 ) could improve the resolution from the genetic differentiation of strictly related isolates in an haplo-group or clonal linage [62, 63]. The multiplex 15-MS assay is the best available tool to characterize *T. gondii* from genetically different or identical isolates during an outbreak, laboratory contamination and from mixed infections. The limitation of this assay is the request of an automatized sequencer with the 'gene scan' tool. The disadvantage is that samples with poor DNA can cause low intensity signals, generating non-specific PCR products [61, 62].

### 4.6. High-resolution melting (HRM)

In homogeny sample, the HRM method can analyse genetic variations, which allows to characterize polymorphisms based on the melting temperature generated by the DNA length and GC content [62]. On the base of only one SNP from gene B1 which is found in multiple copies, the HRM can classify correctly three different types of strains of *T. gondii* [63]. This assay was developed to determine the genotype of *T. gondii* directly from biological samples, with a better genotyping when use multiple copy genes in comparison to one copy genes, avoiding a cellular culture or bioassay.

## Author details

María de la Luz Galván Ramírez[1*], Laura Verónica Sánchez Orozco[2*] and Cynthia Guadalupe Temores Ramírez[3]

*Address all correspondence to: mlgalvanr@gmail.com and sanchezorozco.cucs.udg@gmail.com

1 Department of Physiology, University Center of Health Sciences, University of Guadalajara, Guadalajara, Jalisco, Mexico

2 Department of Molecular Biology, University Center of Health Sciences, University of Guadalajara, Guadalajara, Jalisco, Mexico

3 Department of Cellular and Molecular Biology, University Center of Biological and Agricultural Sciences, University of Guadalajara, Guadalajara, Jalisco, Mexico

## References

[1] Sabin AV, Elizky PK. *Toxoplasma* and obligate intracellular parasitism. Science. 1937;**85:**(336–8):17815128. DOI: 10.1126/science.85.2205.336.

[2] Chai JY, Lin A, Shin EH, Oh MD, Han ET, Nan HW, Lee SH, Chai JY, Lin A, Shin EH, Oh MD, Han ET, Nan HW, Lee SH. Laboratory passage and characterization of an isolate of *Toxoplasma gondii* from an ocular patient in Korea. J. Parasitol. 2003;**41:**(147–154):PMID: 12972728. DOI: 10.334/kjp.200341.3.147.

[3] Stajner T, Vasiljević Z, Vujić D, Marković M, Ristić G, Mićić D, Pasić S, Ivović V, Ajzenberg D, Djurković-Djaković O. Atypical strain of *Toxoplasma gondii* causing fatal reactivation after hematopoietic stem cell transplantion in a patient with an underlying immunological deficiency. J. Clin. Microbiol. 2013;**51:**(2686–2690):PMID: 23761151. DOI: 10.1128/JCM.01077-13.

[4] Ibebuike K1, Mantanga L, Emereole O, Ndolo P, Kajee A, Gopal R, Pather S. Ibebuike K, Mantanga L, Emereole O, Ndolo P, Kajee A, Gopal R, Pather S. Cerebellar toxoplasmosis in HIV/AIDS infant. Cerebellar toxoplasmosis in HIV/AIDS infant: case report and review of the literature. Neurol. Sci. 2012;**33:**(1423–1428):PMID: 22286317. DOI: 10.1007/s10072-012-0960-x.

[5] Monaco SE, Monaghan SA, Stamm JA, Khalbuss WE, Nichols L, Pantanowitz. Toxopl asmosis in a post-transplant bronchoalveolar lavage: a case report. Diagn. Cytopathol. 2012;**40:**(629–634):PMID: 21591274. DOI: 10.1002/dc.21646.

[6] Değirmenci A1, Döşkaya M, Caner A, Ciçek C, Korkmaz M, Gürüz Y, et al. *Toxoplasma gondii* RH Ankara: production of evolving tachyzoites using a novel cell culture method. Exp. Parasitol. 2011;**128:**(1–8):PMID: 21296077. DOI: 10.1016/j.exppara.2011.01.019.

[7] Mahadevan M, Ramalingaiah AH, Parthasarathy S, Nath A, Ranga U, Krishna SS. Neuropathological correlate of the "concentric target sign" in MRI of HIV associated cerebral toxoplasmosis. J. Mag. Res. Imag. 2013;**38:**(488–495):PMID: 23440973. DOI: 10.1002/jmri.24036.

[8] Garweg JG. Determinants of immunodiagnostic success in human ocular toxoplasmosis. ParasiteImmunol.2005;**27:**(61–68):PMID:15882232.DOI:10.1111/j.1365-3024.2005.00747.x.

[9] Miller D, Davis J, Rosa R, Diaz M, Perez, E. Utility of tissue culture for detection of *Toxoplasma gondii* in vitreous humor of patients diagnosed with toxoplasmic retinochoroiditis. J. Clin. Microbiol. 2000;**38:**(3840–3842):PMID: 11015415.

[10] Peyron F, Lobry JR, Musset K, Ferrandiz J, Gomez-Marin JE, Petersen E,et al. Serotyping of *Toxoplasma gondii* in chronically infected pregnant women: predominance of type II in Europe and types I and III in Colombia (South America). Microbes Infect. 2006;**8:**(2333–40): PMID: 16938480. DOI: 10.1016/j.micinf.2006.03.023.

[11] Fuentes I, Rubio JM, Ramírez C, Alvar J. Genotypic characterization of *Toxoplasma gondii* strains associated with human toxoplasmosis in Spain: direct analysis from clinical samples. J. Clin. Microbiol. 2001;**39**(4):(1566–1570). DOI: 10.1128/JCM.39.4.1566-1570.2001

[12] Sabin A, Feldman HA. Dyes as microchemical indicators of a new immunity phenomenon affecting a protozoan parasite (*Toxoplasma*). Science. 1948;**108:**(660–3). DOI: 10.1126/science.108.2815.660

[13] Jacobs L, Lunde MN. Hemoaglutination test for toxoplasmosis. J. Parasitol. 1957;**43:**(308–314):PMID: 13439469.

[14] Desmonts G, Remington JS. Direct agglutination test for diagnosis of *Toxoplasma* infection: method for increasing sensitivity and specificity. J. Clin. Microbiol. 1980;**11:**(562–568):PMID: 7000807.

[15] Montoya JG, Berry A, Rosso F, Remington JS. The differential agglutination test as a diagnostic aid in cases of toxoplasmic lymphadenitis. J. Clin. 2007;**45:**(1463–1468).

[16] Yamamoto YI, Hoshino-Shimizu S, Camargo ME. A novel IgM-indirect hemagglutination test for the serodiagnosis of acute toxoplasmosis. J. Clin. Lab. Anal. 1991;**5:**(127–132):PMID: 2023058.

[17] Fulton JD, Turk JL. Direct agglutination test for *Toxoplasma gondii*. Lancet. 1959;**12:**(1068–1069):PMID: 13825641.

[18] Garin JP, Ambroise TP, Cornet AM, Dien-Truong T, Despeinges J. Interet de la fluoresence et de l'inmnofluoresence dans le diagnostic Parasitologique et serologique de la Toxoplasmosis. Revue de 1' Institut Pasteur de Lyon. 1967;**68:**(179–205).

[19] Engvall E, Perlmann P. Quantitative assay of immunoglobulin G. Immunochemistry. 1971;**9:**(871–4):PMID: 5135623.

[20] Liu Q, Wang Z-D, Huang S-Y, Zhu X-Q. Diagnosis of toxoplasmosis and typing of *Toxoplasma gondii*. Parasites & Vectors. 2015;**8:**(292):PMID: 26017718. DOI: 10.1186/s13071-015-0902-6.

[21] Kotresha D, Noordin R. Recombinant proteins in the diagnosis of toxoplasmosis. APMIS. 2010;**118:**(529–542):PMID: 20666734. DOI: 10.1111/j.1600-0463.2010.02629.x.

[22] Aubert D, Maine GT, Villena I, Hunt JC, Howard L, Sheu M, et al. Recombinant antigens to detect *Toxoplasma gondii* -specific immunoglobulin G and immunoglobulin M in human sera by enzyme immunoassay. J. Clin. Microbiol. 2000;**38:**(1144–1150):PMID: 10699010.

[23] Hill D, Coss C, Dubey JP, Wroblewski K, Sautter M, Hosten T, et al. Identification of a sporozoite-specific antigen from *Toxoplasma gondii*. J Parasitol. 2011;**97:**(328–37):PMID: 21506817. DOI: 10.1645/GE-2782.1.

[24] Hedman K, Lappalainen M, Seppaia I, Makela O. Recent primary *Toxoplasma* infection indicated by a low avidity of specific IgG. J. Infect. Dis. 1989;**159:**(736–740):PMID: 2926163.

[25] Pfrepper KI, Enders G, Gohl M, Krczal D, Hlobil H, Wassenberg D, et al. Seroreactivity to and avidity for recombinant antigens in toxoplasmosis. Clin. Diagn. Lab. Immun. 2005;12(8):(977–982):PMID: 16085916. DOI: 10.1128/CDLI.12.8.977-982.2005.

[26] de Ory F, Casas I, Domingo CJ, Echevarria J. Application of fluoroimmunoassay to the identification of low avidity specific IgG against pathogenic human viruses and *Toxoplasma gondii*. Clin. Diagn. Virol. 1995;**3:**(323–332).

[27] Deshpande PS, Kotresha D, Noordin R, Yunus MH, Saadatnia G, Golkar M, et al. IgG avidity Western blot using *Toxoplasma* gondii rGRA-7 cloned from nucleotides 39–711 for serodiagnosis of acute toxoplasmosis. Rev. Inst. Med. Trop. Sao Paulo. 2013;**55:**(79–83):PMID: 23563759. DOI: http://dx.doi.org/10.1590/S0036-46652013000200003.

[28] Gutierrez J, Rodriguez M, Piedrola G, del Carmen MM. Detection of IgA and low-avidity IgG antibodies for the diagnosis of recent active toxoplasmosis. Clin. Microbiol. Infect. 1997;**3**(658-662):PMID: 11864209. DOI: http://dx.doi.org/10.1111/j.1469-0691.1997.tb00474.x

[29] Ali-Heydari S, Keshavarz H, Shojaee S, Mohebali M. Diagnosis of antigenic markers of acute toxoplasmosis by IgG avidity immunoblotting. Parasite. 2013;**20:**(18):PMID: 23688778. DOI: 10.1051/parasite/2013017.

[30] Ashburn D, Joss AW, Pennington TH, Ho-Yen DO. IgA, IgE, and IgG avidity tests have any value in the diagnosis of *Toxoplasma* infection in pregnancy? J. Clin. Pathol. 1998;**51:**(312–315):PMID: 9659246.

[31] Lefevre-Pettazzoni M, Le Cam S, Wallon M, Peyron F. Delayed maturation of immunoglobulin G avidity: implication for the diagnosis of toxoplasmosis in pregnant women. Eur. J. Clin. Microbiol. Infect. Dis. 2006;25:(687–693):PMID: 17024503. DOI: 10.1007/s10096-006-0204-1.

[32] Meek B, Diepersloot RJ, van Gool T, Speijer D, Peek R. IgM recognition of recombinant *Toxoplasma gondii* antigens by sera of acutely or latently infected humans. Diag. Microbiol. Infect. Dis. 2003;**45:**(45–52):PMID: 12573550.

[33] Galván RML, Guillen VC, Saavedra DR, Islas RA. Analysis of *Toxoplasma* gondii antigens with sera from toxoplasmosis. Rev. Soc. Bra. Med. Trop. 1998;**31:**(271–277):PMID: 9612018.

[34] de Morais Oliveira AC, Silva Borges DS, Reis Carvalho F, Gomes de Macêdo A, Mota CM, de Morais Oliveira AM. Evaluation of colostrum as an alternative biological sample for the diagnosis of human congenital toxoplasmosis. BMC Infect. Dis. 2015;**15**:(519):PMID: 26573138. DOI: 10.1186/s12879-015-1242-z.

[35] Stroehle A, Schmid K, Heinzer I, Naguleswaran A, Hemphill A. Performance of a Western immunoblot assay to detect specific anti-*Toxoplasma gondii* IgG antibodies in human saliva. J. Parasitol. 2005;**91:**(561–563):PMID: 16108547. DOI: 10.1645/GE-423R.

[36] Lang W, Miklossy J, Deruaz JP, Pizzolato GP, Probst A, Schaffner T, Gessaga E, Kleihues P. Neuropathology of the acquired immune deficiency syndrome (AIDS): a report of 135 consecutive autopsy cases from Switzerland. Acta Neuropathol. 1989;**77:**(379–90):PMID: 2540610.

[37] Budka H, Costanzi G, Cristina S, Lechi A, Parravicini C, Trabattoni R, Vago L. Brain pathology induced by infection with the human immunodeficiency virus (HIV). Neuropathology. 1987;**75:**(185). DOI: 10.1007/BF00687080

[38] Miyamoto C, Mattos Neto RB, Cesare SD, Belfort Junior R, Burnier MN. Use of CD25 as an immunohistochemical marker for acquired ocular toxoplasmosis. Arq. Bras. Oftalmol. 2010;**73:**(443–446):PMID: 21225130. DOI: dx.doi.org/10.1590/S0004-27492010000500011.

[39] Anselmo LM, Vilar FC, Lima JE, Yamamoto AY, Bollela VR, Takayanagui CM. Usefulness and limitations of polymerase chain reaction in the etiologic diagnosis of neurotoxoplasmosis in immunocompromised patients. J. Neurol. Sci. 2014;**346:**(231–234):PMID: 25240445. DOI: 10.1016/j.jns.2014.08.034.

[40] http://protists.ensembl.org/Toxoplasma_gondii/Info/Annotation/)

[41] http://www.toxodatabase.org/

[42] http://www.jcvi.org/cms/home/.

[43] Yamagish J, Suzuki Y. The genome-wide identification of promoter regions in *Toxoplasma gondii*. Methods Mol. Biol. 2015;**1201:**(193–205):PMID: 25388115. DOI: 10.1007/978-1-4939-1438-8_11.

[44] Jalal S, Nord CE, Lappalainen M, Evengard B, on behalf of the ESCMID Study Group on toxoplasmosis. Rapid and sensitive diagnosis of *Toxoplasma gondii* infection by PCR. Clin. Microbio.l Infect. 2004;**10**(937-939):PMID: 15373893 . DOI: 10.1111/j.1469-0691.2004.00948.x

[45] Kasper DC, Sadeghi K, Prusa AR, Reischer GH, Kratochwill K, Förster-Waldl E,et al. Quantitative real-time polymerase chain reaction for the accurate detection of *Toxoplasma gondii* in amniotic fluid. Diagn. Microbiol. Infect. Dis. 2009;**63**:(10–15):PMID: 18990529. DOI: 10.1016/j.diagmicrobio.2008.09.009

[46] Blay EA, Ghansah A, Otchere J, Koku R, Kwofie KD, Bimi L, et al. Congenital toxoplasmosis and pregnancy malaria detection post-partum: effective diagnosis and its implication for efficient management of congenital infection. Parasitol. Int. 2015;**64:**(603–608). DOI: dx.doi.org/10.1016/j.parint.2015.08.004

[47] Belaz S, Gangneux JP, Dupretz P, Guiguen C, Robert-Gangneux F. A 10-year retrospective comparison of two target sequences, REP-529 and B1, for *Toxoplasma gondii detection* by quantitative PCR. J. Clin. Microbiol. 2015;**53:**(1294–1300):PMID: 25653416. DOI: 10.1128/JCM.02900-14.

[48] Robert-Gangneux F, Sterkers Y, Yera H, Accoceberry I, Menotti J, Cassaing S, et al. Molecular diagnosis of toxoplasmosis in immunocompromised patients: a 3-year multicenter retrospective study. J. Clin. Microbiol. 2015;**53:**(1677–1684):PMID: 25762774. DOI: 10.1128/JCM.03282-14.

[49] Switaj K, Master A, Skrzypczak M, Zaborowski P. Recent trends in molecular diagnostics for *Toxoplasma gondii* infections. Clin. Microbiol. Infect. 2005;**11:**(170–176):PMID: 15715713. DOI: 10.1111/j.1469-0691.2004.01073.x.

[50] Bretagne S. Molecular diagnostics in clinical parasitology and mycology: limits of the current polymerase chain reaction (PCR) assays and interest of the real-time PCR assays. Clin. Microbiol. Infect. 2003;**9:**(6). DOI: 10.1046/j.1469-0691.2003.00677.x

[51] Zainodini N, Zare-Bidaki M, Abdollahi SH, Afrooz M, Ziaali N, Ebrahimian M, et al. Molecular and serological detection of acute and latent toxoplasmosis using real-time PCR and ELISA techniques in blood donors of rafsanjan city. Iran. Iran J. Parasitol. 2014 ;**9:** (336–341):PMC4316564.

[52] Notomi T, Okayama H, Masubuchi H, Yonekawa T, Watanabe K, Amino N. Loop-mediated isothermal amplification of DNA. Nucleic Acids Res. 2000;**28:**(e63):PMID: 10871386 PMCID.

[53] Lau YL, Meganathan P, Sonaimuthu P, Thiruvengadam G, Nissapatorn V, Chen Y. Specific, sensitive, and rapid diagnosis of active toxoplasmosis by a loop-mediated rsothermal amplification method using blood samples from patients. J. Clin. Microbiol. 2010;**48:**(3698–3702). DOI: 10.1128/JCM.00462-10

[54] Zhang H, Thekisoe OM, Aboge GO, Kyan H, Yamagishi J, Inoue N, et al. *Toxoplasma gondii*: sensitive and rapid detection of infection by loop mediated isothermal amplification (LAMP) method. Exp. Parasitol. 2009;**122:**(47–50):PMID: 19545521. DOI: 10.1016/j.exppara.2009.01.012.

[55] Howe DK, Sibley LD. *Toxoplasma gondii* comprises three clonal lineages: correlation of parasite genotype with human disease. J. Infect. Dis. 1995;**172:**(1561–1566). DOI: doi.org/10.1093/infdis/172.6.1561

[56] Ajzenberg D, Cogne N, Paris L, Bessieres MH, Thulliez P, Filisetti D, et al. Genotype of 86 *Toxoplasma gondii* isolates associated with human congenital toxoplasmosis, and correlation with clinical findings. J. Infect. Dis. 2002;**186:**(684–689). DOI: doi.org/10.1086/342663

[57] Khan A, Su C, German M, Storch GA, Clifford DB, Sibley LD. Genotyping of *Toxoplasma gondii* strains from immunocompromised patients reveals high prevalence of type I strains. J. Clin. Microbiol. 2005;**43:**(5881–5887). DOI: 10.1128/JCM.43.12.5881-5887.2005J

[58] Su C, Zhang X, Dubey JP. Genotyping of *Toxoplasma gondii* by multilocus PCR-RFLP markers: a high resolution and simple method for identification of parasites. Int. J. Parasitol. 2006;**36:**(841–848):PMID: 16643922. DOI: 10.1016/j.ijpara.2006.03.003.

[59] Ferreira IM, Vidal JE, Costa-Silva TA, Meira CS, Hiramoto RM, de Oliveira AC P,et al. *Toxoplasma gondii*: genotyping of strains from Brazilian AIDS patients with cerebral toxoplasmosis by multilocus PCR-RFLP markers. Exp. Parasitol. 2008;**118:**(221–227):PMID: 17950282. DOI: 10.1016/j.exppara.2007.08.006.

[60] Ajzenberg D, Collinet F, Mercier A, Vignoles P, Darde ML. Genotyping of *Toxoplasma gondii* isolates with 15 microsatellite markers in a single multiplex PCR assay. J. Clin. Microbiol. 2010;**48:**(4641–4645):PMID: 20881166. DOI: 10.1128/JCM.01152-10.

[61] Ajzenberg D, Banuls AL, Tibayrenc M, Darde ML. Microsatellite analysis of *Toxoplasma gondii* shows considerable polymorphism structured into two main clonal groups. Int. J. Parasitol. 2002;**32:**(27–38):PMID: 11796120.

[62] Ferreira Ade M, Vitor RW, Carneiro AC, Brandao GP, Melo MN. Genetic variability of Brazilian *Toxoplasma gondii* strains detected by random amplified polymorphic DNA-polymerase chain reaction (RAPD-PCR) and simple sequence repeat anchored-PCR (SSR-PCR). Infect. Gen. Evol. 2004;**4:**(131–142). DOI: dx.doi.org/10.1016/j.meegid.2004.03.002

[63] Costa JM, Cabaret O, Moukoury S, Bretagne S. Genotyping of the protozoan pathogen *Toxoplasma gondii* using high-resolution melting analysis of the repeated B1 gene. J. Microbiol. Meth. 2011;**86:**(357–363). DOI: http://dx.doi.org/10.1016/j.mimet.2011.06.017

# 3

# Congenital Toxoplasmosis: *In Vivo* Impact of *Toxoplasma gondii* Infection on Myogenesis and Neurogenesis

Alessandra F. Gomes and Helene S. Barbosa

**Abstract**

Congenital toxoplasmosis (TC) from *Toxoplasma gondii* positive mother to child transmission results in fetal death, abortion, or infantile neurologic and neurocognitive deficits as well as chorioretinitis. This study aims to analyze the morphological changes in brain and skeletal muscle cells of Swiss mouse embryos during experimental congenital toxoplasmosis. Swiss mice, before mating, were gavage inoculation infected with approximately 25 or 50 cysts of ME-49 strain *T. gondii*. Eighteen day postcoitus maternal and embryonic muscle and brain samples were collected and processed for histopathological analysis. The muscle tissue from embryos of infected mothers, in comparison with healthy muscle myofibers, exhibited discontinuous and shorter myofibrils, more interfibrillar space and immature cells with fewer stained and poorly defined striated profiles. These *in vivo* findings might be related to an adhesion protein decrease, observed *in vitro*, where myogenesis was completely affected during *Toxoplasma* infection. The neurogenesis was severely affected with irregularly arranged cells, reduced cell density, and a significant intercellular space increase. The brain tissue presented ischemia, cell death, necrosis, and thrombi, increasing according to the degree of the acute infection, which compromised the neurogenesis, thereby justifying brain size decrease in these embryos.

**Keywords:** *Toxoplasma gondii*, experimental toxoplasmosis, myogenesis, neurogenesis

## 1. Introduction

*Toxoplasma gondii* is a parasite that persists during the chronic phase of the disease in the form of tissue cysts mainly in brain and skeletal muscle. *T. gondii* has been implicated in the pathogenesis of inflammatory myopathies and brain diseases, which are of great medical importance due to congenital toxoplasmosis (CT) [1, 2]. Prevention is an essential measure against *T. gondii* infection from mother to child [3, 4].

The ability to transmigrate through the placenta to replicate in various fetal tissues, evading the immune system of the fetus, makes Toxoplasma a major cause of prenatal complications. This infection can seriously interfere with the development of the fetus, possibly leading to abortion or serious pathologies after birth with severe consequences in childhood, adolescence, or adulthood [3–7]. Among the most common brain afflictions are encephalitis, altered mental status, seizures, weakness, cranial nerve disorders, sensory abnormalities, movement disorders, psychomotor or mental retardation, and behavioral alterations. Acute retinocorioidite is a severe condition, which may develop, involving vitreous hypervascularization and retinal necrosis with a total loss of vision [6, 8–12]. With regard to muscle tissue, the *T. gondii* infection can decrease and even inhibit the formation of new fibers by negatively modulating adhesion proteins such as cadherin [13–15]. Toxoplasmosis also causes myocarditis and polymyositis either by recent infection or by reactivation of tissue cysts in immunosuppressed, immunodeficient, and even immunocompetent individuals [1]. The study of conditions resulting from Toxoplasma infection in brain and muscle tissue has been developed from infected adult mice [7, 16–20]. The influence of Toxoplasma in these tissues during embryonic development in the murine model has yet not been explored despite the predilection of this parasite for these tissues in the chronic phase of the disease. The focus on skeletal muscle as a model for experimental toxoplasmosis opens new prospects for parasite biology understanding during interaction with one of the *T. gondii* target cells for parasite establishment in the chronic phase of the disease [13, 21–29]. Therefore, we decided to investigate the role of *T. gondii* in myogenesis and neurogenesis processes in murine embryos from adult females, that were infected before mating.

## 2. Experimental design

Three experimental protocols were developed in an attempt to establish trans-chromosome (TC) in mice, premating infection, imminently postmating, and during pregnancy. Swiss mice during the mating period (five females and one male per experiment, $n = 5$) were divided into two groups and inoculated via gavage with approximately 25 (Group 1) or 50 cysts (Group 2) of ME-49 strain *T. gondii* (type II). After infection, the mice were placed in cages for 24 h with a suitable male of the same species and age. Thereafter, the animals were visually monitored daily (morning, afternoon, and evening) on the general aspects of lethargy, vaginal bleeding, and mortality. The dead animals were collected immediately and their embryos examined for macroscopic aspects of the peritoneum, spleen, liver, and lung. Pregnant females that sustained pregnancy underwent cesarean section approximately 18 days postcoitus, their embryos, alive or not, collected.

For the diagnosis of possible morphological changes in muscular and cerebral tissue caused by parasite presence in embryos from *T. gondii* cyst-infected mothers, embryonic thighs and brains were collected, sectioned longitudinally, and fixed in Millonig-Rosman solution

(10% formaldehyde in phosphate buffer). The tissues were then processed for impregnation in paraffin, and 3 μm thick sections were stained as routine with hematoxylin and eosin (H&E) for the analysis of morpho-structural and parasitological parameters. Alternatively, part of the material was processed by freezing in liquid nitrogen (−196°C). Five-micrometer thick sections were obtained at −25°C in Leica CM1800 cryostat (Germany), attached to slides treated in poly-L-lysine and fixed in 4% PFA in PBS.

## 3. Results

From three experimental protocols for *T. gondii* cyst mouse infection, postcoitus and during pregnancy promoted 100% in the number of abortions, embryo reabsorption, or adult female death. The most successful protocol was premating adult female mouse infection. However, some animals did not carry the pregnancy to term and this complication arose soon after conception.

The severity of the *T. gondii* infection in adult females and embryos was directly proportional to the concentration of parasites (cysts) inoculated. Group 1 displayed fetal reabsorption, miscarriages, and stillbirths with a loss rate of over 50% (**Figure 1A**). This group was separated from animals with clinical signs of TC according to the increasing severity scale (**Figure 1B**). The stillborns presented different degrees of morphological impairment. The live embryos of this group were born underdeveloped and with little reaction to external stimuli (**Figure 1B**). They presented extensive liver disease characterized by necrosis, abdominal bloating with high fluid retention, and apparent swelling of the spleen as well as cutaneous and pulmonary hemorrhaging (data not shown).

In addition, by macroscopic analysis, besides the swelling of some organs, there was malformation of the anterior and posterior limbs as well as significant decrease in skull size characterizing microcefalia in these animals (**Figure 1B**). These embryos from infected mothers were extremely swollen, both brain and muscle tissues retaining so much fluid that it was impossible to obtain samples for histological analysis (**Figure 1B**). Some of these embryos exhibited a very committed development such as malformation of the trunk (**Figure 1C**) and even total absence of hindlimb formation (**Figure 1C** and **D**).

Group 2 females inoculated with 50 cysts, although fertilized, did not terminate pregnancy, dying in few days. Many embryos were reabsorbed. In this experimental condition, there was nearly a total loss of females and their embryos.

Longitudinal sections of pregnant mouse muscle tissue infected with 25 cysts of *T. gondii* (Group 1), showed similar cyst structures between muscle fibers (**Figure 2A**). In various sections, the images suggested that parasites were evading the cysts and invading other cells (**Figure 2B** and **C**). The healthy mouse embryo leg muscle tissue demonstrated high density of mature myofibers arranged lengthwise, reduced interfibrillar space, and a well-organized striated profile (**Figure 3A**, **C**, and **E**). Even where these fibers were spaced, the amount of mononuclear cells from the connective tissue or inflammatory infiltrate was markedly small

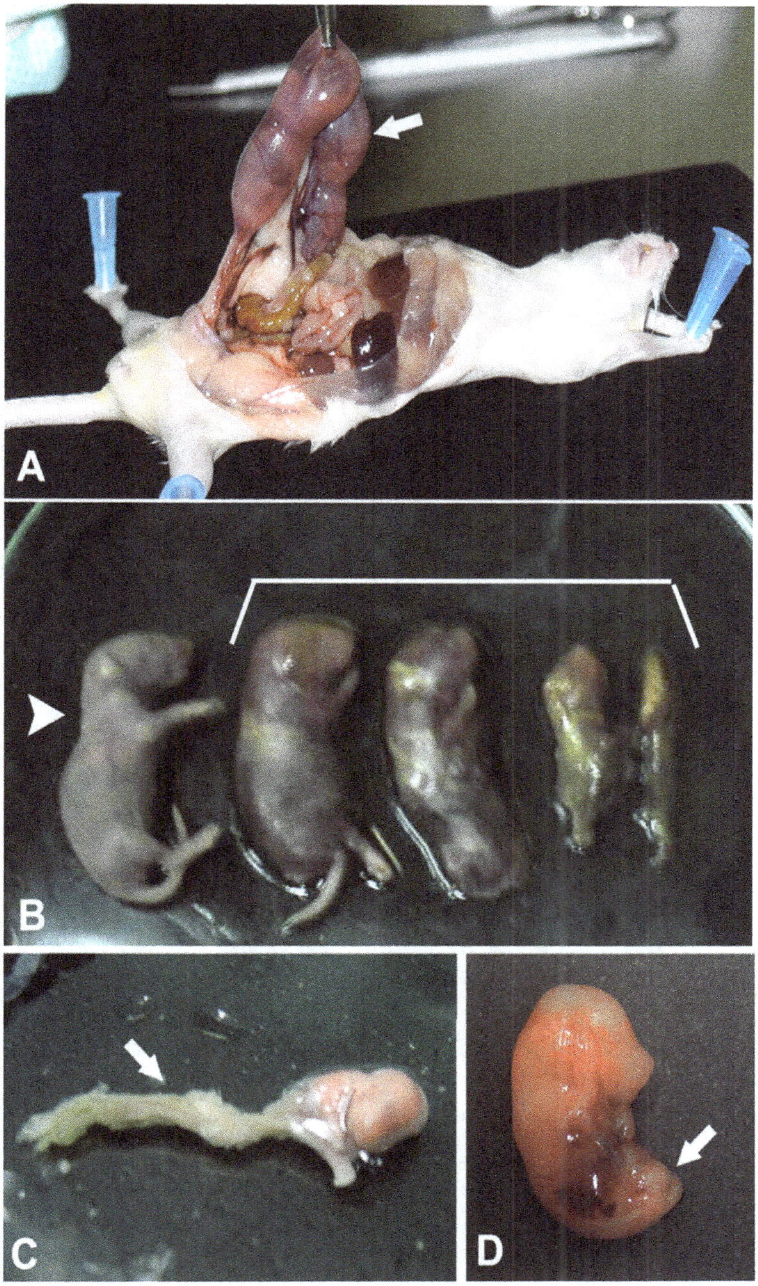


**Figure 1.** Swiss mouse embryos from experimentally infected mothers with *T. gondii*. (A) Harvesting of embryos by cesarean section (arrow). (B) The infection differentially affected pups in the same litter. In the extreme left of this picture is shown one pup apparently unaffected by the infection, whereas its littermate present different degrees of morphological alterations and decrease of skull size characterizing microcephaly in these animals. (C) Stillborn embryos show congenital malformation, including compromise of the trunk and hindlimbs (arrow). (D) Embryo present atrophy of the hindlimbs (arrow).

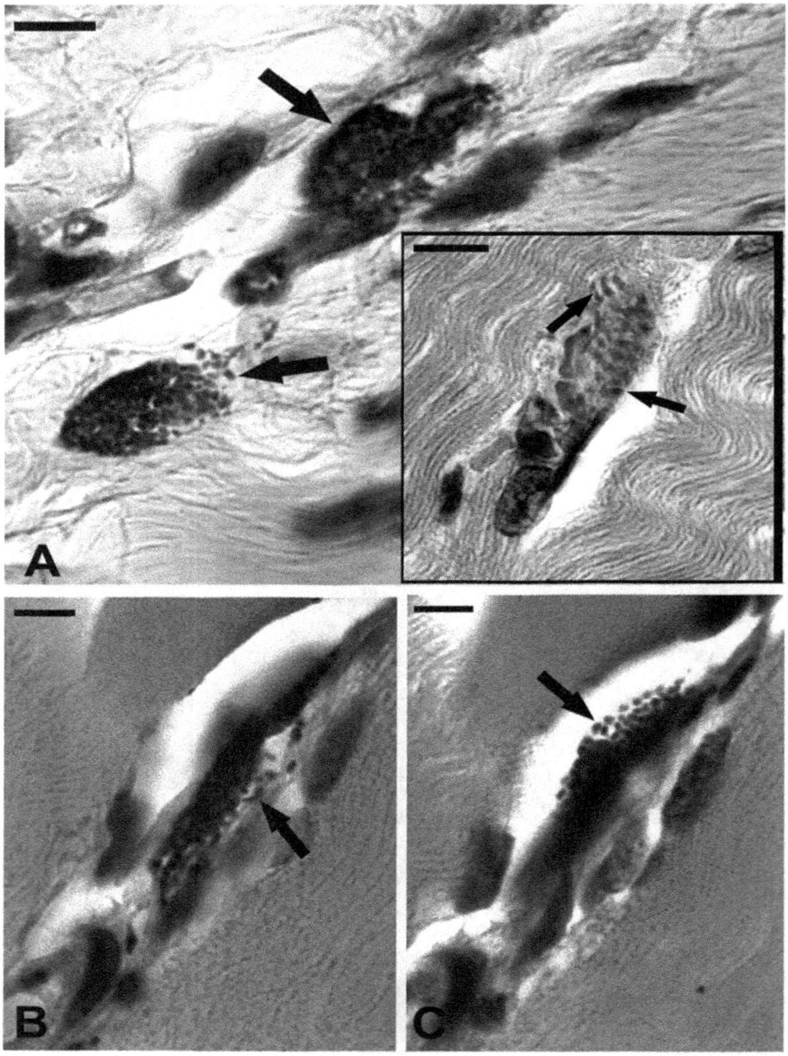


**Figure 2.** By light microscopy, longitudinal sections of adult muscle tissue of pregnant female infected with 25 cysts of *T. gondii* (Group 1). (A) Cyst-simile structures can be seen between myofibers (arrows), Bar: 15 μm. Note that the parasites seem to evade these structures (inset), Bar: 20 μm. (B and C) The same cell can be seen in two distinct focal planes showing small structures similar to Toxoplasma (arrows), Bars: 10 μm.

(**Figure 3A**, **C**, and **E**). However, the thigh muscles of embryos from *T. gondii* cyst-infected mothers, as compared to tissue from uninfected mice, contained a significant reduction in myofiber density and a great enlargement of the interfibrillar space (**Figure 3B**). Connective tissue cells filled this space, probably mononuclear cell inflammatory infiltrates such as macrophages, lymphocytes, mast cells, and eosinophils (**Figure 3B**, **D**, and **F**). Besides the shortening of mainly mature myofibers, muscle tissue analyzed of embryos born from infected mice presented several bipolar cells possessing small and elongated nuclei characterizing myoblasts

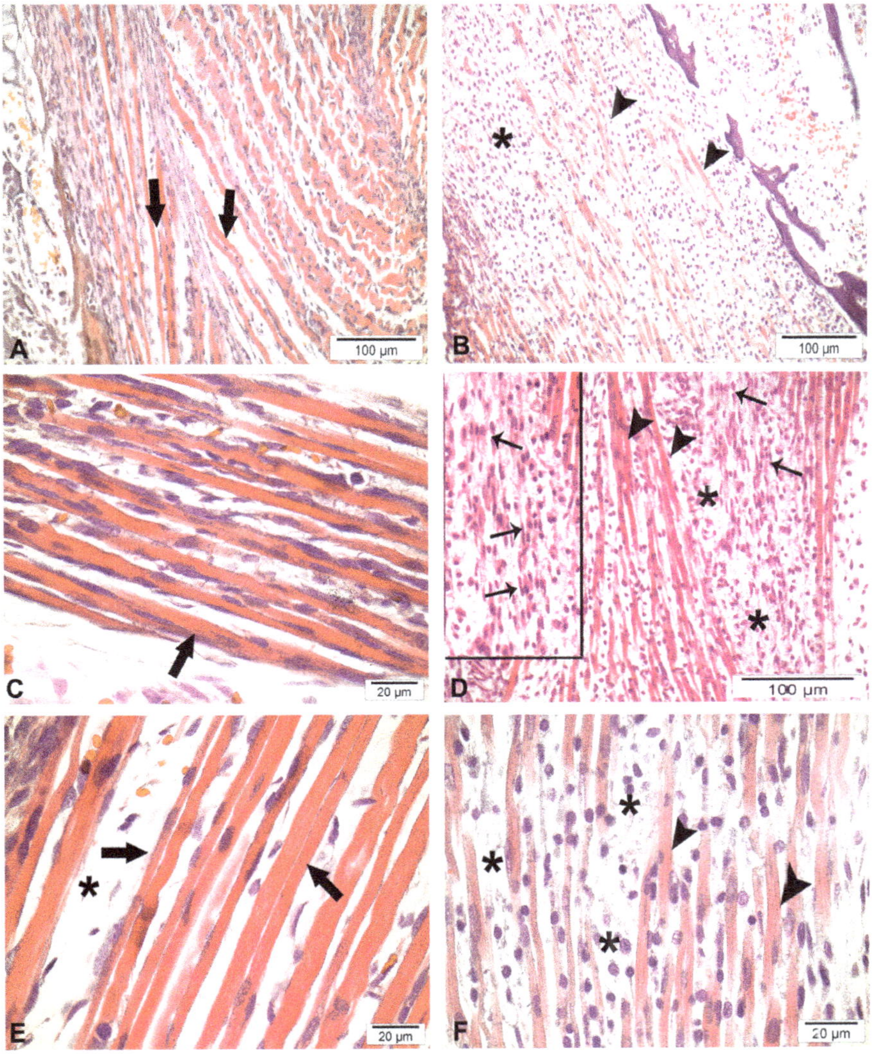


**Figure 3.** Longitudinal sections of the muscle tissue of thighs of murine embryos normal and from infected mother. (A, C, and E) Healthy embryo: note the high density of mature myofibers and small interfibrillar space (arrows). (B) Embryo muscle from infected mother: smaller density of myofibres (arrowhead) and greater spacing between them, probably filled by cells of connective tissue and cell inflammatory infiltrates such as: macrophages, lymphocytes, mast cells, and eosinophils (asterisks). (C) Healthy embryo: at higher magnification, dense and mature myofibres are observed with parallel arrangement and many nuclei. Note limited interfibrillar space and few mononuclear cells between myofibers. (D) Embryo from infected mother: muscle with scarcity of myofibers (arrowhead). Besides greater interfibrillar space, presence of a large number of mononuclear cells (asterisks). Note several bipolar cells with nuclei small and elongated (fine arrows). Inset: more detail these of aligned cells (myoblasts in the process of alignment and fusion). (E) Detail of healthy embryo myofibers. Higher cytoplasmic density of the myofibres with a striated profile and more organized. Interfiber space with number of cells, mononuclear cells markedly smaller (asterisk). (F) Embryo from infected mother: myofibers are smaller, less dense, less stained, and more spaced (asterisk). Apparently they are immature cells (less nuclei and cytoplasmic) and discontinuous in their extension (arrowhead).

in the process of alignment and fusion (**Figure 3D**). These embryos presented discontinuous, shorter, less dense, and slightly colored myofibrils with more interfibrillar space and immature cells with fewer stained and poorly defined striated profiles (**Figure 3B**, **D**, and **F**).

Brain samples of control embryos and infected mothers were examined. All control embryo brain tissues did not show any changes, the brain tissue normal and cell density characteristics of healthy tissue. Tissue section showed arranged cells in a pink color with the cytoplasm unaltered in purple, the nuclei with no visible changes in the chromatin arrangement and almost no intercellular space (**Figure 4A**). In contrast, the brains of embryos from infected mothers exhibited irregularly arranged cells with higher concentrations at apparently less injured points, reduced cell density, and a significant increase of intercellular space, possibly due to the decrease of the adherent junctions (**Figure 4B–D**). In addition, there was weak

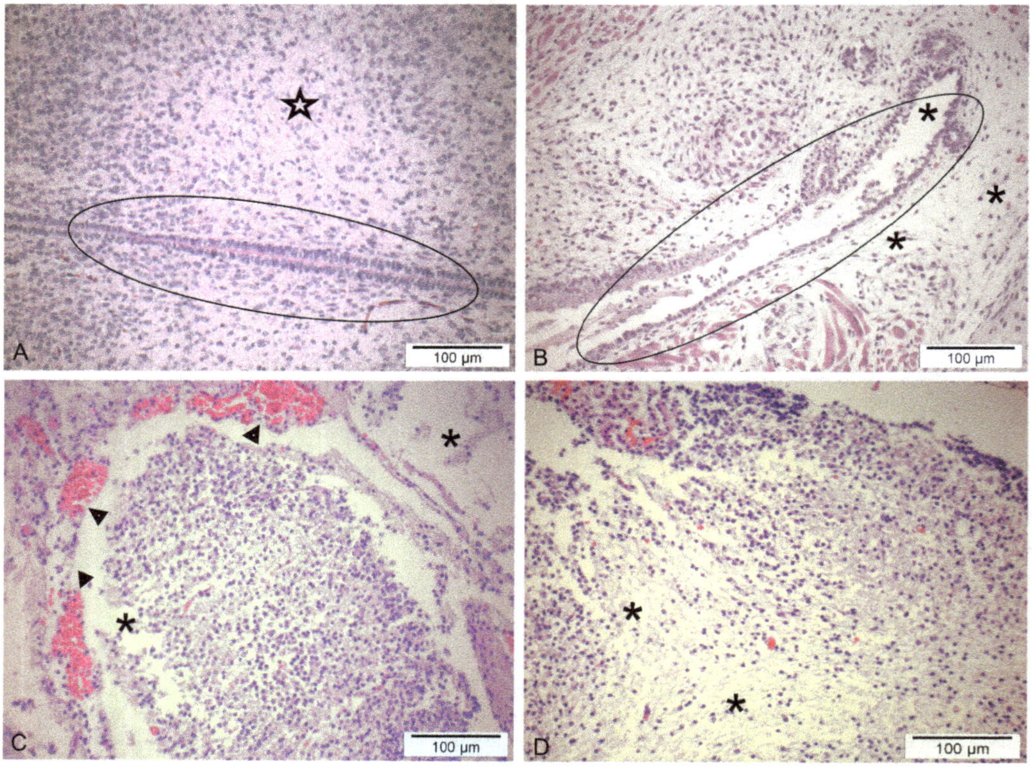


**Figure 4.** Using H&E staining, brain samples were examined for histopathological damages caused by Toxoplasma in embryos from infected mother. (A) Brain of an uninfected control, histology without any pathological changes. Regularly arranged cells of similar size (circle), cell density characteristic of healthy tissue, well stained, cells arranged in a pink color, with the cytoplasm unaltered in purple, the nuclei with no visible changes in the chromatin arrangement and almost no intercellular space (star). (B–D) The neurogenesis was severely affected and cerebral cortex of these embryos was compromised. Irregularly arranged cells, more concentrated at a point apparently less injured, reduced cell density, with a significant increase of intercellular space (asterisks). Note several points with recent thrombi of different sizes due to the massive presence of red blood cells (arrowhead).

cytoplasmic labeling and nuclear marking disparity, some larger nuclei almost transparent, others much smaller, marked. The presence of mononuclear cell inflammatory infiltrates was noted, such as macrophages, lymphocytes, mast cells, and eosinophils. There were several points with massive presence of red blood cells, implying recent thrombi in all analyzed sections (**Figure 4B** and **C**). In addition, different levels of brain tissue impairment were apparent (**Figure 4D**), such as presence of cells similar to astrocytes and neurons, which possibly suffered karyolysis (weak nuclear staining) and eosinophilia (**Figure 5B** and **C**). Some of these cells presented nearly transparent cytoplasm resulting from the loss of basophilia and others an apoptotic process characteristic (**Figure 5C**). No analyzed sections revealed parasites.

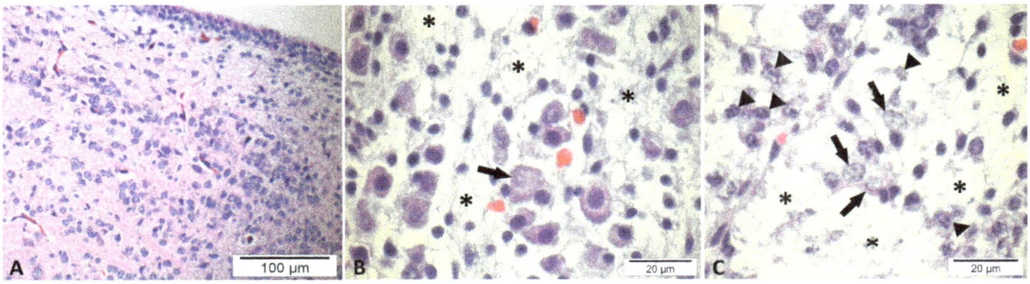


**Figure 5.** Using H&E staining and light microscopy embryonic brain cell lesions with CT was analyzed. (A) General aspects of normal embryonic brain tissue. (B and C) Observe the lower density and cellular organization in the brains of embryos from *T. gondii*-infected mothers (asterisk). Some cells, similar to astrocytes, possibly suffered karyolysis (weak nuclear staining) (arrow) and eosinophilia (asterisk), with the almost transparent cytoplasm resulting from the loss of basophilia (asterisk). (C) Presence of cells with a nucleus characteristic of the apoptotic process (arrowhead).

## 4. Discussion

This study investigated the role of *T. gondii* infection in neurogenesis and myogenesis of skeletal muscle tissue of murine embryos from infected mothers. Our previous results *in vitro* disclosed significant parasite interference in the myogenesis process, hence the motivation for the development of this work.

Our first experimental strategy was gavage infection of the female with cysts aiming to mimic *T. gondii* primary transmission in nature through ingestion of raw or poorly cooked meat containing these cysts [30]. The developmental commitment of embryos from Toxoplasma-infected mothers was incontestable, and the *T. gondii* pathogenicity degree is determined by many factors such as susceptibility of host species, infection stage (acute or chronic), and parasite strain virulence [17, 30, 31]. Macroscopic images clearly expose the malformation or not of anterior and posterior limbs as well as other malformations during the development of ME-49 strain *T. gondii*-infected mice.

Our experimental model with Swiss mice involving infection of the female prior to mating demonstrated that during the first week of pregnancy, there was significant fertility reduction, embryos with low birth weight, fetal reabsorption, miscarriages, and stillbirths, presenting a loss rate of over 50% for Group 1 (inoculated with 25 cysts) and almost 100% in Group 2 (inoculated with 50 cysts). However, since each cyst can vary in bradyzoite numbers (which may die or survive), it was not possible to define the parasite concentration that generated a certain vertical transmission rate. This would explain the loss of more than 70% of the embryos, considering that bradyzoites differentiate to tachyzoites that can damage the placenta, leading to loss of the embryo by spontaneous abortion or absorption, as proposed by Vargas-Villavicencio et al. [20]. These data confirm that the severity of Toxoplasma infection in females and embryos depends upon the concentration of parasites [18–20, 31]. TC is one of the most serious consequences of acute Toxoplasma infection, the greatest severity observed in early pregnancy as demonstrated experimentally in this study.

Embryos from infected mothers presented brain tissue with possible levels of ischemia and morphological aspects compatible with cell death mechanisms. Inflammatory reactions were apparent suggesting the focal presence of mononuclear cell infiltrates, necrosis, and thrombi, which increased according to the degree of infection development, compromising the neurogenesis. It is known that during apoptosis, the cells lose their adherent junctions [32], and lesions, due to ischemia or hypoxia together with other stimuli, also triggering cell death (necrosis and apoptosis) [33, 34]. Some cells, similar to astrocytes and neurons, underwent karyolysis (weak nuclear staining) and eosinophilia with the nearly transparent cytoplasm resulting from the loss of basophilia [35, 36]. The results described here during the cerebral histological analysis point to neuropathogenesis induced by the *T. gondii* infection. Sun et al. [37] demonstrated that this infection in early gestation might inhibit the proliferation, differentiation, and migration of neural stem cells in rats. It has been reported that *T. gondii* induces apoptosis of neural stem cells via the endoplasmic reticulum stress pathway [38]. Although we did not detect the presence of the parasite at the lesion site, some authors suggest that parasite proteins may directly interfere with neuronal function, either in infected or neighboring cells [18, 39–41]. These data corroborate our observations implying a *T. gondii* proapoptotic effect in cerebral cells and also justify the embryonic brain size decrease as described here.

The systemic inflammatory response induced by the parasite (toxoplasmosis sepsis) witnessed in our experiments may have caused multiple organ failure of these embryos, as proposed earlier [17]. Despite the already known involvement of muscle tissue in the development of the toxoplasmosis chronic phase [42], no studies involving embryos from *T. gondii*-infected mothers have ever investigated the influence of this infection in muscle tissue development. Our histological analysis demonstrated that muscle tissue from such embryos, in comparison with the healthy muscle myofibers, possessed lower density and higher interfibrillar space. Connective tissue cells and probably mononuclear cell inflammatory infiltrates such as macrophages, lymphocytes, mast cells, and eosinophils fill this space [1, 16]. Besides the shortening of myofibers and absence of mature myofibers, muscle tissue from *T. gondii*-infected embryos presented several bipolar cells with small, elongated nuclei characterized as myoblasts, still in the process of alignment and fusion (myogenesis). Myofibers from these embryos displayed, besides small size, lower density of cytoplasmic material (characterized by a slight staining, H&E), discrete striation, and a discontinuous profile. These apparently immature cells with few nuclei directly influenced the length of myofibrils thus interfering with the myogenesis process. Healthy embryos have the muscle tissue with many satellite cells attached to the myofibers, myoblasts in the process of fusion, and mature myofibers parallelly aligned dense and continuous [43]. The histological staining technique of H&E showed well-defined myofibers with striated characteristics of this cell type, dense cytoplasmic material, and greater proximity between them. This high cytoplasmic density characterized by intense staining of myofibers must be associated with an increased myocyte fusion process in the early development of the muscle fiber. However, it has been well established that *T. gondii* can cause myositis either by recent infection or reactivation of tissue cysts, affecting the homeostasis of muscle tissue [1]. Regarding the perspective of this study, our results confirm that *T. gondii* primary infection of premated mouse females affects the embryonic development, inhibiting the process of in the skeletal muscle *in vitro* model myogenesis [13]. In this study was demonstrated that *T. gondii* infection in skeletal muscle cells downregulate the M-cadherin mRNA expression, leading to molecular modifications on the host cell surface that disarray at the contact sites between myoblasts and myoblasts-myotubes, promoting the instability of the junctions. This progressive process interferes with membrane fusion and consequently inhibits the myogenesis process. This set of data justifies the results by histology that point out significant changes in the formation of embryonic myofibers from infected females before mating, corroborated by macroscopic images, showing some embryos with no formation of anterior and posterior members. These changes could lead to the modulation of other molecules contributing to toxoplasmosis pathogenesis in the murine muscle tissue as described here in the *in vivo* system. Additionally, recent research has reported that a virulence factor secreted by *T. gondii* rhoptries (ROP18) may contribute to neuronal apoptosis through the ER stress-mediated apoptosis pathway, which result in neurological diseases by reduction of these cells [41]. In rat brain cells with the same *T. gondii* ME49 strain the apoptosis induction was described, but the cell type involved in this process was not specified [39]. Therefore, we believe that the disorders in muscle tissue during our assays *in vivo* may be also related to a program of cell death, for example, apoptosis with the decrease of the adherent junctions, as also observed in the brain cells of embryos from infected mothers. More detailed histopathological studies are in progress considering that our preliminary analyses clearly indicated that embryos from the same litter had a differentiated influence in the degree of embryo development commitment induced by Toxoplasma.

## Acknowledgements

The authors thank Sandra Maria Oliveira Souza for technical support. English review and revision by Mitchell Raymond Lishon, native of Chicago, Illinois, USA-UCLA 1969.

## Funding

Our work was supported by grants from Conselho Nacional de Desenvolvimento Científico e Tecnológico (CNPq), Fundação Carlos Chagas Filho de Amparo à Pesquisa do Estado do Rio de Janeiro (FAPERJ), Fundação Oswaldo Cruz (Programa Estratégico de Apoio à Pesquisa em Saúde—PAPES IV e VI), Pronex—Programa de Apoio a Núcleos de Excelência—CNPq/FAPERJ and Instituto Oswaldo Cruz/Fiocruz.

## Author details

Alessandra F. Gomes and Helene S. Barbosa*

*Address all correspondence to: helene@ioc.fiocruz.br

Laboratory of Structural Biology, Oswaldo Cruz Institute, Oswaldo Cruz Foundation, Rio de Janeiro, RJ, Brazil

## References

[1] Hassene A, Vital A, Anghel A, Guez S, Series C. Acute acquired toxoplasmosis presenting as polymyositis and chorioretinitis in immunocompetent patient. Joint Bone Spine. 2008;**75**:603–605. DOI: 10.1016/j.jbspin.2007.08.009

[2] Habib FS, Ali NM, El-Kadery AA, Soffar SA, Abdel-Razek MG. Sequential recognition of antigenic markers of *Toxoplasma gondii* tachyzoite by pooled sera of mice with experimental toxoplasmosis. Parasitology Research. 2011;**108**:151–160. DOI: 10.1007/s00436-010-2046-0

[3] Shet A. Congenital and perinatal infections: Throwing new light with an old TORCH. Indian Journal of Pediatrics. 2011;**78**:88–95. DOI: 10.1007/s12098-010-0254-3

[4] Vauloup-Fellous C, Bouthry E. Diagnosis of maternofetal infections. Presse Medicale. 2015;**44**:621–630. DOI: 10.1016/j.lpm.2015.04.016

[5] Ambroise-Thomas P, Pelloux H. Toxoplasmosis—Congenital and in immunocompromised patients: A parallel. Parasitology Today. 1993;**9**:61–63. DOI: org/10.1016/0169-4758(93)90038-H

[6] Jones J, Lopez A, Wilson M. Congenital toxoplasmosis. American Family Physician. 2003;**67**:2131–2138

[7] Senegas A, Villard O, Neuville A, Marcellin L, Pfaff AW, Steinmetz T, Mousli M, Klein JP, Candolfi E. *Toxoplasma gondii*-induced foetal resorption in mice involves interferon-gamma-induced apoptosis and spiral artery dilation at the maternofoetal interface. International Journal for Parasitology. 2009;**39**:481–487. DOI: 10.1016/j.ijpara.2008.08.009

[8] Holland GN. Ocular toxoplasmosis in the immunocompromised host. International Ophthalmology. 1989;**13**:399–402

[9] Morhun PJ, Weisz JM, Elias SJ, Holland GN. Recurrent ocular toxoplasmosis in patients treated with systemic corticosteroids. Retina. 1996;**16**:383–387

[10] Weiss LM, Dubey JP. Toxoplasmosis: A history of clinical observations. International Journal For Parasitology. 2009;**39**:895–901. DOI: 10.1016/j.ijpara.2009.02.004

[11] Kaye A. Toxoplasmosis: Diagnosis, treatment, and prevention in congenitally exposed infants. Journal of Pediatric Health Care. 2011;**25**:355–364. DOI: 10.1016/j.pedhc.2010.04.008

[12] Del Grande C, Galli L, Schiavi E, Dell'Osso L, Bruschi F. Is *Toxoplasma gondii* a trigger of bipolar disorder? Pathogens. 2017;**10**:6. DOI: 10.3390/pathogens6010003

[13] Gomes AF, Guimarães EV, Carvalho L, Correa JR, Mendonça-Lima L, Barbosa HS. *Toxoplasma gondii* down modulates cadherin expression in skeletal muscle cells inhibiting myogenesis. BMC Microbiology. 2011;**11**:110. DOI: 10.1186/1471-2180-11-110

[14] Gherardi R, Baudrimont M, Lionnet F, Salord JM, Duvivier C, Michon C, Wolff M, Marche C. Skeletal muscle toxoplasmosis in patients with acquired immunodeficiency syndrome: A clinical and pathological study. Annals of Neurology. 1992;**32**:535–542. DOI: 10.1002/ana.410320409

[15] Montoya JG, Jordan R, Lingamneni S, Berry GJ, Remington JS. Toxoplasmic myocarditis and polymyositis in patients with acute acquired toxoplasmosis diagnosed during life. Clinical Infectious Diseases. 1997;**24**:676-683

[16] Tonino P, Finol HJ, Marquez A. Skeletal muscle pathology in mice experimentally infected with *Toxoplasma gondii*. Journal of Submicroscopic Cytology and Pathology. 1996; **28**:521–526

[17] Stahl W, Sekiguchi M, Kaneda Y. Multiple organ dysfunction in congenital murine toxoplasmosis. Tokai Journal of Experimental and Clinical Medicine. 2004;**29**:53–63

[18] Tonin AA, Da Silva AS, Thomé GR, Sangoi MB, Oliveira LS, Flores MM, Schetinger MR, Fighera RA, Moresco RN, Camillo G, Vogel FS, Lopes ST. Influence of toxoplasmosis on acetylcholinesterase activity, nitric oxide levels and cellular lesion on the brain of mice. Pathology Research and Practice. 2014;**210**:526–532. DOI: 10.1016/j.prp.2014.04.025

[19] Vargas-Villavicencio JA, Besné-Mérida A, Correa D. Vertical transmission and fetal damage in animal models of congenital toxoplasmosis: A systematic review. Veterinary Parasitology. 2016;**223**:195–204. DOI: 10.1016/j.vetpar.2016.04.024

[20] Vargas-Villavicencio JA, Cedillo-Peláez C, Rico-Torres CP, Besné-Mérida A, García-Vázquez F, Saldaña JI, Correa D. Mouse model of congenital infection with a non-virulent *Toxoplasma gondii* strain: Vertical transmission, "sterile" fetal damage, or both? Experimental Parasitology. 2016;**166**:116–123. DOI: 10.1016/j.exppara.2016.04.002

[21] Andrade EF, Stumbo AC, Monteiro-Leal LH, Carvalho L, Barbosa HS. Do microtubules around the *Toxoplasma gondii*-containing parasitophorous vacuole in skeletal muscle cells form a barrier for the phagolysosomal fusion?. Journal of Submicroscopic Cytology and Pathology. 2001;**33**:337–341

[22] Barbosa HS, Ferreira-Silva MF, Guimarães EV, Carvalho L, Rodrigues RM. Absence of vacuolar membrane involving *Toxoplasma gondii* during its intranuclear localization. Journal of Parasitology. 2005;**91**:182–184. DOI: 10.1645/GE-276R

[23] Guimarães EV, de Carvalho L, Barbosa HS. Primary culture of skeletal muscle cells as a model for studies of *Toxoplasma gondii* cystogenesis. Journal of Parasitology. 2008;**94**:72–83. DOI: 10.1645/GE-1273.1

[24] Guimarães EV, Carvalho Ld, Barbosa HS. Interaction and cystogenesis of *Toxoplasma gondii* within skeletal muscle cells in vitro. Memórias do Instituto Oswaldo Cruz. 2009; **104**:170–174

[25] Ferreira da Silva M da F, Barbosa HS, Gross U, Lüder CG. Stress-related and spontaneous stage differentiation of *Toxoplasma gondii*. Molecular BioSystems. 2008;**4**:824–834. DOI: 10.1039/b800520f

[26] Ferreira-da-Silva M da F, Takács AC, Barbosa HS, Gross U, Lüder CG. Primary skeletal muscle cells trigger spontaneous *Toxoplasma gondii* tachyzoite-to-bradyzoite conversion at higher rates than fibroblasts. International Journal of Medical Microbiology. 2009;**299**:381–388. DOI: 10.1016/j.ijmm.2008.10.002

[27] Ferreira-da-Silva Mda F, Rodrigues RM, Andrade EF, Carvalho Ld, Gross U, Lüder CG, Barbosa HS. Spontaneous stage differentiation of mouse-virulent *Toxoplasma gondii* RH parasites in skeletal muscle cells: An ultrastructural evaluation. Memórias do Instituto Oswaldo Cruz. 2009;**104**:196–200

[28] Gomes AF, Magalhães KG, Rodrigues RM, de Carvalho L, Molinaro R, Bozza PT, Barbosa HS. *Toxoplasma gondii*—Skeletal muscle cells interaction increases lipid droplet biogenesis and positively modulates the production of IL-12, IFN-g and PGE2. Parasites & Vectors. 2014;**7**:47. DOI: 10.1186/1756-3305-7-47

[29] Souto XM, Barbosa HS, Menna-Barreto RF. The morphological analysis of autophagy in primary skeletal muscle cells infected with *Toxoplasma gondii*. Parasitology Research. 2016;**115**:2853–2861. DOI: 10.1007/s00436-016-5040-3

[30] Dubey JP. Toxoplasmosis—A waterborne zoonosis. Veterinary Parasitology. 2004;**126**:57–72. DOI: 10.1016/j.vetpar.2004.09.005

[31] Rorman E, Zamir CS, Rilkis I, Ben-David H. Congenital toxoplasmosis—Prenatal aspects of *Toxoplasma gondii* infection. Reproductive Toxicology. 2006;**21**:458–472. DOI: 10.1016/j.reprotox.2005.10.006

[32] Gulisano W, Bizzoca A, Gennarini G, Palmeri A, Puzzo D. Role of the adhesion molecule F3/Contactin in synaptic plasticity and memory. Molecular and Cellular Neuroscience. 2016;**28**:30276–30277. DOI: 10.1016/j.mcn.2016.12.003

[33] Zhao M, Zhu P, Fujino M, Zhuang J, Guo H, Sheikh I, Zhao L, Li XK. Oxidative stress in hypoxic-ischemic encephalopathy: Molecular mechanisms and therapeutic strategies. International Journal of Molecular Sciences. 2016;**17**:E2078. DOI: 10.3390/ijms17122078

[34] Danese A, Patergnani S, Bonora M, Wieckowski MR, Previati M, Giorgi C, Pinton P. Calcium regulates cell death in cancer: Roles of the mitochondria and mitochondria-associated membranes (MAMs). Biochimica et Biophysica Acta. 2017;**10**:30004-X. DOI: 10.1016/j.bbabio.2017.01.003

[35] Shen Y, Wang Z, Li F, Sun L. Morphological characteristics of eosinophilic neuronal death after transient unilateral forebrain ischemia in Mongolian gerbils. Neuropathology. 2016;**36**:227–236. DOI: 10.1111/neup.12264

[36] Zhou CX, Zhou DH, Elsheikha HM, Zhao Y, Suo X, Zhu XQ. Metabolomic profiling of mice serum during toxoplasmosis progression using liquid chromatography-mass spectrometry. Science Report. 2016;**6**:19557. DOI: 10.1038/srep19557

[37] Sun XN, Liu ZJ, Guan ZY, Liang RW, Zhang HY, Wu XY, Yu L, Guan YJ. Effect of *Toxoplasma gondii* infection on the embryonic neural stem cells in rats. Zhongguo Ji Sheng Chong Xue Yu Ji Sheng Chong Bing Za Zhi. 2012;**30**:253–257

[38] Wang T, Zhou J, Gan X, Wang H, Ding X, Chen L, Wang Y, DU J, Shen J, Yu L. *Toxoplasma gondii* induce apoptosis of neural stem cells via endoplasmic reticulum stress pathway. Parasitology. 2014;**141**:988-995. DOI: 10.1017/S0031182014000183

[39] Shen DF, Matteson DM, Tuaillon N, Suedekum BK, Buggage RR, Chan CC. Involvement of apoptosis and interferon-gamma in murine toxoplasmosis. Investigative Ophthalmology & Visual Science. 2001;**42**:2031–2036.

[40] Haroon F, Händel U, Angenstein F, Goldschmidt J, Kreutzmann P, Lison H, Fischer KD, Scheich H, Wetzel W, Schlüter D, Budinger E. *Toxoplasma gondii* actively inhibits neuronal function in chronically infected mice. PLoS One. 2012;**7**:e35516. DOI: 10.1371/journal.pone.0035516

[41] Wan L, Gong L, Wang W, An R, Zheng M, Jiang Z, Tang Y, Zhang Y, Chen H, Yu L, Shen J, Du J. *T. gondii* rhoptry protein ROP18 induces apoptosis of neural cells via endoplasmic reticulum stress pathway. Parasites & Vectors. 2015;**8**:554. DOI: 10.1186/s13071-015-1103-z

[42] Remington JS, Cavanaugh EN. Isolation of the encysted form of *Toxoplasma gondii* from human skeletal muscle and brain. The New England Journal of Medicine. 1965;**273**:1308–1310. DOI: 10.1056/NEJM196512092732404

[43] Tajbakhsh S. Skeletal muscle stem cells in developmental versus regenerative myogenesis. Journal of Internal Medicine. 2009;**266**:372–389. DOI: 10.1111/j.1365-2796.2009.02158.x

# 4

# Effects of Nanoparticles in Cells Infected by *Toxoplasma gondii*

Sprakel-Leyke Silja, Paulke Bernd-Reiner and Presber Wolfgang

**Abstract**

Core-shell model drug carriers on two nanoscale size levels have been applied in cell culture studies and focused on Toxoplasmosis therapy. In synthesis, a seed of rhodamin B-labelled polystyrene latex particles was coated by polybutyl cyanoacrylate under physical inclusion of two different new drugs against Toxoplasmosis. Drug-loaded and drug-free core-shell model drug carriers were added to a cell culture of human macrophages, infected by ***Toxoplasma gondii***, following an infection plan. Drug release from the carriers had been studied before by enzymatic degradation by means of pork liver esterase. Particle size decrease by degradation was investigated in a UV/VIS spectrometer via transmission measurements. Drug release profiles were obtained by HPLC studies. The dynamics in the population of infected human macrophages, *T. gondii* as well as model drug carrier numbers were registered by an FACS (fluorescence-activated cell sorter). As main result, the drug-free references in the two series of core-shell model drug carriers achieved ca.85% of the observed maximum in Toxoplasmosis therapy efficiency. These data were correlated with an immune stimulant effect on the side of the human macrophages, caused by the cell uptake of colloidal substrate, foreign to the body.

**Keywords:** toxoplasmosis, nanoparticles, model drug carriers, human macrophages, cell culture, infection, therapy efficiency, immune stimulation

## 1. Introduction

Nanoparticles (NPs) are a tool for specifically targeting drugs or diagnostics to selected tissues or cell types [1–3]. Their use in cancer research and therapy is of special interest [4–9] as well as to overcome the blood-brain barrier [10, 11]. At least in theory, they are a tool to optimise pharmacological data such as drug release, tissue specificity and even cell specificity [2].

In some cases, drug crystals have been used successfully as nanocarriers [12, 13]. NPs composed of polymers may be loaded with drugs which they release in a controlled manner, or they are coated with molecules which give them specific surface characteristics to bind and be taken up by certain cells. Despite these attractive goals and 30 years of research, there are no polymeric nanoparticles in practical, pharmaceutical use. There is hope to apply nanoparticles to deliver drugs across the blood-brain barrier [10, 14, 15].

The reasons for this obvious failure include following: first, the unresolved problem of cytotoxicity of several nanocarrier types [16], low drug loading and insufficient delivery of the bound drug and lack of production facilities to supply demand.

The problem of toxicity could be overcome at least partially by high selectivity with regard to the cells by which the NPs are taken up. Such a strategy is especially interesting in the case of cells, infected with microbes which only multiply intracellularly, such as viruses and some parasites, as these often alter the surface of the host cell, thereby offering the specific targets needed. In this case, even toxic NPs could be useful, as they would exert their toxicity mainly or even better only in or against infected cells which would inhibit the multiplication of the pathogens and destroy them.

At the moment, there are some data showing that tissue specificity may be achieved. One of the interesting targets is the endothelial barrier of the brain. Despite the big potential [17], there are no data concerning infected cells. As it is important to develop drugs against intracellular parasites such as *Toxoplasma* or *Leishmania*, therefore the goal is to establish a system which would allow to trace the fate of nanoparticles in infected cell cultures. It should be possible to evaluate the cell and parasite proliferation and the differential uptake of NPs.

A fluorescence-activated cell sorter (FACS) represents a useful tool to measure particles which differ in size and more importantly, in fluorescence [18]. Thus, it is possible to count extracellular parasites and their host cells separately, if they differ in size. To find the intracellular parasites and to differentiate between infected and non-infected cells, green fluorescent protein-transfected parasites were used. In the past, it was shown that it is possible to follow the fate of *Leishmania* in a cell culture which is conventionally treated (by adding drugs at the necessary concentration) [19].

Because the FACS is able to discriminate between fluorescences of different wave lengths, the purpose of this study was to establish a system with stained NPs as an additional reacting partner [20]. In the case of *Leishmania*, only phagocytic cells, mainly macrophages, act as host cells and the parasite becomes internalised through phagocytosis. There are some data that NPs without drugs may even interfere with normal white blood cell functions, including phagocytosis.

As NPs are recognised as foreign structures, they are eliminated by phagocytising cells [21, 22]. Thus, it should be easier to treat microorganisms which multiply within macrophages, because the nanoparticles would be concentrated automatically in the desired target cells. An example for this strategy is *Leishmania* [23]. Another interesting goal of nanoparticle research is targeting NPs to the brain [11, 14, 24]. *Toxoplasma gondii* offers a possibility to combine these aims. *T. gondii* is a parasite which multiplies in different cell types including macrophages and phagocytising cells in the brain [25]. The main problems in treatment of toxoplasmosis are infections during pregnancy and *Toxoplasma* encephalitis in the case of immunocompromised patients [25–28]. In normal *Toxoplasma* infections, the multiplication of the parasites is stopped by the immune system, but cysts remain in all formerly infected tissues including the brain, serving as a source for exacerbations. Therefore, efficient treatment of all infected cells to prevent cyst formation would be an interesting goal. Thus, we started our experiments with NPs in *T. gondii*-infected cultures, knowing that *T. gondii* has a completely different mode of penetration which is mostly independent of the support of the host cell [29].

To come closer to in vivo conditions and to make it easy to observe an effect, the culture should work for at least 3 days to allow several cycles of multiplication.

Initially, all experiments with FACS should be controlled by microscopy, to prove that the interpretation of the FACS data is consistent with the images seen under the microscope.

## 2. Results and discussion

The established and considered system consisted of three components: nanoparticles, parasites and cells which differed in size and shape. However, there were also infected cells, cells loaded with nanoparticles and infected cells with nanoparticles which should be differentiated as well. To trace the fate of parasites and nanoparticles with FACS, they had to be stained with dyes which are distinguishable from each other. Because the green fluorescent protein, *Toxoplasma* was transfected with, shows fluorescence in green and yellow [33, 34] a red dye to stain the nanoparticles gave sufficient results. Of the dyes tested, rhodamine B gave the best results. The intensity of fluorescence corresponds with the amount of dye, fixed inside the core of the NPs and should increase exponentially (to the third) with the increasing radius of the NPs. In larger particles, however, there seems to be a quenching, as light is unable to penetrate from the core of the particle to the surface.

Next, a broader spectrum of NPs of different sizes was tested to see, which gave the best results. To be able to compare the FACS data with microscopical counting, the NPs had to be larger than 100 nm; otherwise, microscopical identification, especially of intracellular particles, would be impossible. In **Table 1**, one of the two best candidates is shown. As the results obtained with the two different NPs in these experiments were identical, only data with MC81cs are shown here.

The nanoparticle suspensions were homogeneous in size, checked by electron microscopy—data not shown—and were shown to be non-toxic, by measuring growth of cell cultures in their presence.

**Figure 1A** shows an infected cell in the presence of NPs. NPs with diameters between 200 and 300 nm were focused on as they were perfect for these purposes, being visible under a microscope, and therefore allowing the opportunity to compare microscopically the results, obtained with FACS with the situation in the cell culture.

| **MC81** | | | **Core** | | **Core-shell (cs)** | | **Cs + pentamidine** | |
|---|---|---|---|---|---|---|---|---|
| Z-ave (nm) | | | 133.1 | | 213.4 | | 221 | |
| PI | | | 0.065 | | 0.046 | | 0.071 | |
| ZP (mV) | pH | Distilled water | −93.20 | 5.52 | −84.79 | 5.5 | −79.70 | 5.55 |
| | | 10E-3M NaCl | −70.33 | 5.53 | −63.40 | 5.51 | −61.66 | 5.51 |
| | | 10E-2M NaCl | −50.85 | 5.54 | −30.60 | 5.51 | −29.00 | 5.45 |
| Surface charge density ($\mu C/cm^2$) | | | −2.54 | | −0.93 | | −0.96 | |
| **MC81c** | | | **MC81cs** | | | | | |
| | | | No drug | | Pentamidine | | Spiramycin | |
| Size (nm) | | 133.1 | 213.4 | | 222.1 | | 198.1 | |
| PI | | 0.065 | 0.046 | | 0.071 | | 0.04 | |

**Table 1.** Nanoparticle properties (mean particle diameter [z-average] and polydispersity index from dynamic light scattering, zetapotential [ZP] from particle electrophoresis).

The same area photographed using different filters: the arrow points to a macrophage cell infected with one *Toxoplasma* cell.

a. Three channel photography (FITC/PI/neutral): NPs are attached to the macrophage, and some are scattered around.

b. Two channel photography (FITC/PI): the parasite inside the cell is clearly visible.

c. One channel photography (FITC): only the parasite (green) is visible.

d. One channel photography (PI): the parasite is invisible, the cell appears red as a result of uptaken NPs, and some extracellular NPs are visible.

**Figure 1B–D** demonstrates how different filters are able to distinguish the dyes used. In a first series of experiments, different amounts of NPs added to cell culture were tested with the result that approximately 60,000 particles per cell gave measurable and reproducible results in this system. Most of the NPs were phagocytised by the cells within the first few hours.

As parasites not only infect cells and multiply—increasing in number in an unpredictable way— they will also destroy host cells, thereby diminishing their number.

To calibrate the exact increase or decrease in the different components, 'Perfect Counting Beads' (Caltag Laboratories) were added before FACS scan and all data were adjusted to the beads count.

The particle size (FSC-x-axis) and granularity (SSC-y-axis) were determined. In A, toxoplasmas'and in B, macrophages were counted in relation to beads in order to calculate absolute numbers. The beads are always seen in the same position. In parallel, the particles were characterised by fluorescence (see **Figure 3**).

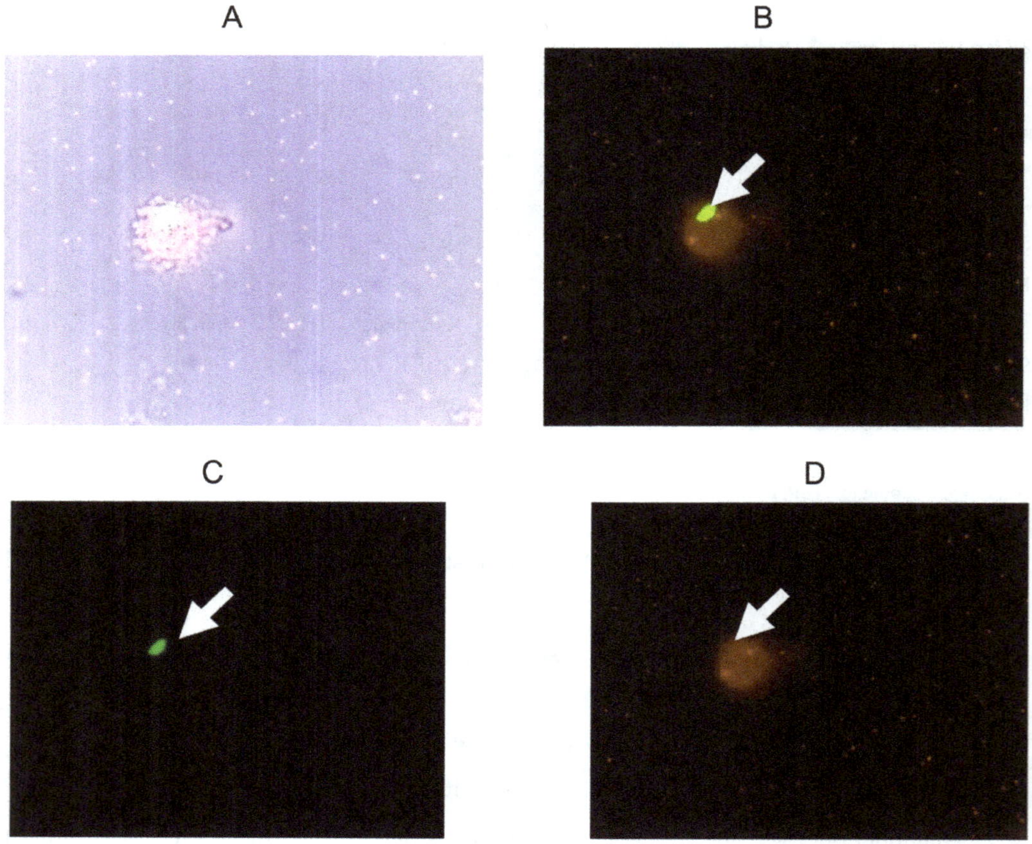


**Figure 1.** Situation in cell culture: macrophages, parasites and nanoparticles (NPs).

**Figure 2** shows an example of data obtained with a culture of J744-A1 cells infected with *T. gondii*. Each sample had to be measured twice: once to count the free parasites (**Figure 2A**) and a second time to count the cells (**Figure 2B**) separated by their size (FSC) and their granularity (SSC).

For analysis, the counted cells were sorted by fluorescence then. The series of dot blots in **Figure 3** compares uninfected, untreated control cells (A), infected cells (B), infected cells treated with unloaded nanoparticles (C), uninfected cells treated with unloaded NPs (D) and infected cells treated with pentamidine-loaded NPs (E).

The dot blots show changes in green fluorescence and granularity. In addition, the mean values of the particles in the gates are given in **Table 2**, as the numbers are hard to calculate from the images. The shift in the mean values is often more impressive than the density or position of the dots.

A

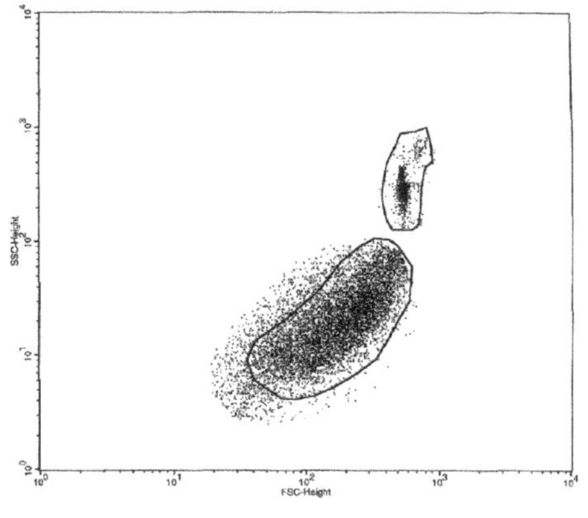


Tube 2 Infection control

| Region | Events | % Gated | % Total | X Mean | X Geo Mean | Y Mean | Y Geo Mean |
|---|---|---|---|---|---|---|---|
| R1 | 1846 | 18.46 | 18.46 | 546.01 | 543.77 | 329.01 | 313.71 |
| R2 | 7183 | 71.83 | 71.83 | 214.94 | 178.95 | 24.96 | 19.97 |

B

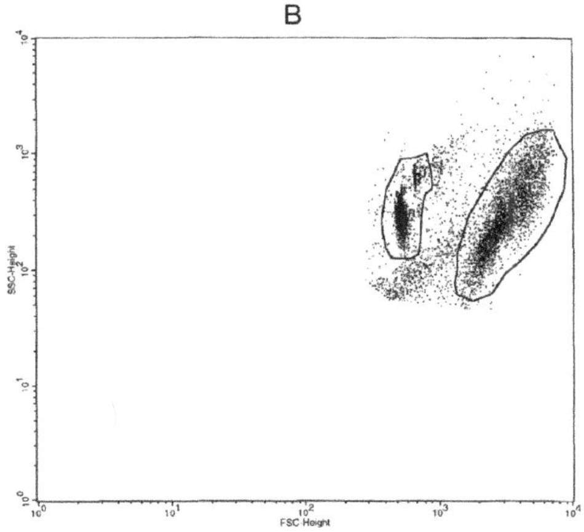


Tube 1 Cell control

| Region | Events | % Gated | % Total | X Mean | X Geo Mean | Y Mean | Y Geo Mean |
|---|---|---|---|---|---|---|---|
| R1 | 4933 | 49.33 | 49.33 | 540.11 | 537.92 | 344.53 | 329.27 |
| R2 | 3968 | 39.68 | 39.68 | 3343.07 | 3134.86 | 362.81 | 286.31 |

**Figure 2.** Particle size (FSC-x-axis) and granularity (SSC-y-axis) of (A) Toxoplasma cells and (B) macrophages population.

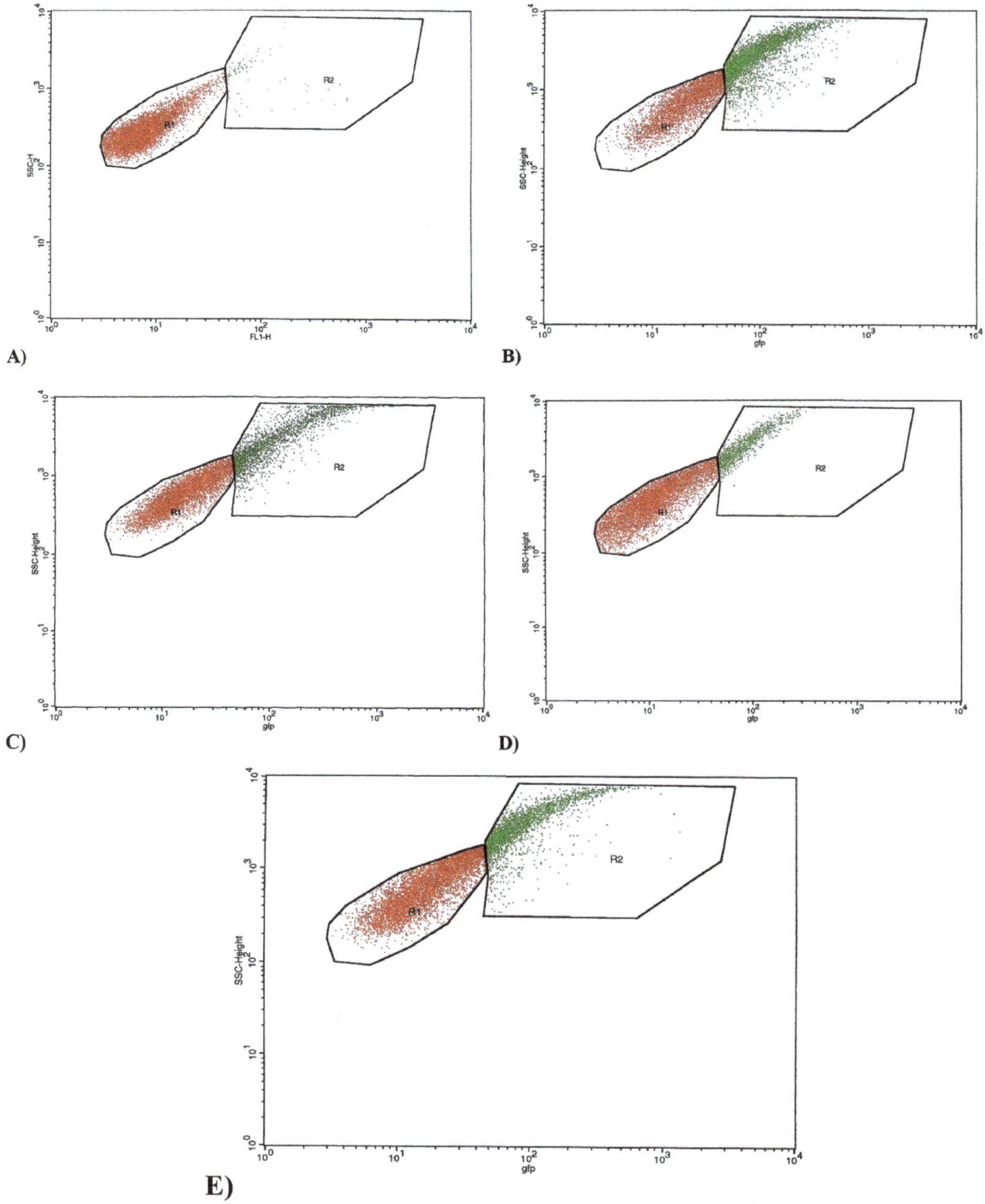


**Figure 3.** Granularity (SSC) and green fluorescence (FL1) of non-infected, untreated cells (A), infected, untreated cells (B), infected and treated with pure nanoparticles (C), uninfected cells, treated with nanoparticles (D) and infected cells, treated with pentamidine-loaded nanoparticles (E), given after 1 day of incubation.

**Figure 3A** illustrates the fluorescence of the macrophages of the cell control with its characteristic unspecific autofluorescence. The presence of *Toxoplasma* and/or NPs induces a movement into the area of higher fluorescence (**Figure 3B–E**). Whereas the *Toxoplasma* induces a stronger shift into the green fluorescence (**Figure 3B**), the NPs induced a smaller one (**Figure 3D**) which is an effect of an unspecific stimulation of the cells resulting in an increased autofluorescence [30].

The corresponding **Table 2** shows the percentage of particles in the gate for non-infected cells (R1) and the percentage in the gate of infected cells (R2) as well as the corresponding mean values (mean) and geometrical mean values (G-M).

Green fluorescence is represented on the x-axis and granularity on the y-axis.

Macrophages, activated by nanoparticles, have a basic fluorescence which is at least partially an indicator of their activity [36]. Thus, controls of cells, treated only with nanoparticles, are essential. For data processing, other combinations may be selected, such as granularity or red fluorescence. There is always an overlap of data however, and the interpretation of the blots must be proofread against the mean values of the particles within the gates—here given in the corresponding tables.

In the following series of experiments, a cell system was established in a manner that after infection on day zero, there is a continuous multiplication of Toxoplasma at least until day three. Defined concentrations of cells were put into wells, and parasites in different ratios were added for this purpose. The ratio parasite to cell is given as MOI (multiplicity of infection). All tests were carried out in three wells in parallel, and all experiments were carried out at least twice. The most promising results were obtained with MOI's of 1–10.

**Figure 4** shows the results of one of these experiments. MOI's of 10, 5, 2 and 1 were used, and free parasites (A), total cells (B) and infected cells (C) were determined at the first, second and third day after infection. There was a large increase in free parasites over the 3 days with MOI's of 10 and 5, a moderate increase with an MOI of 2 and almost no increase with an MOI of 1 (**Figure 4A**). In parallel, there was no such strong increase in total cell number as with the uninfected controls (**Figure 4B**). With the high MOI's of 10 and 5, there was a decrease at day two and an increase at day three. Only with MOI's of 1 and 2, there was a slight increase in cells over the 3 days. The number of infected cells indicates that with a MOI of 10 and 5, almost all cells were infected, whereas with MOI'of 2 and 1, many cells remained uninfected until day three (compare **Figure 4B** and **C**).

It was shown that MOI 2 is most appropriate for these tests, because there was an increase in the parasites and of the cells over the 3 days.

In a culture of infected cells, running for at least 3 days, there will be individual death of cells and parasites. Some of the free *Toxoplasma* in the culture will die and—as the infected cells disintegrate after liberating multiplied parasites—will shift into the debris. Thus, there will be an unpredictable increase or decrease in cell counts. To differentiate between an increase of non-infected cells and a loss of infected cells, both of which result in an increase in the percentage of non-infected cells, it was necessary to determine the total number of cells and the proportion of infected and non-infected cells in relation to the cell input on day zero. Before measuring, cells were fixed with paraformaldehyde, and after 'Perfect Counting Beads' (Caltag Laboratories) were added, the samples were counted.

| Experiment | R1 % | R1 X mean | R1 X G–M | R2% | R2 X mean | R2 X G–M |
|---|---|---|---|---|---|---|
| **A** C | 98.84 | 8.35 | 7.35 | 1.16 | 102.68 | 77.60 |
| **B** C+T | 50.83 | **23.42** | **20.62** | 49.17 | **108.24** | **91.94** |
| **C** C+T+NPs | 73.05 | **18.68** | **16.16** | 26.95 | **165.08** | **116.78** |
| **D** C+NPs | 85.46 | 13.72 | 11.16 | 14.54 | 88.33 | 80.10 |
| **E** C+T+NPs+P | 69.55 | **19.58** | **16.84** | 30.45 | **103.65** | **86.43** |

Exp.: part of the experiment corresponding to **A** to **E**; R%: percent of counts in this gate; R1 X mean: mean value of counts in gate 1; R1 X G-M: geometrical mean value of counts in gate 1; R2 X mean: mean value of counts in gate 2; R2 X G-M: geometrical mean value of counts in gate 2.

**Table 2.** Granularity (SSC) and green fluorescence (FL1) with the corresponding values of **Figure 3**.

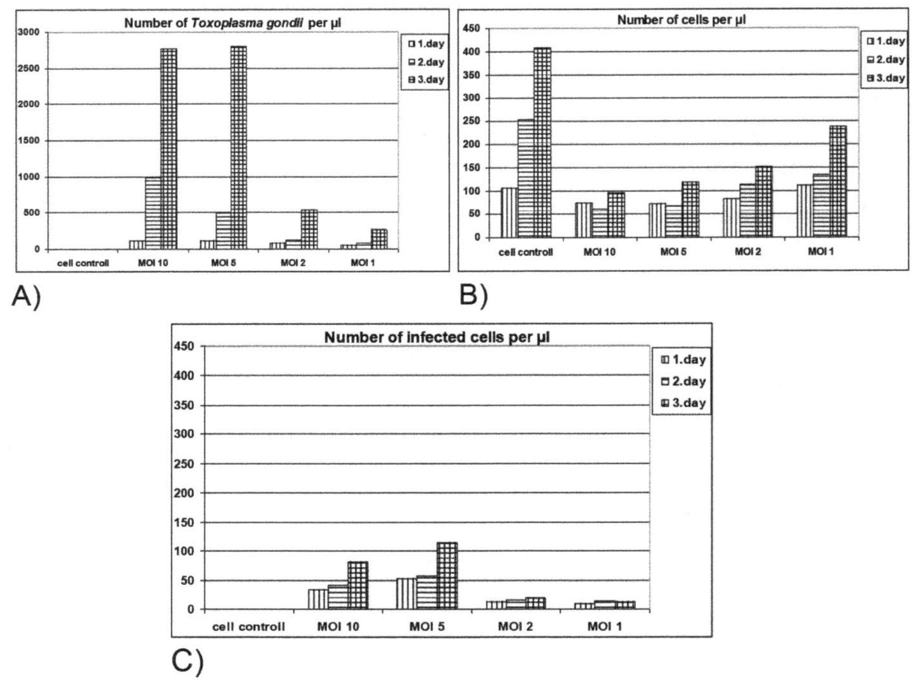


**Figure 4.** Influence of multiplicity of infection (MOI) $1.36 \times 10^5$ cells per ml was infected with different multiplicities of infection (10, 5, 2 and 1). A number of free parasites (A), total cell number (B) and number of infected cells (C) were determined over 3 days.

There was an indication that even unloaded NPs have an inhibitory effect. To prove this, the influence of pentamidine-loaded and unloaded nanoparticles on Toxoplasma-infected cell cultures was determined. **Figure 5** shows the histograms in each case for day 2 of non-infected cells (A), infected untreated cell controls (B), cells only treated with NPs (C), infected cells treated with unloaded NPs (D) and pentamidine-loaded NPs (E). The histograms show the changes in green fluorescence (FL1) and number of counts. One table with all data obtained (**Figure 5A**) is shown as an example of how CellQuest® analyses data. Data of corresponding tables, with the mean values of the gates for all 3 days, are given in **Table 3**. It is shown that the presence of Toxoplasma induced a shift to higher fluorescence. Comparing the data of infected cells, treated with pentamidine-loaded nanoparticles with those treated with unloaded nanoparticles, demonstrates that nanoparticles alone had an effect on *T. gondii* multiplication.

Simply comparing the mean values of M2 (the gate with the infected cells) would lead to a misinterpretation: the geometrical mean value would indicate that NPs even enhance Toxoplasma multiplication (106.69 vs. 86.41-labelled with '1' in **Table 3**), and the median would also suggest this (84.26 vs. 77.04 labelled with '2' in **Table 3**).

By looking at the percentage, one sees that with NPs, there was an increase in cells in the gate of non-infected cells (M1: 71.0 vs. 49.5% labelled with '3' in **Table 3**) and as the mean value of all cells indicates, there was an inhibition by unloaded NPs visible as reduction in green fluorescence (57.48 vs. 63.41 labelled with '4' in **Table 3**). The median indicates that the inhibition was substantially (22.27 vs. 43.32 labelled with '5' in **Table 3**).

The mean value of the green fluorescence marker reflects the parasitic load, as fluorescence is proportional to parasite number. Thus, few cells with high numbers of parasites may increase the mean value despite the fact that there were lots of non-infected cells. The median indicates the shift of the population towards infected or non-infected cells. The closer the median of infected, treated cells come to non-infected control cells, the better the treatment success. The geometrical mean gives some information, concerning the heterogeneity, but avoids the overestimation of exceptionally heavy infected single cells.

By measuring 10,000 cells, FACS offered the opportunity to statistically treat these data in different ways, resulting in a more complex interpretation. In addition to this evaluation of data, one had to take into account that nanoparticles are known to stimulate the macrophages [30–32]. As an increase in unspecific fluorescence was seen, an inhibition of Toxoplasma growth by unloaded nanoparticles was not surprising.

The explanation was that the nanoparticles counteracted the suppression of activities caused by the parasites [33], and this unspecific stimulation of macrophages by nanoparticles was more effective than the inhibition of parasites within downregulated host cells.

As cells, treated with nanoparticles, were always used as controls to estimate the unspecific increase in fluorescence, it was realised that there was a substantial inhibition by unloaded nanoparticles in all experiments.

In an additional series of experiments, the effect of nanoparticles without any drug was specifically proven. Data of an experiment to determine the effect of particle number on the multiplication of *T. gondii* during a period of 3 days are given in **Figure 6**.

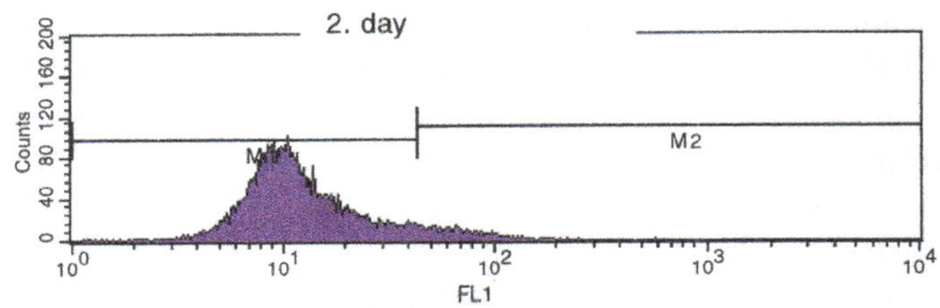


A)

| Marker | Left, Right | Events | % Gated | % Total | Mean | Geo Mean | CV | Median | Peak Ch |
|---|---|---|---|---|---|---|---|---|---|
| All | 1, 9910 | 10000 | 100.00 | 100.00 | 16.77 | 12.57 | 111.60 | 10.75 | 10 |
| M1 | 1, 43 | 9311 | 93.11 | 93.11 | 12.73 | 11.11 | 58.92 | 10.37 | 10 |
| M2 | 43, 9910 | 697 | 6.97 | 6.97 | 71.02 | 66.29 | 47.17 | 61.53 | 63 |

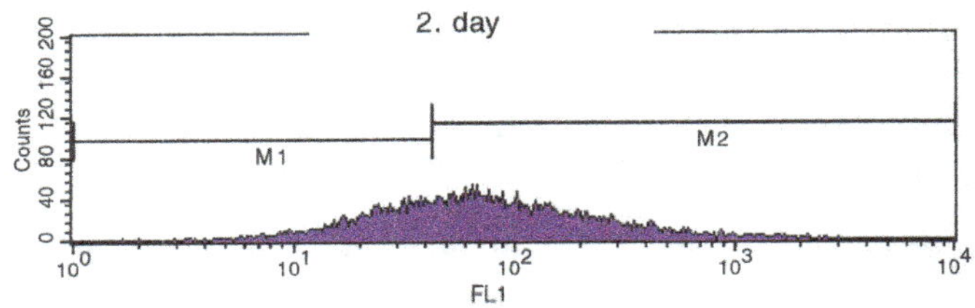


B)

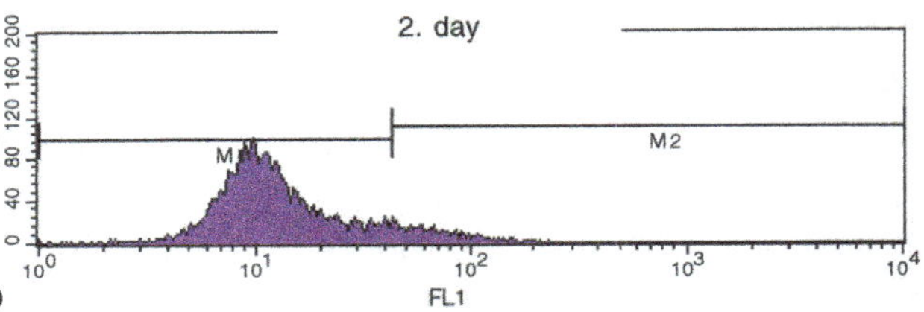


C)

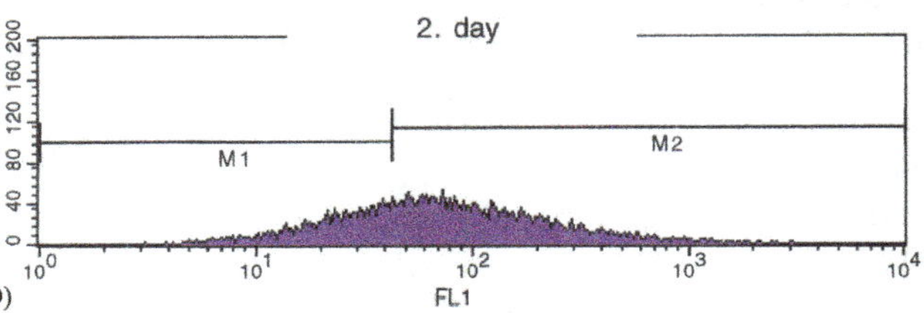


D)

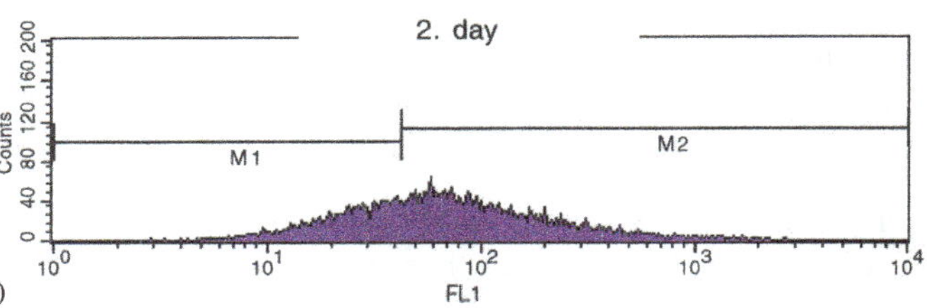


E)

**Figure 5.** FACS counts of non-infected, infected and NPs-treated cell. Histograms are shown in each case for day 2 of non-infected cells (A), infected untreated cell controls (B), cells only treated with NPs (C), infected cells treated with unloaded NPs (D) and pentamidine-loaded NPs (E). The histograms show the changes in green fluorescence (FL1) and number (counts). M1 indicates the non-infected cells and M2 the infected ones. (T = *Toxoplasma gondii*).

| | 1. day | | | 2. day | | | 3. day | | |
|---|---|---|---|---|---|---|---|---|---|
| | All | M1 | M2 | All | M1 | M2 | All | M1 | M2 |
| Cell control [%] | | *98.6* | *1.4* | | *93.0* | *7.0* | | *92.0* | *8.0* |
| Mean | 9.29 | | | 16.77 | | | 16.14 | | |
| Geomean | 7.30 | 7.08 | 70.91 | 12.57 | 11.11 | 66.29 | 10.23 | 8.68 | 65.62 |
| Median | 6.79 | 6.73 | 57.25 | 10.75 | 10.37 | 61.53 | 9.22 | 8.58 | 59.89 |
| Infected cells [%] | | *35.0* | *65.0* | | *33.0* | *67.0* | | ***49.5***[3] | *50.5* |
| Mean | 160.49 | | | 127.46 | | | **63.41**[4] | | |
| Geomean | 75.89 | 18.78 | 156.81 | 70.30 | 23.32 | 121.25 | 42.25 | 20.27 | **86.41**[5] |
| Median | 73.63 | 19.81 | 145.90 | 66.12 | 25.71 | 103.66 | **43.32**[5] | 22.07 | **77.04**[2] |
| Cells + NPs [%] | | *93.0* | *7.0* | | *90.5* | *9.5* | | *85.5* | *15.5* |
| Mean | 14.63 | | | 18.76 | | | 22.96 | | |
| Geomean | 10.06 | 8.77 | 67.19 | 13.70 | 11.60 | 65.49 | 13.21 | 9.81 | 74.96 |
| Median | 8.28 | 7.99 | 62.08 | 11.44 | 10.84 | 61.53 | 11.44 | 9.91 | 69.16 |
| Cells + Toxopl. + NPs [%] | | *34.0* | *66.0* | | *33.5* | *66.5* | | ***71.0***[3] | *29.0* |
| Mean | 159.64 | | | 118.23 | | | **57.48**[4] | | |
| Geomean | 76.71 | 19.57 | 156.14 | 142.73 | 23.22 | 117.34 | 27.56 | 15.92 | **106.69**[1] |
| Median | 72.34 | 21.29 | 143.30 | 64.94 | 25.71 | 101.82 | **22.27**[5] | 15.96 | **84.29**[2] |
| Cells + Toxopl.+ NPs (pentamidine-loaded) [%] | | *37.0* | *63.0* | | *35.0* | *65.0* | | *69.0* | *31.0* |
| Mean | 157.60 | | | 115.67 | | | 43.75 | | |
| Geomean | 73.90 | 20.18 | 158.34 | 65.71 | 23.49 | 113.57 | 27.49 | 27.49 | 79.96 |
| Median | 67.93 | 21.48 | 144.60 | 61.80 | 25.71 | 95.60 | 25.95 | 17.31 | 68.54 |

[1,2,3,4] and [5] refer to numbers in discussion.

**Table 3.** Mean values of total cells and gates of **Figure 5**. In addition to the mean values, the percentage of M1 and M2 of total cells for each part is given.

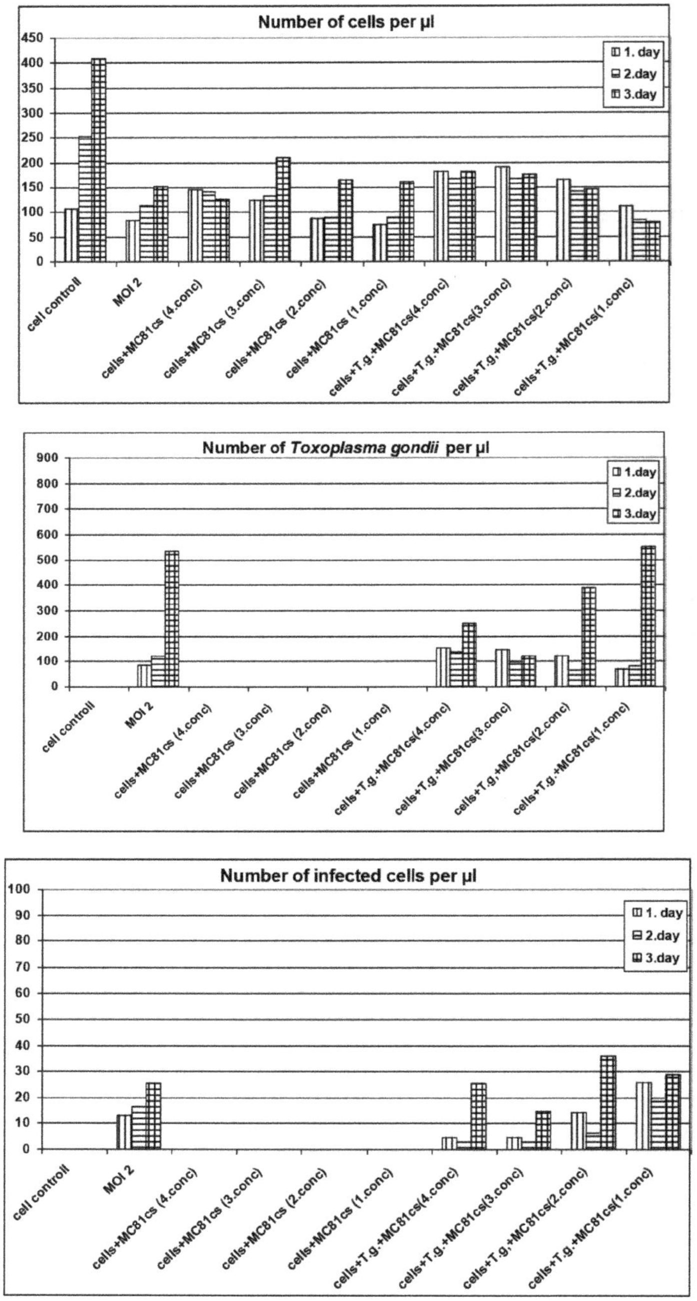


**Figure 6.** Effect of different concentrations of NPs (MC81cs) on cell proliferation and of *Toxoplasma gondii* (T. g) growth. (A) A number of all remaining cells (infected and non-infected) after 1, 2 and 3 days of infection and treatment. (B) A number of free (extracellular) *Toxoplasma gondii*. There are no *Toxoplasma* in NPs-treated, non-infected cells. (C) A number of infected cells after treatment with different concentrations of NPs.

Part A shows the increase in the infected and non-infected cells with different NPs concentrations. As can be seen, NPs in a high concentration (conc.4) inhibited proliferation over the 3 days. The lower concentrations led to a small increase on day two and a larger increase on day three. With infected cells, there was no difference between conc. 4 and 3, and only a slight decrease in cells with conc. 2. But with the lowest concentration, conc. 1, there was a decrease over the 3 days.

Part B shows the increase in *Toxoplasma* in the presence of NPs. Concentrations 4 and 3 suppressed the propagation of *Toxoplasma*. There was a reduced number of free *Toxoplasma* compared with the infection control. At concentrations 1 and 2 on the third day, there was a large increase in free *Toxoplasma* with concentrations even higher than in the untreated control.

Part C shows the number of infected cells which decreased at all NPs concentrations on day two and increased on the third day. The third concentration led to the smallest number of infected cells over the 3 days.

Cells were infected with an MOI of 2. The concentrations of NPs were as follows:

| | |
|---|---|
| Conc 1: 118,000 NPs/cell | Conc 3: 24,000 NPs/cell |
| Conc 2: 60,000 NPs/cell | Conc 4: 12,000 NPs/cell |

As discussed above, the effect of NPs was interpreted as activating the functions suppressed by Toxoplasma. On the other hand, there may be negative effects on macrophage functions, too [34]. Thus, in other cases (with other cells or with other parasites), the effect could be different. If there is stimulation, a treatment with nanoparticles alone could have some influence on a Toxoplasma infection, as drug-loaded particles have.

One way to prove this is to repeat these experiments in other, non-phagocytising host cells. The problem is that they will not take up the nanoparticles as easily as the macrophages do. As there are other microorganisms which also multiply within macrophages, there could be other indications for this type of treatment.

In all experiments described so far, Toxoplasma and NPs were added simultaneously to the cells. When nanoparticles influence the activities of phagocytising cells, and *T. gondii* alters the host cell activities, it is interesting to ask, whether the presence of NPs or *T. gondii* interferes with the taking up of the other, is there some type of mutual exclusion? Thus, experiments were carried out with NPs, added four hours after infection with *T. gondii*, or cells were infected 4 h after treatment with NPs. There were no differences in the taking up of NPs or parasites or in the effect of treatment after 3 days. The slope of the parameters was simply shifted (data not shown).

In the future, one will see, whether Leishmania major which in contrast to *T. gondii* are able to grow only in macrophages and are also inhibited by unloaded NPs. A few reports indicate that this should be true [21]. With Leishmania, first data in animal models were published [35, 36]. The fact that Leishmania major multiplies only in phagocytising cells makes them even more interesting for a further use of nanoparticles.

A question to be answered is, whether there is disintegration of nanoparticles by the host cells. There was fluorescence on the third day, what could be the result of dye released after disintegration? Microscopical observation revealed that nanoparticles were still present, at least the non-degradable, fluorescence-labelled polystyrene cores of these core-shell nanoparticles.

With the methods used, a disintegration of the nanoparticles could not be demonstrated in detail as it should start with the cleavage of the ester groups of the polymer shell by esterases which would not alter the structure in a way that could be seen with a microscope. As it only happens inside the cells, this alteration cannot be found with FACS, as there is no change in granularity.

As the core particles remain undigested, granularity will indicate the presence of particles. In the case that there would be no disintegration, this may be an advantage of an in vitro system using phagocytising cells, as the activation will persist. The consequences for in vivo conditions remain to be determined. Allen showed in 1988 that repeated application of liposomes could led to an impairment of Kupffer cells in the liver and fixed macrophages in the spleen which remove most of these NPs [37].

Our aim was to establish a system which allows the observation of the interaction of nanoparticles and microorganisms, infecting a cell culture, because there should be difference between infected and non-infected cells which could be used for targeting. The results are very promising. As various cell lines are able to produce interleukins or other modulators, there is the possibility to characterise the influence of nanoparticles in even more detail.

The data that NPs without any drugs have the same effect as drug-loaded NPs offer the opportunity to use NPs directly for treatment. Perhaps part of the effect of Atovaquone crystal nanoparticles in a Toxoplasma-mouse model should be attributed to the effect of nanoparticles [13], rather than to the direct effect of the drug against the parasite.

## 3. Experimental part

### 3.1. Colloid and polymer chemistry

#### *3.1.1. Preparation of nanoparticles*

Core-shell latex nanoparticles (MC81cs see **Table 1**) were synthesised by seeded, aqueous polymerisation of butyl cyanoacrylate onto polystyrene cores. Polystyrene cores were prepared by emulsion polymerisation of styrene in a water/ethanol mixture (16:1; v/v) in the presence of rhodamine B and purified by dialysis against deionised water. One gram of these core particles in water with a pH of 2 was used as seed for the polymerisation of 2 g butyl cyanoacrylate [38]. In the case of pentamidine loading, 5 mg pentamidine/g polymer was added to the polymerisation medium. Resulting core-shell nanoparticles were purified by dialysis against de-ionised water after neutralisation with sodium hydroxide (1 M aqueous solution).

*3.1.2. Characterisation of nanoparticles*

The particle size, determined as $Z_{ave}$ (average particle diameter) and the polydispersity index (PI), was measured by photon correlation spectroscopy (PCS), using a Zetamaster S (Malvern Instruments). Electrophoretic mobilities were measured to reflect the effective surface charge (Zetamaster S, Malvern Instruments). For transformation into zeta potential, the Smoluchowski model for ideal smooth spheres was used. Measurements were carried out in ultra-pure water (Millipore), 0.01 M NaCl solution and in 0.001 M NaCl solution.

Surface charge density was titrated by means of 0.1 mM PDADMAC solution (MW approx. 100,000) at a combination of particle charge detector PCD-03 pH (MÜTEK) and automatic titrator Titrino 716 (Metrohm). Purified, aqueous nanoparticle suspensions were stored in the refrigerator until use.

*3.1.3. Beads*

'Perfect Counting Beads' (Caltag Laboratories) were used to adjust the cell and *T. gondii* number. Immediately before counting with FACS, a defined number of beads were added and for calculation of inhibition and growth, all cells and *T. gondii* were adjusted to the known bead concentration.

### 3.2. Biology of Infections

*3.2.1. T. gondii GFP growth and experimental infection:*

Tachyzoites of the RH (CAT-GFP) strain of *T. gondii* (obtained from D. Soldati; Centre of Molecular Biology, Heidelberg University, Germany) were maintained in vitro in human epitheloid carcinoma cells (HELA) by serial passage into RPMI medium supplemented with 10% FCS (Gibco-BRL) twice a week (Gibco-BRL).

Macrophages and parasites were counted in a Fuchs-Rosenthal chamber and adjusted to the concentrations indicated. In most cases, macrophages of a concentration of $1.36 \times 10^5$ per ml were used and the multiplicity of infection (MOI) in most experiments was 2.

### 3.3. Cell culture work

*3.3.1. Cell lines*

Macrophages: The intracellular Toxoplasma infection studies were performed on J 774-A1 cells (mouse monocyte macrophages, ACC 170; German Collection of Microorganisms and Cell Cultures). The macrophages were grown in Dulbecco's MEM containing 10% heat-inactivated foetal calf serum (Boehringer, Germany) at 37°C in 5% $CO_2$ atmosphere.

*3.3.2. FACS-analysis*

Parasites, infected cells and non-infected cells were counted with FACS-scan analytical flow cytometry and equipped with a 15 mV, 488 nm air-cooled argon ion laser (Becton Dickinson). Multiparametric data were analysed using CellQuest® Software. Ten thousand 'particles', defined by size and granularity, were measured for each analysis.

The optimised instrument parameters for the assay were as follows: forward scatter (E 00, log mode), side scatter (319 voltage, log mode) fluorescence 1 (FL1; 613 voltage, log mode) and fluorescence 2 (FL2; 528, log mode).

Each experiment was carried out in a triple manner and performed in a special laboratory. The equipment was decontaminated with FACS-safe solution (1% active chlorine, Becton Dickinson).

Adding formaldehyde to a final concentration of 0.2% resulted in a preservation of the samples. Samples could be stored for days in a refrigerator and be measured at a more convenient time.

### 3.3.3. *Microscopy and photography*

An epifluorescence microscope (Axioskop; Zeiss) was used to view the infection fate of J774 A1 cells with *T. gondii* GFP. The microscope was equipped with a 50 W high-pressure mercury lamp (HB050; Osram) and 10×, 40× and 100× objectives (Zeiss). Narrow band filter sets HQ-F41-007 and HQ-F41-001 (AHF Analysentechnik) were used to analyse the GFP and red signals, respectively, at a magnification of 1000×. Image processing was performed with a standard software package delivered with the instrument (Zeiss Axiovision 3.1).

## Author details

Sprakel-Leyke Silja[1], Paulke Bernd-Reiner[2] and Presber Wolfgang[1*]

*Address all correspondence to: wolfgang.presber@charite.de

1 Institute of Microbiology and Hygiene, University of Medicine Berlin (Charité), Berlin, Germany

2 Fraunhofer Institute for Applied Polymer Research, Potsdam-Golm, Germany

## References

[1] Kreuter J. Eur. J. Drug. Metab. Pharmacokinet. 1994; 19: 253.

[2] Akerman ME, Chan WC, Laakkonen P, Bhatia, SN, Ruoslahti E. *Proc. Natl. Acad. Sci. USA*. 2002; 99: 12617.

[3] Bala I, Hariharan S, Kumar MN. *Crit. Rev. Ther. Drug Carrier Syst.* 2004; 21: 387.

[4] Brigger I, Dubernet C, Couvreur P. *Adv. Drug Deliv. Rev.* 2002; 54: 631.

[5] Sullivan DC, Ferrari M. *Mol Imaging*. 2004; 4: 364.

[6] Brannon-Peppas L, Blanchette JO. *Adv. Drug Deliv. Rev.* 2004; 56: 1649.

[7] Gradishar WJ. *Breast Cancer Res. Treat.* 2005; 89(Suppl. 1): p.17.

[8] Steiniger SC, Kreuter J, Khalansky AS, Skidan IN, Bobruskin AL, Smirnova ZS, Severin SE, Uhl U, Kock M, Geiger KD, Gelperina SE. *Int. J. Cancer*. 2004; 109: 759.

[9] Couvreur P, Vauthier C. *J. Controlled Release*, 1991; 17: 187.

[10] Kreuter J. *Adv. Drug. Deliv. Rev.* 2001; 47: 65.

[11] Kabanov AV, Batrakova EV. *Curr. Pharm. Des.* 2004; 10: 1355.

[12] Sordet F, Aumjaud Y, Fessi H, Derouin F. *Parasite.* 1998; 5: 223.

[13] Schöler N, Krause K, Kayser O, Müller R.H, Borner K, Hahn H, Liesenfeld O. *Antimicrob. Agents Chemother.* 2001; 45: 1771.

[14] Alyautdin R, Gothier D, Petrov V, Kharkevich D, Kreuter J. *Eur. J. Pharm. Biopharm.* 1995; 41: 44.

[15] Kreuter J. *Curr. Med. Chem. Central Nervous System Agents.* 2002; 2: 241.

[16] Lherm C, Müller RH, Puisieux F, Couvreur P. *Int. Pharm.* 1992; 84: 13.

[17] Kayser O, Olbrich C, Croft SL, Kiderlen AF. *Parasitol. Res.* 2003; 90: 6.

[18] Abdullah S, Flath B, Presber W J. *Microbiol. Methods.* 1999; 37: 123.

[19] Plock A, Nimtz M, Wray V, Sokolowska-Köhler W, Presber W. *Clin. Microbiol. Infect.* 2001; 7(Suppl.1): 263.

[20] Härtig W, Paulke B.-R, Varga S, Seeger J, Harkany T, Kacza J. *Neurosci. Lett.* 2003; 338: 174.

[21] Gaspar R, Preat V, Opperdoes FR, Roland M. *Pharm Res.* 1992; 9: 782.

[22] Müller RH, Rühl D, Lück M, Paulke B.-R. *Pharm. Res.* 1997; 14: 18.

[23] Deniau M, Durand R, Bories C, Paul M, Astier A, Couvreur P, Houin R. *Ann. Parasitol. Hum. Comp.* 1993; 68: 34.

[24] Debanjan D, Senshang L. *J. Pharm. Sci.* 2005; 94/95: 1343.

[25] Montoya JG, Liesenfeld O. *Lancet*, 2004; 363: 1965.

[26] Luft BJ, Remington JS. *J. Infect. Dis.* 1988; 157: 1.

[27] Luft BJ, Remington JS. *Clin. Infect. Dis.* 1992; 15: 211.

[28] Wong SY, Remington JS. *AIDS.* 1993; 7: 299.

[29] Robibaro B, Hoppe HC, Yang M, Coppens I, Ngo HM, Stedman TT, Paprotka K, Joiner KA. *Int J Parasitol.* 2001; 12: 1343.

[30] Heintzelman DL, Lotan R, Richards-Kortum RR. *Photochem. Photobiol.* 2007; 71: 237.

[31] Gamazo C, Blanco-Prieto M, Lecaroz C, Vitas A, Gander B, Irache JM, Prior S. *Curr. Med. Chem. Anti Canc Agents,* 2004; 3: 43.

[32] Prior S, Gander B, Lecároz C, Irache JM, Gamazo C. J. *Antimicrob. Chemother.* 2004; 53: 981.

[33] Butcher B, Denkers E. *Infect. Immun.* 2002; 70: 5216.

[34] Olbrich C, Schöler N, Tabatt K, Kayser O, Müller RH. *J. Pharm. Pharmacol.* 2004; 56: 883.

[35] Durand R, Paul M, Rivollet D, Houin R, Astier A, Deniau M. *Int. J. Parasitol.* 1997; 27: 1361.

[36] Basu MK, Lala S. *Curr. Mol. Med.* 2004; 4: 681.

[37] Allen TM. *Adv. Drug Deliv. Rev.* 1988; 2: 55.

[38] Scherer D. 1992 Einfluß von Polybutylcyanoacrylat-Nanapartikeln auf die orale Absorbtion von Arzneistoffen, PhD Thesis, Johann Wolfgang Goethe-Universität, Frankfurt am Main.

# 5

# Modulation of Host Programmed Cell Death Pathways by the Intracellular Protozoan Parasite, *Toxoplasma gondii* — Implications for Maintenance of Chronic Infection and Potential Therapeutic Applications

Sandra K. Halonen

**Abstract**

Programmed cell death (PCD) pathways are genetically programmed mechanisms that can trigger the cell to die or commit "cell suicide". There are three major forms of pro-grammed cell death that are now recognized: apoptosis (type I), autophagy (type II) and necrotic cell death or necroptosis (type III). While these cell death processes were once thought to occupy discrete cell states, evidence suggests that apoptosis, autophagy and necrosis are often regulated by similar pathways and share initiator and effector mole-cules and some subcellular compartments indicating that crosstalk exists between these three main forms of cell death pathways, resulting in a balanced interplay by which the cell decides its fate. PCD pathways have important roles in many cellular processes such as development and oncogenic transformation, but PCD pathways also play important roles in host defense and elimination of pathogens. *Toxoplasma gondii* is a microbial patho-gen for which programmed cell death pathways are a key part of the host defense. *T. gon-dii* is an obligate intracellular protozoan parasite that infects approximately one-third of the world's population. In most immunocompetant individuals, the chronic infection is asymptomatic due to an effective immune response that eliminates active parasite repli-cation. The parasite has evolved immune evasion strategies that enable it to survive and persist long enough in the host however to establish a chronic infection in which the cyst stage persists within neurons in the brain and skeletal muscle in the periphery. *T. gondii* has evolved multiple mechanisms to resist killing by apoptotic, autophagic and necrotic cell death pathways, and the parasite's manipulation of host PCD pathways plays a cru-cial role in host–parasite interactions and maintenance of the chronic infection. While most individuals chronically infected with *T. gondii* are asymptomatic, severe disease can occur in immunocompromised individuals where the infection reactivates from the brain causing severe necrotizing encephalitis, and increasing evidence indicates chronic cere-bral toxoplasmosis in some individuals may lead to neuropsychiatric disorders such as schizophrenia and suicidal behavior. This review will focus on the role of PCD pathways in host defense of *T. gondii* and the parasite manipulation of these PCD pathways. A better understanding of the molecular components underlying the PCD pathways and the parasite manipulation of these pathways may yield new therapeutic targets for treatment of clinical sequelae of cerebral toxoplasmosis.

**Keywords:** Apoptosis, autophagy, necroptosis, necrosis, toxoplasmosis

## 1. Introduction

### Overview of Programmed Cell Death (PCD) pathways and applications to *Toxoplasma gondii* infection

Programmed cell death (PCD) pathways are genetically programmed mechanisms that can trigger the cell to die or commit "cell suicide". There are three major forms of programmed cell death which are now recognized: apoptosis (type I), autophagic cell death (type II) and necrotic cell death or necroptosis (type III) [1–4]. Apoptosis, the best-characterized and dominant form of PCD, is a controlled physiological process of cellular self-destruction that removes dead cells without damage to the host. Apoptosis is critically important during development and morphogenesis and eliminates damaged cells such as cancerous cells or infected cells that may interfere with normal function. Necrosis, conversely, is a cell death process that is observed in response to severe stresses such that occurs after physical injury or prolonged ischemia and has been long thought to be an unregulated process. However, a programmed form of necrotic death, called necroptosis, is now recognized that can occur during physical traumas, in neurodegeneration, in cell death due to ischemia or infection and that, in contrast to unordered necrosis, has dedicated molecular pathways controlling necrotic cell death. Autophagy is predominantly a strategy for survival and not death, serving as a housekeeping mechanism of normal turnover of long-lived proteins and whole organelles and crucial to maintenance of healthy cells. However, autophagy can promote cell death during normal development and excessive autophagy, stimulated in times of stress such as nutrient deprivation and some diseases, can lead to what is now recognized as autophagic cell death [5–7]. While these cell death processes were once thought to occupy discrete cell states, evidence suggests apoptosis, autophagy and necroptosis are often regulated by similar pathways, share initiator and effector molecules and some subcellular compartments indicating a complex crosstalk exists between these three main forms of cell death pathways, resulting in a balanced interplay by which the cell decides its fate [8].

PCD pathways are also an important part of host defense against intracellular pathogens. The intracellular protozoal pathogen, *Toxoplasma gondii,* is a common infection that causes a chronic infection of central nervous system that persists for the lifetime of the individual. PCD pathways are a key part of the host defense against *T. gondii,* but the parasite has evolved multiple mechanisms to resist killing by host cell death pathways. Parasite manipulations of host cell death pathways are essential components leading to successful establishment of infection and for maintenance of the chronic infection in the host. In this review, the molecular components and signaling pathways of each of the three main types of PCD pathways will be discussed with the role of these PCDs in the pathogenesis of the intracellular pathogen, *T. gondii*, and potential therapeutic targets for toxoplasmosis and other diseases, the focus of this review.

## 2. Apoptosis, necroptosis and autophagic cell death pathways: Morphological features and molecular components

Apoptosis, necroptosis and autophagic cell death pathways operate via distinct genetically programmed molecular mechanisms containing dedicated molecular components and leading to characteristic morphological features (Figure 1). Apoptosis operates via a caspase-dependent mechanism while necroptosis and autophagic cell death are caspase-independent processes, with autophagic cell death being cathepsin-dependent and necroptosis mediated via the receptor interacting protein kinase 3 (RIP3) and its substrate, the mixed lineage kinase-like domain protein, MLKL [8]. Apoptosis results in mitochondrial membrane permeabilization, chromatin condensation and DNA fragmentation, resulting in cells become smaller (pknotic) and membrane blebbing into apoptotic bodies. Phagocytes, such as macrophages, subsequently engulf apoptotic cells and hence apoptosis is considered a noninflammatory form of programmed cell death. Necrotic cell death, in contrast to apoptosis, is marked by swelling of ER and mitochondrial organelles, increase in cell size, rapid rupture of the plasma membrane resulting in lysis of the cell and release of danger-associated molecular patterns (DAMPs) which stimulate inflammation. While necrosis has traditionally been considered to be "pathological cell death", necroptosis is now recognized to occur via a regulated mechanism that is inhibited by caspases [9, 10]. Autophagy is the process by which cells recycle cellular constituents and involves engulfment of cytoplasmic material and intracellular organelles within double-membrane vesicles called autophagosomes that fuse with lysosomes to make autophagolysosomes that degrade the cellular cargo via cathepsins located in the autolysosomes. The molecular components and signaling pathways of each cell death processes are reviewed below, followed by the current understanding of the crosstalk that exists between these PCD pathways.

### 2.1. Apoptosis

The term apoptosis was first used in 1972 by Kerr, Wyllie and Currie [11] to describe a form of cell death morphologically distinct from necrosis. Apoptosis has since been well studied and is now understood to be a regulated energy-dependent process mediated via cysteine-dependent aspartate-directed enzymes called caspases [3]. Apoptosis is a homeostatic process that balances cell numbers and plays a crucial role in several physiological processes including embryogenesis to shape morphological structures such as fingers, in the establishment of functional synaptic connections in the nervous system, in development of the immune response to remove self-reactive lymphocytes and at the termination of the immune response to remove antigen-specific lymphocytes. Apoptosis is also used to rid the body of cells in various pathological conditions such as removal of cancerous cells, infected cells or cells damaged by noxious agents [12].

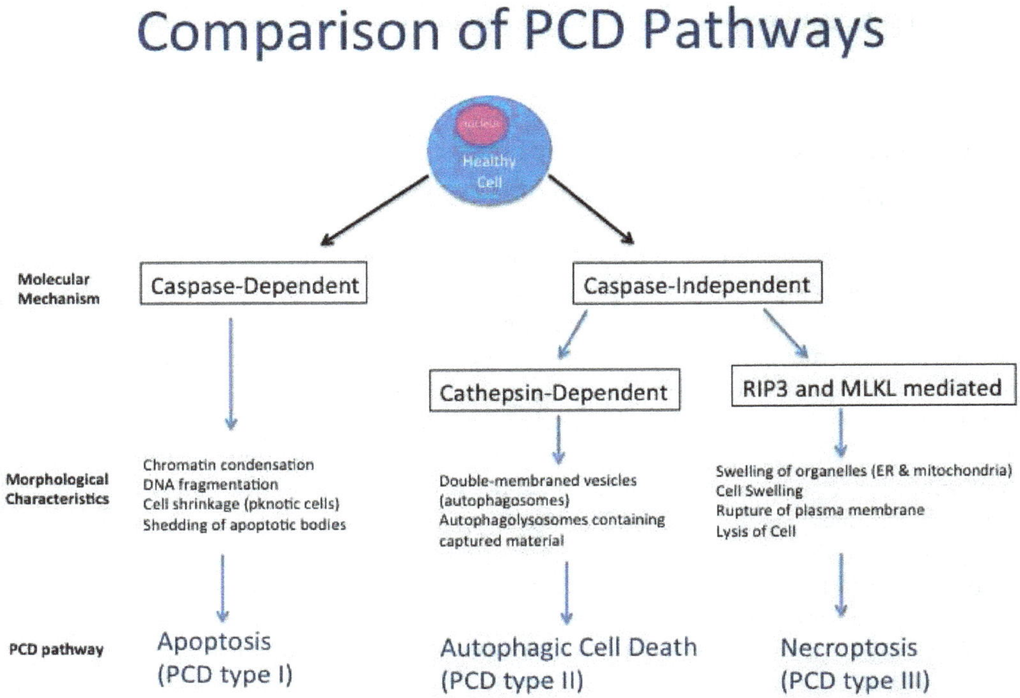


**Figure 1. Comparison of three types of Programmed Cell (PCD) Pathways.** The molecular mechanisms and morphological characteristics of Apoptosis, Autophagic Cell Death and Necroptosis cell death pathways, so-called PCD types I, II and III, respectively, are indicated. RIP3 = receptor-interacting protein kinase 3; MLKL = mixed lineage kinase-like domain protein

### 2.1.1. *Signaling pathways and molecular components of apoptosis*

Apoptosis is mediated via caspases which are present in the cytoplasm as pro-enzymes and when activated initiate a proteolytic cascade that results in apoptosis of the cell. There are three activation pathways that can initiate apoptosis: the extrinsic (death receptor) pathway, the intrinsic (mitochondrial) pathway and the granzyme pathway (Figure 2). There are about 14 known caspases which are divided into initiator and effector caspases. Initiator caspases, caspases 8, 9 and 10, are triggered by either the extrinsic, intrinsic or granzyme pathway, respectively. All three pathways converge on caspase 3, which activates effector caspases 6 and 7 that lead to apoptosis. A major target of effector caspases is poly-ADP-ribose polymerase (PARP) which is involved in DNA repair, cell survival, proliferation and differentiation.

The extrinsic pathway is initiated by binding of cell membrane receptors of Fas (CD95) or tumor necrosis factor (TNF) family receptor (TNFR), which after binding its relevant ligand of FasL or TNF$\alpha$, respectively, trimerizes and attracts the docking proteins Fas-associated death domain (FADD) and TNF receptor-associated death domain (TRADD), respectively. FADD

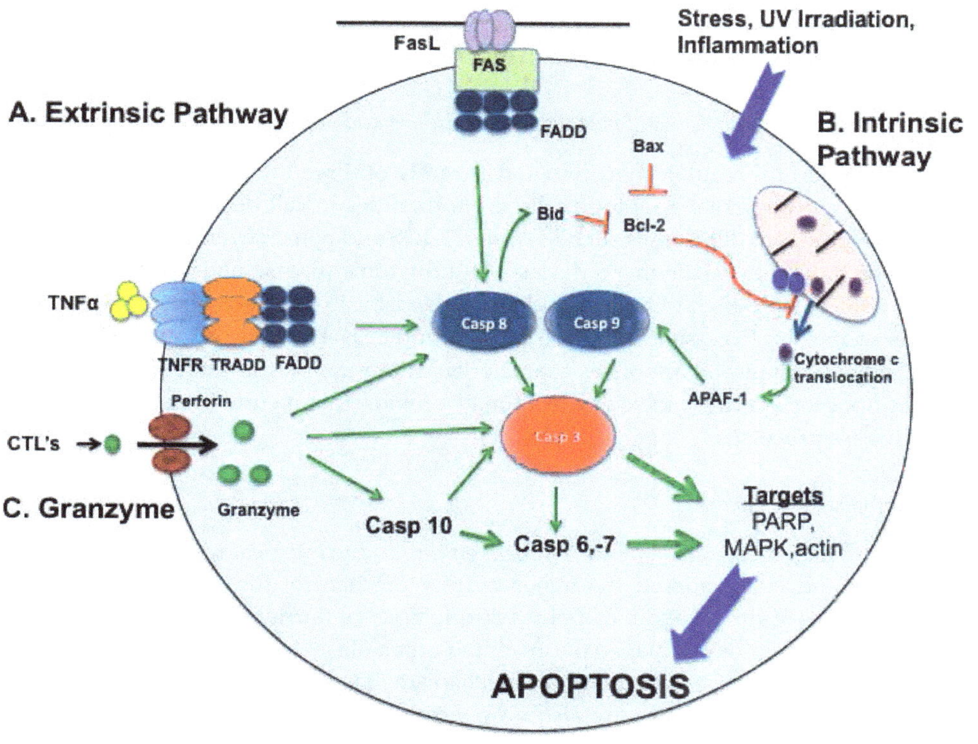


**Figure 2. Signaling Pathways of Apoptosis.** Apoptosis is induced through either the extrinsic pathway (A), intrinsic pathway (B) or the granzyme pathway (C). Activation of initiator caspases 8 and 9 (Casp 8,-Casp9), leads to apoptotic cell death through activation of Caspase 3 (Casp3) and subsequent activation of effector caspases 6 and 7 (Casp 6-Casp7). The extrinsic pathway (A) is initiated via extracellular molecules, FasL and TNFα, which bind to TNFR family members, Fas and TNFR respectively which activate Casp8 (green lines). The intrinsic pathway (B) is initiated by stress, UV irradiation and inflammation which act on the mitochondria through the pro-apoptotic Bcl-2 family members, such as Bax, resulting in the blockage of the anti-apoptotic activity of Bcl-2 (red lines). As a result, Cytochrome c is released into the cytoplasm and activates Casp9 through APAF-1 (green lines). Casp8 may also trigger the intrinsic pathway through activation of Bid, which inhibits the anti-apoptotic activity of Bcl-2. The granzyme pathway (C) is activated via cytotoxic T cells (CTLs) that introduce granzyme molecules into the target cells via secretion of perforin, which through a multimerization process forms a pore in the cell membrane allowing granzyme into the target cell. Granzymes cleave multiple caspases, including Caspase 10.

contains two death effector domains that can bind and cleave caspase 8. TRADD lacks death effector domains but binds FADD that then cleaves caspase 8. Activated caspase 8 then activates caspase 3. The intrinsic pathway is activated via changes in the mitochondria membrane potential which can be triggered via stress, toxic reagents, UV irradiation and inflammation. Changes in mitochondria membrane result in translocation of cytochrome c from the inner mitochondrial membrane into the cytoplasm. Cytochrome c binds to apoptosis protease activating factor 1 (APAF-1) which in the presence of ATP cleaves caspase 9. The intrinsic pathway is regulated by Bcl-2 which localizes to the outer mitochondria membrane. Bcl-2 members (Bcl-2 and Bcl-x) are anti-apoptotic while others such as Bax and Bad are pro-apoptotic. The granzyme activation pathway is stimulated by cytotoxic T lymphocytes (CTLs) or NK cell secretion of perforin, which creates pores in the target cell membrane allowing granzymes into the cytoplasm activating caspase 10 which can then activate caspase 3.

*2.1.2. Apoptosis in physiological and pathological conditions and potential therapeutic application*

Apoptosis is a tightly regulated process and is rarely observed in healthy animals because phagocytes rapidly remove apoptotic cells. Abnormalities in cell death regulation can be a significant component of diseases such as cancer, AIDS and neurodegenerative diseases such as Parkinson's disease, Alzheimer's disease, Huntington's disease and amyotrophic lateral sclerosis. Some of these conditions are characterized by insufficient apoptosis and others excessive apoptosis. Excessive apoptosis, for example, is a feature of neurodegenerative diseases while resistance to apoptosis characterizes many cancers. Understanding the mechanisms of apoptosis at the molecular level may provide therapeutic interventions in these diverse disease processes.

*2.1.2.1. Autophagic cell death*

Autophagy, which means literally to "eat oneself", is a physiological response to stress such as starvation and is considered the major cellular mechanism for generating the needed metabolic sources of energy and metabolites during times of nutrient deprivation. Autophagy can also be used to remove damaged or unwanted organelles, such as mitochondria and long-lived proteins. Autophagy is a homeostatic mechanism that is predominantly a cytoprotective process [7, 13]. Other substrates are also now recognized as potential cargo for autophagy including lipids, nucleic acids, reticulocytes and intracellular pathogens and viruses. The concept of autophagic cell death has been a matter of debate, but it is now recognized as a type of programmed cell death mechanism that can lead to both apoptotic and necrotic cell death in certain circumstances such as extreme stress conditions [14, 15]. Autophagic cell death or type II programmed cell death is now used to refer to cell death process distinct from apoptosis that is caspase-independent and occurs with accumulation of double-membrane organelles called autophagosomes.

*2.1.3. Signaling pathways and molecular components of autophagy*

Autophagy delivers cytosolic materials to the interior of the lysosomes for degradation via a process involving the "*de novo*" formation of cytoplasmic double-membrane vacuoles called autophagosomes which then fuse with lysosomes forming an autolysosome that degrades the cellular cargo (Figure 3). Autophagy is regulated by a genetic program with a number of autophagy-related genes (Atg) whose gene products (ATG proteins) regulate distinct steps in autophagy. The autophagic pathway proceeds through the following defined steps: (i) initiation phase involves the formation of an isolation membrane or phagophore, (ii) elongation of the phagophore, (iii) maturation of an autophagosome with accumulation of cytosolic cargo, (iv) fusion of the mature autophagosome with the lysosome and (v) degradation of the contents via lysosomal proteases (i.e., cathepsins) in the autolysosome. The initiation phase involves formation of an initiation complex comprised of the class III PI3 kinase, VSP34, which converts phosphatidylinositol to phosphatylinositol-3-phosphate (PI3P). The activity of VSP34, which binds to beclin 1, requires the activity of VSP15, the regulator beclin 1 and ATG14L (Figure 3a). Elongation of the autophagosome membrane requires action of two ubiquitin-like conjugation systems, the Atg5–Atg12 conjugation system and the microtubule-associated protein-1 light chain (LC3). The phosphatidylethanolamine-conjugated form of LC3, LC3-PE (also called LC-II) is generated by ATG4-dependent proteolytic cleavage of LC3 and the action of the E1 ligase, ATG7, the E2 ligase, ATG3 and the E3 ligase complex, ATG12/ATG5/ATG16L. LC3-PE stably associates with the autophagosome and is commonly used as a marker for autophagosomes.

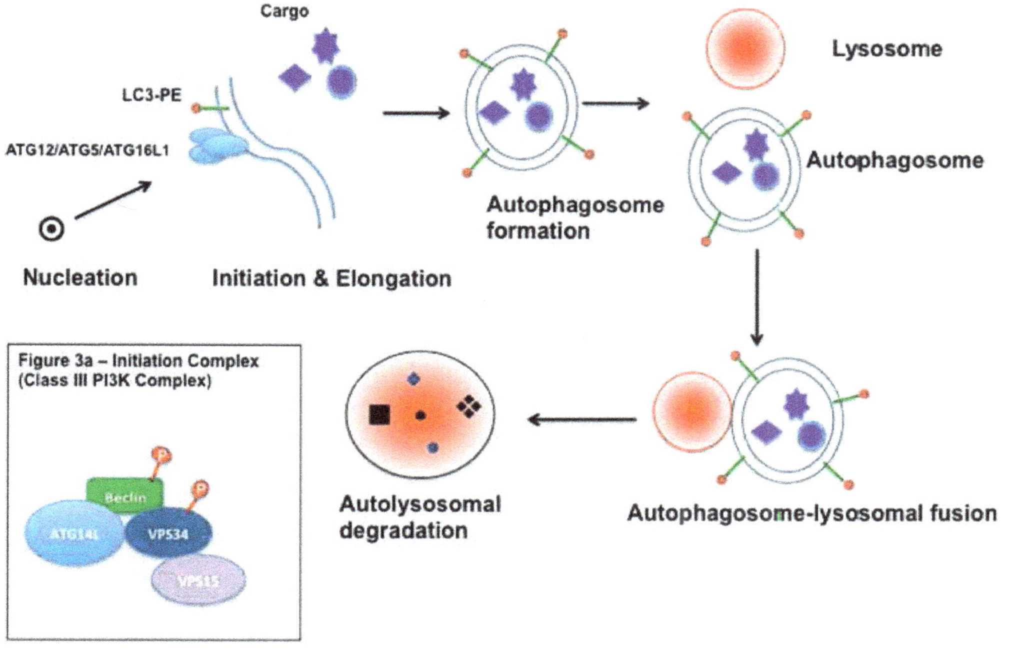


**Figure 3. Autophagy Pathway**. Autophagy is a membrane-dependent pathway that involves a series of defined steps beginning with a nucleation step which then leads to: 1). Initiation of the isolation membrane or phagophore, 2). Formation of the autophagosome around cellular cargo, 3). Fusion of autophagosome with lysosomes, and 4). Degradation of cargo by lysosomal proteases in autolysosomes. Formation of the initiation complex (also called Class III PI3K Complex) as shown in Figure 3a, consists of Beclin-1, ATG14L, VPS34 and VPS15. Activation of the initiation complex requires disruption of binding of Bcl-2 to Beclin-1. The Class III PI3K complex generates PI3P at the site of nucleation of the isolation membrane, which leads to binding of PI3P-binding proteins and the subsequent recruitment of proteins involved in the 'elongation reaction' of the isolation membrane. These proteins contribute to membrane expansion resulting in the formation of a double-membrane structure, the autophagosome that surrounds cellular cargo. The phosphatidylethanolamine-conjugated form of the LC3 (LC3-PE) is generated by the ATG4 dependent proteolytic cleavage of LC3 and the action of E1 ligase, E2 ligase and the E3 ligase ATG12/ATG5/ATG16L. LC3-PE stably associates with the autophagosome and is a marker of autophagosomes and therefore LC3 is commonly used as a marker of autophagy pathway.

While the autophagy pathway is primarily a homeostatic process promoting cell survival, increased autophagosomal formation can occur coincidentally with cell dying indicating autophagy may be involved in regulated cell death pathways, most notably apoptosis [7, 13]. For example, in apoptosis-comprised cells, cells die via a caspase-independent mechanism characterized by autophagosome accumulation, implicating a role for autophagy in the cell death process. Autophagy and apoptosis may also be regulated coordinately as anti-apoptotic proteins that downregulate apoptosis can also downregulate autophagy. For example, members of the Bcl-2 family can bind to beclin-1, thus inhibiting the formation of initiation complex that is necessary to stimulate autophagy. Other studies indicate once apoptosis is activated, apoptosis effector molecules may suppress autophagy as beclin-1 is cleaved and inactivated by caspases. Finally, studies also indicate autophagy proteins may play a dual role in regulation of apoptosis and autophagy. For example, Atg5 may affect the extrinsic apoptotic pathway through interaction with FADD proteins, while Atg12 is an effector of intrinsic apoptotic pathway with both Atg5 and Atg12 acting as pro-apoptotic regulators.

Autophagy pathway has also been implicated in necrosis and necroptosis cell death. Evidence indicates autophagy may be able to act as an inhibitor of necrosis/necroptosis by preserving cellular functions, removing toxic products and maintaining cellular energy. For example, knockdown studies of components of autophagy pathways, such as beclin-1, have found cytotoxicity is exacerbated suggesting that autophagy has a cytoprotective role. Autophagy may be able to act as a buffer to metabolic stress, providing a mechanism to generate ATP to maintain metabolic viability and thus prevent necrotic cell death. Conversely, studies using a specific inhibitor of necroptosis, necrostatin-1, found both necroptosis and autophagy were inhibited, indicating autophagy may be induced by necrosis. Molecular components underlying the relationship between autophagy and necroptosis/necrotic cell death at this point are poorly understood.

#### *2.1.4. Physiological and pathological roles of autophagic cell death and therapeutic implications*

Thus, while autophagy is now recognized to play a role in apoptotic and necrotic cell death programs, this process is complex and incompletely understood. However, increasing evidence indicates autophagic cell death may be necessary for cell death in certain circumstances. It has been suggested autophagic cell death represents a failed adaptive mechanism that may have prevented death under milder conditions. Understanding of the relationships of autophagic cell death with other programmed cell death modalities will require further study. The study of autophagy in disease is an emerging area of research. Autophagy pathway and/or autophagic cell death pathways which result in failure to remove damaged organelles and/or damaged cells are now thought to contribute to various diseases such as cancer, neurodegenerative diseases such as Parkinson's disease, aging and inflammation. Elucidation of the influence of autophagy with other cell death programs will be essential to the development of therapeutics targeting autophagy for treatment of these various diseases. In the context of infectious disease, autophagy also is now recognized to play an important role in intracellular pathogen defense, and it has been suggested that intracellular pathogen load could be a factor that disrupts the balance between cell survival and cell death [16].

## 2.2. Necroptosis

Pathologists first used the term "necrosis" in the early 19th century to describe tissue destruction. Necrosis is characterized by organelle swelling and cell lysis, releasing the cellular content of cells and resulting in inflammation. The first indication that necrosis could occur in a regulated manner arose from observation that tumor necrosis factor (TNF$\alpha$) could trigger apoptosis and necrotic forms of cell death. Caspase inhibition strongly exacerbates necrotic cell death, indicating caspase activity negatively regulates necrosis. This accumulating evidence led to the concept of "programmed necrosis" and the coining of the term necroptosis in 2005 to designate regulated necrotic cell death [4, 9]. Receptor-interacting protein kinase 3 (RIP3) and its substrate, the mixed lineage kinase-like domain protein (MLKL), are now recognized as the key activation steps and the molecular hallmarks of regulated necrotic cell death or necroptosis.

### *2.2.1. Signaling and molecular components of necroptosis*

Programmed necrotic cell death can be activated when cells are stimulated by ligation of death receptors including CD95 (also known as FAS), TNF receptors (TNFRs) and TNF-related apoptosis-inducing ligand (TRAIL). Ligation of cell death receptors leads to the formation of complex 1, comprised of TNFR-associated death domain protein (TRADD), TNFR-associated factor 2 (TRAF2), receptor-interacting kinase 1(RIP1) and cellular inhibitors of apoptosis (CIAPs) (Figure 4). Upon the release of second mitochondria-derived activator of caspases (Smac) from the mitochondria, RIP1 is de-ubiquinated and dissociates from the death receptor and induces the formation of FADD-RIP1-caspase 8 pro-apoptosis complex II. Conversion of complex 1 to complex II indicates a change in cell fate from pro-survival to cell death. When caspase 8 is inhibited, RIP1 and RIP3 form the necrotic death domain complex, the necrosome, and their kinase activities become activated. RIP3 recruits it substrate monomeric MLKL from the cytoplasm and phosphorylates it. The phosphorylation destabilizes MLKL and drives its oligomerization which enables it to bind to phosphatidylinositol phosphate lipids (PIPs) and cariolipin (CL). Different PIPs and CLs orchestrate the translocation of MLKL to different membrane compartments including the mitochondria, endoplasmic reticulum, the Golgi, lysosomes and plasma membranes. In addition to activation via death receptors, it is also now clear that necroptosis can also be initiated by pathogen recognition receptors (PRRs) such as toll-like receptors (TLRs) and cytokines via activation of RIP3 through distinct upstream mechanisms.

### *2.2.2. Physiological and pathological roles of necroptosis and potential therapeutic applications*

Programmed necrosis has been found to be important in host antiviral responses and a variety of tissue-damage related diseases such as acute pancreatitis, ischemic reperfusion injury, retinal detachment, atherosclerosis, neuronal loss in Gaucher's disease, amongst others. It has been a paradigm that apoptotic cell death is anti-inflammatory with dead cells cleared by phagocytes while necrotic cell death leads to inflammation and tissue damage. Necrotic cells, however, can be internalized by macrophages although via macropinocytosis and thus in a manner distinct from phagocytosis of apoptotic cells, but they are nonetheless efficiently cleared by professional and nonprofessional phagocytes and hence rarely found in tissues. Large numbers of dying cells such as may occur in excessive tissue injury, autoimmune diseases such as systemic lupus erythematosus or infectious disease may lead to the defective clearance of necrotic cells and contribute to the persistent inflammation and tissue damage. However, smaller number of cells dying via necrosis or necroptosis may not necessarily lead to massive tissue damage and hence controlled necrotic cell death may not necessarily lead to massive tissue damage commonly associated with necrotic cell death.

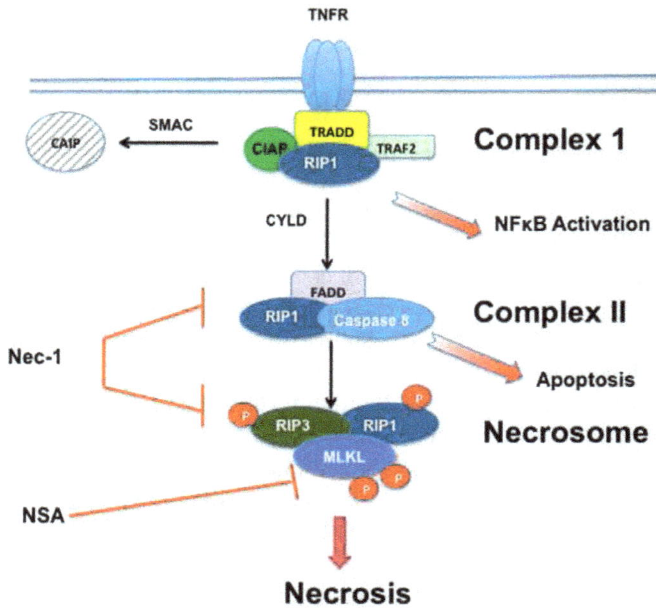


**Figure 4. Necroptosis Signaling Pathway.** Ligation of tumor-necrosis factor 1 (TNFR1) leads to the formation of Complex 1 that is comprised of TNFR-1, TFNR1-associated death domain (TRADD), TNFR-associated factor 2 (TRAF-2), Receptor-interacting kinase 1 (RIP1) and cellular inhibitors of apoptosis (CIAPs). RIP1 is initially modified by ubiquitin chains within Complex I after recruitment to the membrane and serves as the signaling platform for NF-κB activation. Upon release of the second mitochondria-derived activation of caspases (Smac) from the mitochondria, CIAPs are auto-degraded. RIP1 is subsequently de-ubiquinated by CYLD and dissociates from the death receptor, and associates with FADD-RIP1-Caspase8 forming Complex II, which is pro-apoptotic. Within Complex II, Caspase 8 activates Caspase 3/7 to induce apoptosis and blocks necrosis by cleaving and inactivating RIP1 and RIP3. When apoptosis is inhibited, as for example by Z-VAD, RIP1 and RIP3 form the necrotic death complex, the necrosome, and their kinase activities become activated. RIP3 recruits the mixed lineage kinase domain-like protein, MLKL, and phosphorylates MLKL, causing its activation. Activated MLKL then associates with membranes such as the plasma membrane, mitochondrial members and others, causing lysis of these membranes and death of the cell. Inhibitors of necroptosis include, Necrostatin 1 (Nec1) which inhibits RIP1 dependent necrosis by inhibiting the kinase activity of RIP1 to prevent necrosome formation and Necrosulfonamide (NSA), which inhibits MLKL-mediated necrosis.

Knockout of either RIP3 or MLKL genes in mice has been used to assess the physiological and pathological roles of programmed necrosis. These types of studies have confirmed that necroptosis is important in host antiviral responses and in some tissue-damage related diseases. Several inhibitors have been identified that can inhibit necroptosis. Necrostatins, for example, are small molecules that inhibit RIP1 kinase activity and thus inhibit necroptosis (Figure 4). RIP1 also contributes to other processes such as apoptosis and NK-kB activation, however, indicating other processes may also be affected by Nec-1. Targeting RIP3 or MLKL offer more specific inhibitors for study or treatment of necroptosis. A chemical inhibitor of MLKL called necrosulfonamide (NSA), for example, blocks necrosis by preventing oligomerization of MLKL and thus is a specific inhibitor of necroptosis (Figure 4). Use of these specific inhibitors of necroptosis will be essential to elucidate the role of necroptosis in cell death. As the role of programmed necrotic death is now known to occur in several human diseases, development of specific inhibitors of neroptosis could also have therapeutic uses.

### 2.3. Crosstalk between apoptosis, necroptosis and autophagy PCD pathways

As molecular components and regulation of each pathway has become better understood, it has become apparent that significant crosstalk exists between the three major pathways of programmed cell death, the focus of which has been the topic of several recent reviews [3, 8, 10, 13]. Extensive crosstalk exists between apoptosis and autophagy as discussed above in the section on autophagic cell death. The stimuli for apoptosis and autophagy are often the same and evidence indicates instances where they can cooperate, antagonize or assist each other. Caspases, Beclin-1 and/or the TOR kinase pathway have all been implicated in participating in the complex crosstalk between apoptosis and autophagy. Crosstalk between apoptosis and necrosis also appears to exist as receptors that stimulate apoptosis can also stimulate necroptosis. Energy is thought to play a central role in determining the interplay between these two pathways where instances of high ATP levels would enable a cell to undergo apoptosis while low ATP levels would favor necrosis. Other factors such as p53, Bcl-2 proteins and PARP1 are also suggested to play a role. Evidence also suggests a complex interplay between autophagy and necroptosis. Autophagy and necrosis can be activated in parallel or sequentially and can have either opposite or the same effects. Autophagy, for example, can protect against some types of necroptotic cell death with autophagy serving as the last resort before cell death via necrosis. The molecular basis for interlinked processes in autophagy and necroptosis and the impact of autophagy on necroptosis and other cell death pathways [13], however, remain unclear. While the molecular details are not fully understood, it is clear that a complex crosstalk and molecular interplay between apoptosis, autophagy and necroptosis occur and determine the ultimate fate of the cell to survive or die in a given situation or under a given stress signal. A better understanding of the mechanisms of apoptosis, autophagic cell death and necroptosis at the molecular level and the crosstalk between these cell death pathways would provide a deeper insight into different disease processes and may provide novel therapeutic strategies.

## 3. *Toxoplasma gondii:* Manipulation of programmed cell death pathways and impact on host–parasite interactions and maintenance of chronic infection

PCD can be important host cell defense mechanisms to eliminate intracellular pathogens. *Toxoplasma gondii* is an obligate intracellular protozoan parasite that causes a chronic infection with approximately one-third of the world's population chronically infected, making *T. gondii* one of the most prevalent human parasitic infections worldwide [17–19]. In humans, infection with *T. gondii* is characterized by rapid parasite replication and dissemination throughout the body with the parasite capable of infecting all types of nucleated cells. The acute infection is followed by a chronic infection that lasts for the lifetime of the individual with the parasite harbored within neurons in the brain and muscle tissue in intracellular cysts. In most immunocompetant individuals, the infection is asymptomatic due to an effective immune response that eliminates active parasite replication. In immunocompromised individuals such as AIDS patients that are chronically infected, the parasite reactivates from cysts in the brain leading to severe and potentially fatal encephalitis. The parasite can also be transmitted transplacentally and can cause severe neurological complications to the fetus including mental retardation, hydrocephaly and chorioretinitis which can reactivate through the first two decades of life potentially leading to blindness. Finally, increasing evidence indicates that in some immunocompetant individuals, chronic infection with *T. gondii* may lead to development of serious psychiatric disorders such as schizophrenia or suicidal tendencies [20–22].

While the host mounts an effective immune response against *T. gondii*, the parasite has evolved immune evasion strategies that enable it to survive and persist long enough in the host to establish the cyst stage of the infection that can persist for the lifetime of the host. PCD pathways are a key part of the host defense against *T. gondii*, but the parasite has evolved multiple mechanisms to manipulate these pathways. For example, the parasite induces apoptosis in selected immune cell lineages, thus suppressing the host immune response and helping to establish infection but the parasite also has multiple mechanisms to resist killing by apoptotic and, to lesser degree, autophagic and necrotic cell death pathways in different host cell types. Thus, parasite manipulations of host cell death pathways appear to be an essential component to the successful establishment of infection and maintenance of the chronic infection. A brief summary of the mechanisms by which the parasite manipulates these cell death pathways is reviewed below followed by a discussion of the potential therapeutic interventions.

### 3.1. Apoptosis

*T. gondii* has the ability to promote apoptosis of immune effector cells early after infection in selected cell types. In murine models of toxoplasmosis, apoptosis of CD4+, CD8+ T cells, B cells, NK cells and granulocytes is observed in the spleen early after infection [23]. Apoptosis in Peyer's patch T cells in perorally infected mice has also been observed [24]. Acute infection of *Toxoplasma* in both mice and humans induces a state of transient immunosuppression as determined by decreased antibody and T lymphocyte responses. Triggering of apoptosis of T cells and other immune effector cells by *T. gondii* may be one factor by which the parasite restricts the immune response, thus allowing the establishment of infection. Induction of apoptosis of immune effector cells may be somewhat parasite strain-dependent as, in murine models, high levels of apoptosis in T cells was induced when mice were infected with virulent RH strain while this phenomenon was not seen in mice infected with avirulent strains.

Inhibition of apoptosis by infection with *T. gondii* has been found to occur in a wide range of cell types including macrophages and a wide variety of non-immune effector cells such as fibroblasts, endothelial cells, muscle cells and astrocytes [23, 25, 26]. Infected host cells are resistant to induction of apoptosis to a wide range of stimuli including CTL-mediated cytotoxicity, irradiation, growth factor withdrawal, TNF$\alpha$ and several toxic reagents. Blockage of apoptosis in host cells establishes an anti-apoptotic condition of the host cell and favors parasite persistence. Neighboring uninfected cells are also rendered resistant to apoptosis. Inhibition of host cell apoptosis of non-immune effector cells likely ensures the host cell stays alive long enough to facilitate intracellular replication of the parasite in the tissues while suppression of apoptosis of uninfected neighboring cell may help create a microenvironment in different tissues in which the parasite can persist and replicate.

While blockage of apoptosis is known to occur in a wide variety of host cells, modulation of apoptosis in cells of the central nervous system (CNS) is less well studied and results are ambiguous. *T. gondii* can infect neurons, astrocytes and microglia supporting growth of the rapidly replicating tachyzoite form while bradyzoite stage and cysts develop only in neurons and astrocytes. In murine astrocytes, infection blocks apoptosis beginning at 6–24 h after infection, allowing time for the parasite to replicate, egress and initiate infection of a new host cell [26]. Thus, inhibition of apoptosis in astrocyte host cells may allow an increase in parasite numbers in the brain and help establish the chronic infection in the brain. Conversely, several studies indicate the parasite induced apoptosis in neurons. For example, tachyzoites induced apoptosis in mouse brain cells in adult mice including in neurons [27, 28]. Likewise, in a murine model of congenital toxoplasmosis, infection resulted in a decrease in neuron number and markers of apoptosis were found indicating infection induced apoptosis in CNS tissues [29]. In murine neural stem cells, infection was also found to induce apoptosis although only apoptosis of neighboring neurons were assessed in this study [30]. A study in murine brain indicated infected neurons were resistant to apoptosis and apoptosis was only induced in the uninfected neurons [31]. Microglia cells which are activated in the brains of mice infected with *T. gondii* with toxoplasmic encephalitis produced nitric oxide (NO), which induces neuronal apoptosis indicating activated microglia may be part of the mechanism leading to neuronal loss of uninfected neurons [32]. Collectively, the above results are suggestive of a mechanism in which *Toxoplasma* infection of neural tissues induces apoptosis of neurons, thus leading to loss of neurons which could lead to neurological abnormalities. However, it is unclear if apoptosis of infected neurons was induced or, alternatively, if infected neurons are resistant to apoptosis. Suppression of apoptosis of infected neuronal cells may facilitate development of the cysts in neurons and allow persistence of the parasite in the brain. A better understanding of parasite modulation of apoptosis in infected neurons is thus of importance. A better understanding of the modulation of apoptosis in infected neurons could lead to the development of antiparasitic drugs and other therapeutic interventions to control and manage the chronic phase of infection.

### *3.1.1. Parasite mechanisms modulating apoptosis*

The parasite replicates within a membrane-bound compartment called the parasitophorous vacuole (PV), and hence it is not in direct contact with the host cell cytoplasm and regulators or effectors of apoptosis. However, parasite secretory molecules, which are either released into the host cell at invasion, secreted across the PV membrane (PVM) or act at the PVM cytosolic surface, have been identified which can modulate host cell apoptosis [25, 33]. These mechanisms are briefly summarized below.

### *3.1.2. Parasite mechanisms that stimulate apoptosis*

Several mechanisms have been identified by which the parasite can stimulate apoptosis. In parasite-infected murine macrophages, supernatants can induce apoptosis of neighboring uninfected macrophages via nitric oxide [34]. Induction of apoptosis has also been found to occur via nitric oxide secretion from activated microglia. Nitric oxide secretion from activated microglia can lead to neuronal cell death and may be an important mechanism by which infection leads to neuronal loss in the brain. The parasite secretory molecule, GRA1, has been identified as capable of inducing apoptosis of infected monocytes and uninfected bystander cells [35]. Secreted GRA1 from sites of ongoing *T. gondii* replication could also induce apoptosis of monocytes recruited to the site of parasite replication. Given monocytes are essential to control parasite replication at the site of primary infection, inhibition of apoptosis in monocytes could serve to downregulate host responses early in infection, helping to establish the infection in the host.

### *3.1.3. Parasite mechanisms that inhibit apoptosis*

Multiple mechanisms have been identified by which the parasite can inhibit apoptosis [25]. Activation of NF-κB is a mechanism that inhibits apoptosis in fibroblasts and some other host cells [36–38]. Early after infection, the parasite induces rapid translocation of host cell transcription factor, NF-kB, into the nucleus, which activates cell survival pathways and induction of an anti-apoptotic state of the host cell. Nuclear translocation of NF-κB and subsequent gene expression requires activity of the host IκB kinase (IKK). The activation of NF-κB was associated with localization of phosphorylated IκBα subunits to the PVM that was mediated by a parasite-derived IκB kinase (TgIKK). TgIKK is produced as the parasite replicates, and thus allows for a continued phosphorylation of IκB and sustained inhibition of apoptosis. Thus, *T. gondii* modulation of NF-κB gene expression and induction of anti-apoptotic state of the host cell involves both the host cell IKK and TgIKK activity at different phases of infection. NF-kB activation has not been found to occur in infected macrophages. Rather in macrophages, *T. gondii*, inhibits apoptosis by $G_i$-protein-mediated signaling, activating PI 3-kinase leading to phosphorylation of protein kinase B (PKB/AKt) as an inhibitor of apoptosis [39]. A micro-RNA-mediated mechanism has also recently been identified in macrophages that inhibited apoptosis via a reduction in Bim, a pro-apoptotic effector of the Bcl-2 family [40]. Other mechanisms have been identified in various cell types that can inhibit caspase cascade including blockage of caspases 8 and 9 and 3, increased expression of anti-apoptotic molecules of the Bcl-2 family, decreased activity of poly (ADP)-ribose polymerase and inhibition of granzymes [33, 41].

Only a few parasite proteins that modulate apoptosis have been identified. The parasite serine–threonine phosphatase, called TgPP2C, was recently identified which downregulates apoptosis in host cells [42]. TgPP2C is secreted into host cells from the PV and translocates to the host cell nucleus and has been shown to regulate growth and survival of the parasite. Using a yeast two-hybrid system, TgPP2C was found to interact with host cell protein, SSRP1 (structure-specific recognition protein 1), which binds to DNA and regulates DNA repair genes. It is speculated that SSRP1 might also be involved in expression of other genes involved in cell survival and apoptosis. Identification of other parasite molecules by which the parasite manipulates host cell apoptosis would facilitate a deeper understanding of host–parasite relationship and may lead to development of new therapeutic targets and antiparasitic drugs.

#### *3.1.4. Parasite modulation of apoptosis: significance to pathogenesis*

In conclusion, *T. gondii* has the ability to both promote and inhibit apoptosis of its own host cell and of uninfected neighboring cells by multiple mechanisms. The ability to modulate apoptosis varies by host cell type, parasite load and parasite virulence. Manipulation of apoptosis has been proposed to be crucial to promoting a stable parasite–host interaction and allowing establishment of persistent infection [23]. The multitude of anti-apoptosis mechanism that the parasite *T. gondii* employs is likely reflective of its status as an obligate intracellular parasite and the essentiality of maintenance of host cell viability to sustain parasite replication and survival. However, intracellular replication eventually leads to lysis of the host cell and typically occurs between 48 and 72 h post-infection, a temporal scale similar to apoptosis. Given the similar temporal scales of lytic death of the host cell and cell death by apoptosis, it can be argued inhibition of apoptosis of the host cell is not necessary to allow for parasite replication. However, as the parasite needs to obtain purine, cholesterol, tryptophan and other components from the host cell, the parasite inhibition of host cell apoptosis may also serve to maintain the host cell in a pro-survival state to enhance availability of host cell nutrients. Inhibition of apoptosis may also be critical for the chronic phase of infection allowing differentiation of bradyzoites and development of the cyst stage in neurons. A better understanding of manipulation of apoptosis by bradyzoites in host cells and, specifically in neurons, is of great importance as the CNS is the compartment in which the parasite predominantly persists in the chronic infection and the cause of serious clinical sequelae in the CNS of immunocompromised individuals causing reactivated toxoplasmosis, in immature immune system of the fetus and newborns causing congenital toxoplasmosis, and in immunocompetant individuals possibly contributing to the development of serious neuropsychiatric disorders.

### 3.2. Autophagy

Autophagy has been found to play a role in host defense against many intracellular pathogens as the autophagy pathway can degrade intracellular pathogens via autophagolysosomes including *T. gondii* [16]. *T. gondii* replicates within a membrane compartment in the host cell called the parasitophorous vacuole (PV) that is a non-fusogenic compartment and does not fuse with cell lysosomes. However, the PV can be delivered to the lysosomes via autophagy-mediated delivery in IFN-γ-activated macrophages resulting in killing of the parasite [43]. This autophagic-mediated parasite killing is mediated by the immunity-related GTPases (IRGs) which are stimulated by IFN-γ. Engagement of CD40 also has been found to induce killing of *T. gondii* via autophagy in many nonhematopoetic cells including endothelial cells lines, human and mouse retinal pigment epithelial cells as well as in hemopoietic cells such as macrophages [44, 45].

Interestingly, in non-immune-stimulated cells, evidence indicates the parasite can use autophagy to enhance its own survival. In the first 24 h after infection, host cell autophagy is upregulated and the parasite uses autophagy to acquire host cell nutrients, while at 24–36 h after infection when significant parasite replication has occurred, host cell autophagy is suppressed [46, 47]. This biphasic response may be due to the crosstalk that exists between apoptosis and autophagy. That is, inhibition of apoptosis occurs in infected cells during the first 24 h after infection and as a result of crosstalk, it has been suggested that autophagy is stimulated and then, vice versa, during the later stages of the intracellular infection cycle (> 24 h post-infection), as apoptosis inhibition wanes, suppression of autophagy increases. Thus, regulation of host cell autophagy by the parasite may be part of a cell survival mechanism in *T. gondii* infected host cells related to inhibition of apoptosis. Interestingly, parasite-mediated activation of AKt signaling has recently been found to prevent autophagy degradation of the parasite [48]. As AKt activation has also been linked to inhibition of apoptosis in *T. gondii* infected cells, this event suggests AKt signaling may be a pathway by which the parasite can regulate both host cell autophagy and apoptosis pathways [39, 48]. Dual manipulation of host cell apoptosis and autophagy pathways indicates a fine level of control of host PCD pathways by the parasite to promote parasite persistence in the host. Further work on the interplay between apoptosis and autophagy and the parasite modulation of these two processes is needed to further elucidate these mechanisms.

### 3.3. Necrotic cell death

A few *in vitro* studies have reported *T. gondii* inducing necrotic cell death of host cells [49–52]. In IFN-γ stimulated fibroblasts and astrocytes, infection with avirulent parasite strains of the parasite, rather than stimulating autophagic-mediated mechanism of parasite killing, induces disruption of the PV membrane via IRG proteins resulting in parasite death and subsequently triggering of necrotic host cell death [50, 53]. This type of necrotic death of the host cells involved killing of intracellular parasites and thus would promote host survival via elimination of the parasite. In these experiments, the parasite was found to egress within hours after infection, thus limiting replication in host cells which also would promote clearance of the parasite by immune cells. Experiments have similarly found early egress of the parasites in

IFN-γ-stimulated astrocytes, indicating this mechanism may also function in the brain to limit parasite numbers and aid in elimination of the parasite [54].

Conversely, *Toxoplasma*-specific primed T cells were found to be able to induce rapid egress of the parasite, causing necrotic cell death of host cells via ligation of the death receptor or perforin, but as egress was rapid the intracellular parasites escaped killing [55]. These egressed parasites were capable of infecting neighboring cells, thus suggesting that during *Toxoplasma* infection of T cells, death receptor-and perforin-mediated parasite egress may contribute to parasite dissemination of the parasite. Furthermore, as necrotic cell death induced by death receptor or perforin-dependent parasite egress contributes to inflammatory processes, it could also lead to further spread of the parasite due to infection of invading leukocytes. This process may also contribute to the establishment of infection in the brain as infected leukocytes can invade brain. Finally, death receptor-induced or perforin-mediated egress could be involved during the reactivation of *T. gondii* in chronically infected individuals, leading to reinfection of egressed parasites in the brain. Thus, parasite evasion of this cell death pathway may have significant consequences on the clinical sequelae of the chronic infection in the brain. Experiments in fibroblasts found necrotic host cell death was not dependent on the necroptosis mediator RIPK3 or caspases [52]. Further studies are needed to ascertain if necroptosis occurs in other cell types that have been associated with necrotic-type cell death in *T. gondii* infected cells.

## 4. Parasite manipulation of PCD pathways: Conclusions and potential therapeutic implications

A better understanding of the mechanisms by which the parasite modulates apoptosis, autophagic and necrotic host cell death pathways will enhance our understanding of the host/parasite relationship in toxoplasmosis and may yield new therapeutic targets to treat pathological consequences of cerebral toxoplasmosis. For example, while the infection is asymptomatic in immunocompetant individuals, recent evidence indicates chronic infection may lead to psychiatric and other neurological disorders in some individuals. Some of these effects may be due to modifications of processes leading to cell death or resulting in dysregulated cell death, resulting in reduction in CNS cell numbers and specifically of neurons. Conversely, inhibition of apoptosis of astrocytes in the brain could be crucial for establishment of the parasite in this compartment, while inhibition of apoptosis of infected neurons may be essential for development of bradyzoite stage and thus crucial to long-term persistence of the parasite in the brain. The evidence indicates the parasite can manipulate both host cell apoptosis and autophagy pathways, indicating a sophisticated level of parasite control of host PCD pathways and elucidation of the molecular details of these mechanisms could lead to new therapeutic targets with which to control the infection. A better understanding of manipulation of apoptosis and other cell death pathways in the brain cells such as microglia, astrocytes and neurons is of particular importance. The identification of molecular components of PCD pathways crucial to parasite–host interactions in chronic toxoplasmosis could lead to development of new antiparasitic drugs and/or yield new potential therapeutic targets to treat pathological consequences of chronic cerebral toxoplasmosis in immunocompetant individuals and reactivated toxoplasmosis in immunosuppressed individuals. A similar harnessing of apoptotic, autophagic and programmed necrosis cell death pathways has been proposed to treat cancers, neurodegenerative disorders and other diseases, where PCD pathways have been identified as involved in pathogenesis [56]. The dissection of the molecular mechanisms by which *T. gondii* manipulates apoptosis and other cell death pathways thus could also serve as a benefit to probe pathways in normal cells and in diseases in which apoptosis and other cell death pathways play a central role.

## Author details

Sandra K. Halonen*

Address all correspondence to: shalonen@montana.edu

Dept. of Microbiology and Immunology, Montana State University, Bozeman, MT, USA

## References

[1] Tsujimoto Y, Shimizu S. Another way to die: autophagic programmed cell death. Cell Death Differ 2005;12(2):1528–34.

[2] Edinger AL, Thompson CB. Death by design: apoptosis, necrosis and autophagy. Curr Opin Cell Biol 2004;16(6):663–9.

[3] Elmore S. Apoptosis: a review of programmed cell death. Toxicol Pathol 2007;35(4): 495–516.

[4] Vandenabeele P, et al. Molecular mechanisms of necroptosis: an ordered cellular explosion. Nat Rev Mol Cell Biol 2010;11(10):700–14.

[5] Mizushima N, Levine B. Autophagy in mammalian development and differentiation. Nat Cell Biol 2010;12(9):823–30.

[6] Mizushima N, et al. Autophagy fights disease through cellular self-digestion. Nature 2008;451(7182):1069–75.

[7] Green DR, Levine B. To be or not to be? How selective autophagy and cell death govern cell fate. Cell 2014;157(1):65–75.

[8] Nikoletopoulou V, et al. Crosstalk between apoptosis, necrosis and autophagy. Biochim Biophys Acta 2013;1833(12):3448–59.

[9] Sun L, Wang X. A new kind of cell suicide: mechanisms and functions of programmed necrosis. Trends Biochem Sci 2014;39(12):587–93.

[10] Chan FK, Luz NF, Moriwaki K. Programmed Necrosis in the Cross Talk of Cell Death and Inflammation. Annu Rev Immunol 2014; 33:4.1-4.28.

[11] Kerr JF, Wyllie AH, Currie AR. Apoptosis: a basic biological phenomenon with wide-ranging implications in tissue kinetics. Br J Cancer 1972;26(4):239–57.

[12] Norbury CJ, Hickson ID. Cellular responses to DNA damage. Annu Rev Pharmacol Toxicol 2001;41:367–401.

[13] Ryter SW, Mizumura K, Choi AM. The impact of autophagy on cell death modalities. Int J Cell Biol 2014;2014:502676.

[14] Liu Y, Levine B. Autosis and autophagic cell death: the dark side of autophagy. Cell Death Differ 2015;22(3):367–76.

[15] Kroemer G, Levine B. Autophagic cell death: the story of a misnomer. Nat Rev Mol Cell Biol 2008;9(12):1004–10.

[16] Paulus GL, Xavier RJ. Autophagy and checkpoints for intracellular pathogen defense. Curr Opin Gastroenterol 2015;31(1):14–23.

[17] Nath A, Sinai AP. Cerebral Toxoplasmosis. Curr Treat Opt Neurol 2003;5(1):3–12.

[18] Halonen SK, Weiss LM. Toxoplasmosis. Handb Clin Neurol 2013;114:125–45.

[19] Tenter AM, Heckeroth AR, Weiss LM. Toxoplasma gondii: from animals to humans. Int J Parasitol 2000;30(12–13):1217–58.

[20] Okusaga O, Postolache TT. Toxoplasma gondii, the immune system, and suicidal behavior. In: Dwivedi Y. (Ed.) The Neurobiological Basis of Suicide. 2012: Boca Raton (FL).

[21] Niebuhr DW, et al. Selected infectious agents and risk of schizophrenia among U.S. military personnel. Am J Psychiatr 2008;165(1):99–106.

[22] Torrey EF, et al. Antibodies to Toxoplasma gondii in patients with schizophrenia: a meta-analysis. Schizophr Bull 2007;33(3):729–36.

[23] Luder CG, Gross U. Apoptosis and its modulation during infection with Toxoplasma gondii: molecular mechanisms and role in pathogenesis. Curr Top Microbiol Immunol 2005;289:219–37.

[24] Liesenfeld O, Kosek JC, Suzuki Y. Gamma interferon induces Fas-dependent apoptosis of Peyer's patch T cells in mice following peroral infection with Toxoplasma gondii. Infect Immun 1997;65(11):4682–9.

[25] Blader IJ, Koshy AA. Toxoplasma gondii development of its replicative niche: in its host cell and beyond. Eukaryot Cell 2014;13(8):965–76.

[26] Contreras-Ochoa CO, et al. Toxoplasma gondii invasion and replication within neonate mouse astrocytes and changes in apoptosis related molecules. Exp Parasitol 2013;134(2):256–65.

[27] Takahashi J, et al. Bax-induced apoptosis not demonstrated in the congenital toxoplasmosis in mice. Brain Dev 2001;23(1):50–3.

[28] el-Sagaff S, et al. Cell death pattern in cerebellum neurons infected with Toxoplasma gondii. J Egypt Soc Parasitol 2005;35(3):809–18.

[29] Shen DF, et al. Involvement of apoptosis and interferon-gamma in murine toxoplasmosis. Investig Ophthalmol Visual Sci 2001;42(9):2031–6.

[30] Wang T, et al. Toxoplasma gondii induce apoptosis of neural stem cells via endoplasmic reticulum stress pathway. Parasitology 2014;141(7):988–95.

[31] Handel U, et al. Neuronal gp130 expression is crucial to prevent neuronal loss, hyperinflammation, and lethal course of murine Toxoplasma encephalitis. Am J Pathol 2012;181(1):163–73.

[32] Zhang YH, et al. Activated microglia contribute to neuronal apoptosis in Toxoplasmic encephalitis. Parasit Vectors 2014;7:372.

[33] Sinai AP, et al. Mechanisms underlying the manipulation of host apoptotic pathways by Toxoplasma gondii. Int J Parasitol 2004;34(3):381–91.

[34] Nishikawa Y, et al. Toxoplasma gondii infection induces apoptosis in noninfected macrophages: role of nitric oxide and other soluble factors. Parasite Immunol 2007;29(7):375–85.

[35] D'Angelillo A, et al. Toxoplasma gondii dense granule antigen 1 stimulates apoptosis of monocytes through autocrine TGF-beta signaling. Apoptosis 2011;16(6):551–62.

[36] Molestina RE, et al. Activation of NF-kappaB by Toxoplasma gondii correlates with increased expression of antiapoptotic genes and localization of phosphorylated IkappaB to the parasitophorous vacuole membrane. J Cell Sci 2003;116(Pt 21):4359–71.

[37] Molestina RE, Sinai AP. Host and parasite-derived IKK activities direct distinct temporal phases of NF-kappaB activation and target gene expression following Toxoplasma gondii infection. J Cell Sci 2005;118(Pt 24):5785–96.

[38] Payne TM, Molestina RE, Sinai AP. Inhibition of caspase activation and a requirement for NF-kappaB function in the Toxoplasma gondii-mediated blockade of host apoptosis. J Cell Sci 2003;116(Pt 21):4345–58.

[39] Kim L, Denkers EY. Toxoplasma gondii triggers Gi-dependent PI 3-kinase signaling required for inhibition of host cell apoptosis. J Cell Sci 2006;119(Pt 10):2119–26.

[40] Cai Y, et al. Toxoplasma gondii inhibits apoptosis via a novel STAT3-miR-17-92-Bim pathway in macrophages. Cell Signal 2014;26(6):1204–12.

[41] Yamada T, et al. Toxoplasma gondii inhibits granzyme B-mediated apoptosis by the inhibition of granzyme B function in host cells. Int J Parasitol 2011;41(6):595–607.

[42] Gao XJ, et al. Protein phosphatase 2C of Toxoplasma gondii interacts with human SSRP1 and negatively regulates cell apoptosis. Biomed Environ Sci 2014;27(11):883–93.

[43] Martens S, et al. Disruption of Toxoplasma gondii parasitophorous vacuoles by the mouse p47-resistance GTPases. PLoS Pathogens 2005;1(3):e24.

[44] Van Grol J, et al. CD40 induces anti-Toxoplasma gondii activity in nonhematopoietic cells dependent on autophagy proteins. Infect Immun 2013;81(6):2002–11.

[45] Subauste CS. CD40, autophagy and Toxoplasma gondii. Memorias do Instituto Oswaldo Cruz, 2009;104(2):267–72.

[46] Orlofsky A. Toxoplasma-induced autophagy: a window into nutritional futile cycles in mammalian cells? Autophagy 2009;5(3):404–6.

[47] Lee YJ, et al. Proliferation of Toxoplasma gondii suppresses host cell autophagy. Korean J Parasitol 2013;51(3):279–87.

[48] Muniz-Feliciano L, et al. Toxoplasma gondii-induced activation of EGFR prevents autophagy protein-mediated killing of the parasite. PLoS Pathogens 2013;9(12):e1003809.

[49] Liesenfeld O, et al. Association of CD4+ T cell-dependent, interferon-gamma-mediated necrosis of the small intestine with genetic susceptibility of mice to peroral infection with Toxoplasma gondii. J Experiment Med 1996;184(2):597–607.

[50] Zhao YO, et al. Disruption of the Toxoplasma gondii parasitophorous vacuole by IFNgamma-inducible immunity-related GTPases (IRG proteins) triggers necrotic cell death. PLoS Pathogens 2009;5(2):e1000288.

[51] Persson EK, et al. Death receptor ligation or exposure to perforin trigger rapid egress of the intracellular parasite Toxoplasma gondii. J Immunol 2007;179(12):8357–65.

[52] Niedelman W, et al. Cell death of gamma interferon-stimulated human fibroblasts upon Toxoplasma gondii infection induces early parasite egress and limits parasite replication. Infect Immun 2013;81(12):4341–9.

[53] Halonen SK. Role of autophagy in the host defense against Toxoplasma gondii in astrocytes. Autophagy 2009;5(2):268–9.

[54] Melzer T, et al. The gamma interferon (IFN-gamma)-inducible GTP-binding protein IGTP is necessary for toxoplasma vacuolar disruption and induces parasite egression in IFN-gamma-stimulated astrocytes. Infect Immun 2008;76(11):4883–94.

[55] Persson EK, et al. Death receptor ligation or exposure to perforin trigger rapid egress of the intracellular parasite Toxoplasma gondii. J Immunol 2007;179(12):8357–65.

[56] Portt L, et al. Anti-apoptosis and cell survival: a review. Biochim Biophys Acta 2011;1813(1):238–59.

# 6

# Toxoplasmosis and Public Health Genomics

Oymak Sibel, Hız Meliha Merve, Kılıç Sevilay,
Büyük Başak, Halil İbrahim Taş and
Ülken Tunga Babaoğlu

**Abstract**

*Toxoplasma gondii* infection generally causes flu-like symptoms in healthy individuals; however, immunosuppression of the infected individual causes reactivation of the pathogen to its active form and relapse of the toxoplasmosis. Today it is known that toxoplasmosis triggers psychiatric disorders such as schizophrenia as well as behavioral changes such as suicide attempts. Although dermatological manifestations are very rare, the dermatological lesions are not unique. In addition, previous toxoplasma infection also causes congenital infections because of placental infection and causes birth defects and spontaneous abortion. *T. gondii* strains are mainly divided into three main clonal lineages, yet higher recombination rate causes unusual population structure and heterogeneous distribution of the pathogen. Both genetic variations, of the pathogen and the patients, are important for virulence property and success of the therapies. The scientist focuses on the genetic variations of the pathogens and individuals to achieve effective treatment and developed tailor-made medicines. Thus, understanding the molecular basis of the disease and the link of molecular mechanism with host immunity is important to fully know the disease and related disorders. In this chapter, we would like to evaluate the current knowledge on genetic, molecular characteristics of toxoplasmosis in view of public health genomics.

**Keywords:** *Toxoplasma gondii*, schizophrenia, public health genomics

## 1. Introduction

*Toxoplasma gondii* is a life-long infectious protozoan parasite and thus understanding the immunological and molecular pathways during toxoplasmosis is important for effective treatment and vaccine development. *T. gondii* infection and related neurological, behavior, dermatological, and ocular manifestations are an important area of current research. In addition, the molecular life cycle of the pathogen, immunologic, and genetic changes during the infection is also important to diagnose and improve new treatment strategies. The other important research area related to toxoplasmosis is development of safe and efficient diagnostic assays for early detection of pathogens during pregnancy period.

It is thought that *T. gondii* has a role in the etiology of schizophrenia and that parasites have special genes that can be inherited. However, there are some limiting factors. In schizophrenia, it is difficult to show the cause of toxoplasmosis in brain tissue. *T. gondii* can also be found in brain tissue in immunocompetent individuals. Moreover, not all of the *T. gondii*-infected individuals develop schizophrenia. Increased risk of exposure to *T. gondii* has been shown in schizophrenic patients, but the exposure relationship is often studied by case-control studies. Despite the cohort-type studies that show the best relationship between the etiologic agent and the disease, researchers prefer to work in case-control type because of the latent course of the disease, not being a common disease in society, and difficulties in follow-up. It should be kept in mind that genetic factors as well as environmental exposures may increase the risk of this disease and that the presence of the agent before disease development may better explain the causal relationship.

We need a perspective of public health genomics to better understand the relationship between schizophrenia and toxoplasma, which is one of the most frequently used topics in recent years, and also in order to better understand the public health effects of parasites. The clear understanding of the histological, biochemical, and genetic characteristics of parasites can also explain the mechanisms of disease development. For this purpose, in this chapter, genotypic features of *Toxoplasma gondii*, other molecular changes, and mechanisms of schizophrenia development are discussed and suggestions are given in terms of public health.

## 2. Molecular basis of toxoplasmosis

The first line of defense against *T. gondii* compose of dendritic cells (DCs), monocytes, and macrophages, and *Toxoplasma* induces toxoplasmosis-specific $CD4^+$ and $CD8^+$ T cells, which are the secondary defense systems. The ligands expressed by *T. gondii are* recognized by toll-like receptors (TLR) [1–3] and stimulate IL-12 production via MyD88 signaling [4, 5]. GPI-anchored proteins of *T. gondi* is important for both adhesion to host and regulate host immune system via TLR2 and TLR4 on macrophage surface [2, 3] aside profilin that secreted from *T. gondii* binds to TLR11 on dendritic cells [5]. Pro-inflammatory IL-12 secretion triggers IFN-$\gamma$ production by NK cells; thereafter, $CD4^+$ and $CD8^+$ T cells join to release IFN-$\gamma$ [6], and then IFN-$\gamma$ binds to a receptor tyrosine kinase (IFN-$\gamma$-R) and activates the JAK/STAT1 cascade by JAKs phosphorylation (**Figure 1**).

Activation of JAKs phosphorylates the tyrosine residue of STAT1 and cause dimerization of the molecule hence translocate the nucleus [7] then binds to IFN-$\gamma$-responsive gamma-activated site (GAS) consensus sequence and initiate the transcription of IFN$\gamma$-inducible genes Irf-1 and Lrg47 [7, 8]. In addition to T-cell mediated immunity, STAT1 induces nitric oxide (NO) and reactive oxygen species (ROS) production in monocytes and macrophages [9]. Lüder et al. [10]

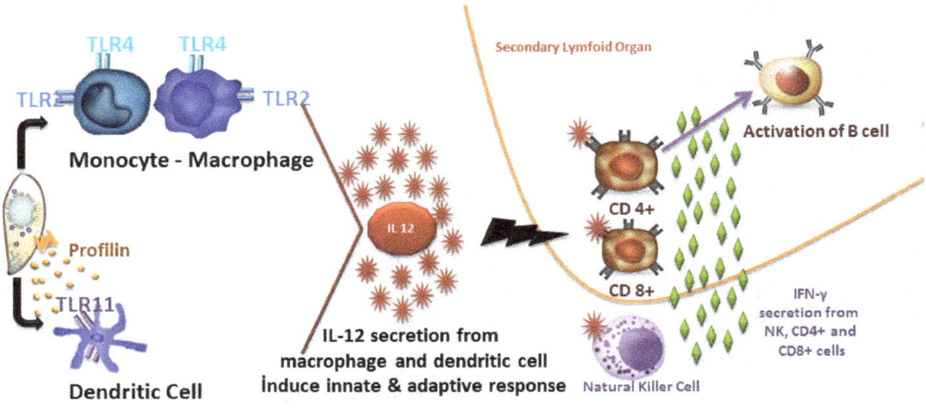


**Figure 1.** Immune response to *Toxoplasma gondii* infection in humans.

have reported the toxoplasma IFN-gamma-induced gene expression via STAT1 pathway. In addition, STAT4-dependent IFN-γ has been reported in dendritic cells and macrophages [11]. Many reports have been shown the *T. gondii* success of toxoplasma's immune evasion strategies [10, 12, 13]. The molecular basis of parasite-host interaction is important in understanding the disease mechanism and developed successful treatment strategy (**Figure 2**).

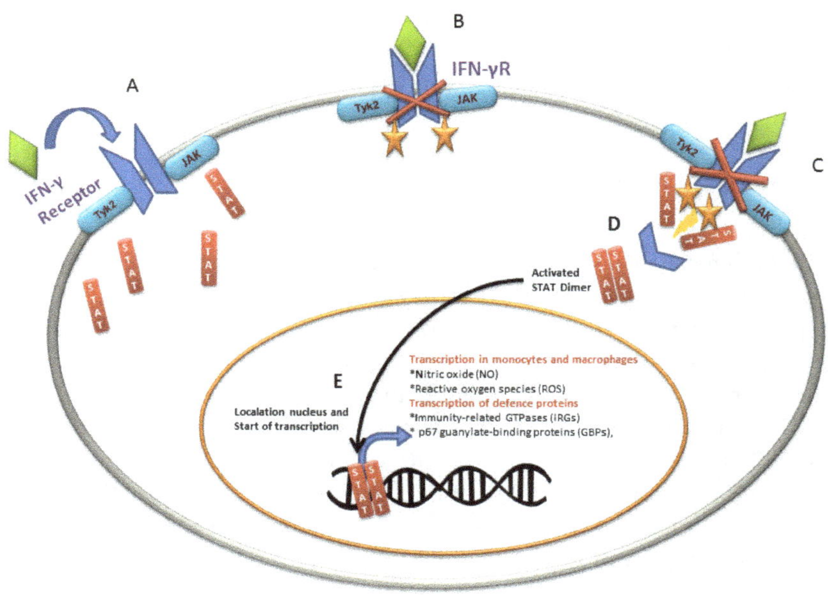


**Figure 2.** JAK-STAT pathway is important to induce toxoplasma-related response genes. INF-γ binds to its receptor (A) and activates the tyrosine kinase activity of receptor (B) and hence the phosphorylate SH2 domain of the STAT (C). Phosphorylation of the STAT triggers dimerization of the molecule (D) and conformational changes cause nuclear localization of the STAT which then binds to the nuclear response sequence on promoter region (E) to induce expression of target genes.

## 3. Genetic variation of *Toxoplasma gondii*

The complexity of an organism is directly related to its genome, and the variation on parasite genome is crucial for their success during evolution. In addition to natural selection, the pharmacy industry also forces parasites for evaluation; thus, genomic diversity also means successful pathogenicity.

*Toxoplasma gondii* consists of three main clonal lineages (types I, II, and III) among North America and Europe [14], and type II is the major strain that causes human infections in North America [14] and Europe [15, 16]. Early studies that performed multilocus enzyme electrophoresis (MLE) had limitations to show biological and epidemiological diversity [17].

Nowadays, high throughput technologies allow the scientist to understand the genetic diversity of *T. gondii*. In contrast, genetic analyses that were performed by multilocus markers have been shown that isolated samples from South America were highly diverse from each other and also from European and North American strains [15–18] due to a higher recombination rate [19]. The recent researchers have been shown that *T. gondii* has unusual population structure with different growth rates [20], frequency of differentiation, motility [21] virulence, persistence, and migration capacity [15, 21–23]. Recent developments in molecular tools allow enhancing their success to identify the genetic diversity of the parasite [24, 25]. Su et al. [25, 26] have analyzed the nuclear and plastid genome of 950 isolates from all over word and reported six major clades dividing 15 haplotypes with 138 unique genotypes. Ning et al. [22] have reported that toxoplasma dense granule protein 20 (GRA20) may be useful for intraspecific phylogenetic analyses. Wang et al. [27] have reported that rhoptry protein 47 may be used as a genetic marker for a phylogenetic relationship. In contrast, genes with low sequence variation such as superoxide dismutase (SOD) are not useful for variation analyses [28, 29].

## 4. Importance of human genetic variation for toxoplasmosis infection

Nowadays, researches are focused on the personalized medicine by using genetic variations of the patients to develop tailor-made therapeutics for appropriate and optimal therapies. The most important part to develop tailor-made therapeutics understands the relation between molecular basis of the disease and phenotypic screening. In addition, genomic variation is also important to understand personal immune response to a specific disease or therapeutic efficiency.

Toll-like receptor (TLR) is a single-pass transmembrane, non-catalytic receptor family, which is crucial for an early innate immune response during evolution. TLR expression differs in the stage of pregnancy, and a different subtype of TLR is activated or deactivated in placental tissues during pregnancy period [30, 31]. Nishimura and Naito have shown that TLR3 expression was the highest in placenta [32]. TLR is linked to infertility [33], pregnancy disorders, and placental dysfunction [34]. In toxoplasmosis TLR2, TLR4, TLR9, and TLR11 have been found important for recognition of ligands expressed by *T. gondii* [1, 35–37]. Andrade et al. [38] have demonstrated *TLR7 and TLR9 sense T. gondii*-associated nucleic acids (DNA or RNA) while TLR11 and TLR12 sense Toxoplasma profiling. Thus, understanding genomic variations in TLR is important to highlight immune defense against *T. gondii* [30, 39, 40]. NOD-like receptor

(NLR) families are important for immediate responses against structures that are present in *T. gondii* like TLR receptors. Dutra et al. [41] have reported that NOD2 gene polymorphism (rs3135499) increases the ocular toxoplasmosis by its effects on IL-17A production. Witola et al. [42] have reported that NALP1, a member of the NLR family of proteins, is crucial for immune responses to *T. gondii* infection and pathogenesis. Variation in immunity-related genes is also associated with toxoplasmosis. Shimokawa et al. [43] have shown that HLA-DQA1 and DQB1 alleles are increasing the risk of congenital toxoplasmosis. In conclusion, human genomic variation influences the defense against *T. gondii* as well as its manifestations of congenital infection and ocular toxoplasmosis.

## 5. Immunohistochemistry of toxoplasmosis

Toxoplasmosis can cause severe fetal conditions during pregnancy, and this fetal influence is related to the trimester of pregnancy. *Toxoplasma gondii* infection in the first trimester of pregnancy (4th week) can cause serious neurological and ophthalmological damage as well as spontaneous termination of pregnancy [44]. Infection of the nervous system leads to central nervous system injuries including hydrocephalus, microcephaly, motor mental retardation, and intracranial calcifications. Microphthalmia can also be observed in the first trimester. *Toxoplasma gondii* infection in the second and third trimester may result in chorioretinitis, visual defects, and mild neurological sequelae [45]. Dermal symptoms of *Toxoplasma gondii* in fetus are nonspecific and differs in each trimester.

Histopathological report attracted attention to especially parasitic infiltration and also inflammatory cell infiltration in affected tissue during toxoplasmosis. Immunosuppressive patients because of reduced inflamatory response due to immunne suppressive agents. Thus, immunohistochemically staining with appropriate antibodies will be helpful in these cases [46, 47]. Pathologic changes especially visible in skin lesions are pseudoepitheliomatous hyperplasia and perivascular lymphohistiocytic infiltration. Parasites can be seen in macrophages by hematoxylin eosin staining or as its single parasitic form by basophilic staining. Bradyzoites form that contains tissue cysts can be visualized by hematoxylin-eosin, Giemsa, Mallory, Biondi, and PAS reagent [48]. Parasites can also be visualized immunohistochemically by marking them with antigen-specific antigens inside the host tissue [49]. Tachyzoites are able to be visualized by light microscopy from samples taken from infected tissues [48, 50]. In addition to light microscopy, immunofluorescence methods can be used to detect parasites and to show them microscopically in samples taken from infected tissues with parasites [50].

## 6. Toxoplasmosis and psychiatric patients

### 6.1. Behavioral changes and toxoplasmosis

Kozar has shown the relationship between toxoplasma infection and psychiatric disorders for the first time [51] *T. gondii*, present in one-third of the world's population, may be associated with an increase in suicide rate [52]. *T. gondii*, a neurotrophic parasite, plays a role in the development of schizophrenia and causes behavioral changes, suicide attempts, and neuropathological degenerations in the brain tissue [53–56, 74]. *T. gondii* has a role in the development of behavioral disorders via changes in neuroimmunomodulation and neurotransmission, yet pathophysiological mechanisms are not fully understood by scientists [57, 58].

### 6.2. Schizophrenia and toxoplasmosis.

Several studies and later metaanalyses have been reported the association between *Toxoplasma gondii* infection with schizophrenia [55, 59, 60]. It has been shown that *T. gondii*-infected individuals increase the risk of schizophrenia when compared to healthy individuals, yet these relationships were only examined by case-control studies. Epidemiologically, the best way to show the relationship between the agent and the disease is to work in cohort type. In contrast, the researchers prefer to work in case-control type studies because of the latent course of the disease, the difficulties encountered in the follow-up, and the life cycle pathogen and rare nature of disease. It should be kept in mind that genetic factors as well as environmental exposures may increase the risk of this disease. Previous toxoplasma infection before neurological disease development may better explain the causal relationship.

Schizophrenia susceptibility genes are associated with life cycle of *T. gondii* [61]. The factors that play a role in the etiology of the disease time of infection, genetic variation of *T. gondii*, and strain of the parasite [60]. In addition to the genetic characteristics of infected individuals, immigration or being the offspring of immigrants is also related with schizophrenia among *T. gondii*-infected humans [62].

*T. gondii* and schizophrenia relations have been linked in many studies [63], and generally it's accepted that *T. gondii* triggers psychiatric disorders via affecting neurotransmitter secretion [54]. It is known that the *T. gondii* genome contains two aromatic amino acid hydroxylases that can directly affect dopamine and/or serotonin biosynthesis [64]. It is unclear how *T. gondii* increased dopamine levels; however, the dopamine is released during inflammation due to the increase of cytokines such as interleukin-2 (IL-2) [65, 66]. Hence, dopamine imbalance in the mesolimbic and mesocortical regions of the brain may play a role in the development of schizophrenia [67].

*T. gondii* modulates host gene expression by secretion of effector molecules [68] or cause post-translational modification such as acetylation of protein residues in neurons and glial cells [69]. The success of the pathogen is its virulence ability to cross biological barriers such as the blood brain barrier [70]. In a study, Du et al. [68] demonstrated that *T. gondii* terminates the NF-κB pathway by its rhoptry protein that causes p65 ubiquitination for proteasomal degradation. In a study, it has been shown that *T. gondii* changes lysine acetylation in astrocytes [69].

TOXO-specific IgG and IgM antibody levels are elevated in schizophrenia [71–75]. In a study in which other demographic variables might affect age, race, sex, and mortality, it was found that the risk of death in serologically positive individuals was five times higher than *Toxoplasma gondii* seronegative ones [75]. Toxo-specific IgG antibody level was found four times higher in patients with schizophrenia than in individuals without [76].

Torrey has shown that *Toxoplasma* seroprevalence in individuals with schizophrenia is 2.73 times higher than the control population [60]. In a study, Emelia et al. [77] have shown significant sero-intensity rates of anti-*T. gondii* IgG antibody in schizophrenic patients when compared to psychiatrically healthy volunteers. Tamer et al. [78] have shown that IgG *T. gondii* antibodies were higher in patients with schizophrenia when compared with controls, and in contrast, Karabulut et al. [79] have reported that there is no association between *T. gondii* IgG positivity and schizophrenia.

## 7. Toxoplasmosis and dermatological disease

Dermatological manifestations are rare and diagnosis of lesion is difficult. Skin lesions in congenital infections are usually exfoliative lesions and hemorrhagic and necrotic papules (small papules in the shape of 'blueberry muffins'). These lesions tend to hold the body. But it can be seen in the entire body, except in the palmoplantar region and face. The skin findings of toxoplasmosis are very varied: the dermatological lesions are reported as roseola, erythema multiforme [80], papular urticaria [80, 84], urticarial, hemorrhagic eruptions, formation of nodules and bullae [81, 82] on palms, soles, hands, legs, trunk, face and chest [83, 84]. Jeffrey and Pollock have shown a 12-year-old boy patient with dermatomyositis and polymyositis and offered to use sulfadiazine, pyrimethamine, and folinic acid for treatment [85]. Fong et al. [81] have reported a 49-year-old HIV-positive Chinese male with hard and painful nodular lesions. Ivanova et al. [86] described a case of 46-year-old male patient with acute toxoplasma lymphadenitis, similar to malignant cervical lymphadenopathy. In another study performed by Marina et al. [87], scientists reported a case of a 43-year-old immunocompetent man who has several erythematous papules and nodules on the body and extremities.

Histopathologic features are common for both acquired and congenital forms. Lymphocytes, macrophages, plasma cells, and superficial and deep perivascular infiltration, which is composed of eosinophils, are seen in the dermis. Tissue forms of *T. gondii* may not always be seen in specimens of biopsy taken from the lesion.

It is important that congenital toxoplasmosis is distinguished from the TORCH group of infectious diseases. Acquired toxoplasmosis may be confused with inflammatory diseases such as viral exanthema, meningococcemia, syphilis, urticarial vasculitis, and erythema multiforme associated with herpes simplex and autoimmune collagen tissue diseases. If active acute infection occurs in organs such as the skin or the eye, or congenital infection occurs, or immunosuppressed patients need treatment, the most effective treatment method is pyrimethamine (from 25 to 50 mg per day followed by 100 mg loading) and sulfadiazine (2–4 mg per day oral, divided into four doses). Patients allergic to sulfonamides may be given clindamycin (300 mg, four times a day).

## 8. Toxoplasmosis and pregnancy

*T. gondii* is an important, warm-blooded pathogen that causes congenital infection during pregnancy which results in cardiovascular, cerebral, and ocular damage in newborns by transplacental infection [87, 88]; *T. gondii* infection also causes birth defects and spontaneous abortion [89–92].

Determination of *T. gondii* infection is crucial during pregnancy to decrease congenital toxoplasmosis [91] and thus companies try to develop new commercial tests. The serologic screening of IgM, IgA, and IgG is important to determine current or past infections of the pregnant women [88, 93]. In addition to serological methods, ELISA IgG avidity is also found safe, efficient, and easy to determine *T. gondii* infection in the first trimester of pregnancy in routine diagnostic treatment [94, 95]. PCR is an effective diagnostic tool to determine the pathogen in a tiny amount of sample with high specificity [96–98]. The scientist's efforts to develop efficient and safe methods to alternates of ELISA, IFA, or modified agglutination test (MAT [88] or to develop these commercial ones to eliminates limitations of previous ones are ongoing [99, 104]. Armengol et al. [100] have compared different commercial assays which use anti-Toxoplasma IgG seroconversion in pregnant women and efficiency of the assays differs.

Pomares et al. [101] have developed new multiplexed *T. gondii* IgG and IgM tests which allow determining the pathogen in ~1 microliter of the serum sample. Mahmoudi et al. [102] have developed ELISA-based interferon-gamma release assay for the early detection of the pathogen. Mohammadpour et al. [103] have been reported that tachyzoites form of *T. gondii* able to detect via its soluble crude antigens by ELISA. Robert-Gangneux et al. [104] have been developed efficient toxoplasmosis assay which able to diagnose from non-cell-rich or non-hemoglobin-rich samples by real time PCR.

The development of diagnostic tests is particularly important in addressing the difficulties encountered during routine follow-ups by the population. Common guidelines are needed to guide both patients and clinicians in the subsequent processes, especially when toxoplasmosis is diagnosed in pregnancies. Sensitive tests to be developed for definite diagnosis are very important because there are problems related to diagnosis in pregnancy. *T. gondii* scans should be done serologically in cats and dogs at the same time. There is a need for regional studies on toxoplasmosis, especially in developing countries because socio-cultural features play a role in the development of the disease. As in many countries, studies in Turkey are continuing. There are studies on seroprevalence of toxoplasmosis and schizophrenia reported from the University and State Hospital in our research area Canakkale [105–108].

## 9. Conclusion

Attention should be paid to veterinary basic health services in combating and protecting zoonoses, which are thought to be an important risk factor in schizophrenia etiology such as *T. gondii*. While the risk of being infected with *T. gondii* by individuals living in urban centers increases risky behaviors such as cat feeding, cleaning of cat external feces, and contact with street cats; these risks are the factors such as contamination of animal products, consumption of raw meat and meat products, general hygiene conditions and inadequate water hygiene in the people living in rural areas and living with agriculture and animal husbandry. Therefore, it is more effective and useful to plan the health trainings and surveys that are to be carried out, considering the socio-demographic and environmental characteristics of these target groups.

Data obtained in screening studies should be recorded with geographic information systems, and risky areas should be identified and individuals at risk (primarily pregnant women, children, people with psychiatric health problems) living in these areas should be regularly monitored. Trainings should be given on healthy lifestyle behaviors, such as personal and environmental hygiene. In clinical practice, in order to prevent *T. gondii* from being missed, in-service trainings should be made to raise awareness and responsibility for health personnel.

In order to overcome the question marks in the schizophrenia mechanism, a gene pool can be created on serum samples obtained from regional and national studies, and the present and changing immunogenetic structure of parasite can be monitored. This important point of public health and genetics is that infectious agents are monitored in a large pool of genes to monitor the changes they show and to help them analyze the distribution of health problems caused by infectious agents in their populations and risk factors. We also believe that the molecular monitoring of parasites such as toxoplasma will help to improve the early diagnosis and treatment of parasitic infections, which are the most important of public health problems, and the prevention and control of these infections.

## Author details

Oymak Sibel[1]*, Hız Meliha Merve[2], Kılıç Sevilay[3], Büyük Başak[4], Halil İbrahim Taş[5] and Ülken Tunga Babaoğlu[6]

*Address all correspondence to: sibeloymakpublichealth@gmail.com

1 Department of Public Health, Faculty of Medicine, Çanakkale Onsekiz Mart University, Canakkale, Turkey

2 Department of Medical Biology, Faculty of Medicine, Çanakkale Onsekiz Mart University, Canakkale, Turkey

3 Department of Dermatology, Faculty of Medicine, Çanakkale Onsekiz Mart University, Canakkale, Turkey

4 Department of Histology and Embriology, Faculty of Medicine, Çanakkale Onsekiz Mart University, Canakkale, Turkey

5 Department of Psychiatry, Faculty of Medicine, Çanakkale Onsekiz Mart University, Canakkale, Turkey

6 Department of Public Health, Faculty of Medicine, Ahi Evran University, Kırsehir, Turkey

## References

[1] Debierre-Grockiego F, Campos MA, Azzouz N, Schmidt J, Bieker U, et al. Activation of TLR2 and TLR4 by glycosylphosphatidylinositols derived from Toxoplasma gondii. Journal of Immunology. 2007;**179**:1129–1137

[2] Wichroski MJ, Ward GE. Biosynthesis of glycosylphosphatidylinositol is essential to the survival of the protozoan parasite *Toxoplasma gondii*. Eukaryotic Cell. 2003;**2**(5):1132–1136

[3] Debierre-Grockiego F, Niehus S, Coddeville B, Elass E, Poirier F, Weingart R, Schmidt RR, Mazurier J, Guérardel Y, Schwarz RT. Binding of *Toxoplasma gondii* glycosylphosphatidylinositols to galectin-3 is required for their recognition by macrophages. Journal of Biological Chemistry. 2010;**285**(43):32744–32750. DOI: 10.1074/jbc.M110.137588

[4] Masek KS, Hunter CA. Pro-Inflammatory Responses in Macrophages during *Toxoplasma gondii* Infection. Austin, TX: Landes Bioscience; 2000–2013. Bookshelf ID: NBK5976

[5] Nathan CF, Murray HW, Wiebe ME, Rubin BY. Identification of interferon-gamma as the lymphokine that activates human macrophage oxidative metabolism and antimicrobial activity. Journal of Experimental Medicine. 1983;**158**(3):670–689. DOI: 10.1084/jem.158.3.670

[6] Hou B, Benson A, Kuzmich L, DeFranco AL, Yarovinsky F. Critical coordination of innate immune defense against *Toxoplasma gondii* by dendritic cells responding via their toll-like receptors. Proceedings of the National Academy of Sciences of the United States of America. 2011;**108**(1):278–283. DOI: 10.1073/pnas.1011549108

[7] Schneider AG, Abi Abdallah DS, Butcher BA, Denkers EY. *Toxoplasma gondii* triggers phosphorylation and nuclear translocation of dendritic cell STAT1 while simultaneously blocking IFNγ-induced STAT1 transcriptional activity. PLoS One. 2013;**8**(3):e60215. DOI: 10.1371/journal.pone.0060215

[8] Lang C, Hildebrandt A, Brand F, Opitz L, Dihazi H, Lüder CG. Impaired chromatin remodelling at STAT1-regulated promoters leads to global unresponsiveness of *Toxoplasma gondii*-infected macrophages to IFN-γ. PLoS Pathogens. 2012;**8**(1):e1002483. DOI: 10.1371/journal.ppat.1002483

[9] Hunter CA, Sibley LD. Modulation of innate immunity by *Toxoplasma gondii* virulence effectors. Nature Reviews Microbiology. 2012;**10**(11):766–778. DOI: 10.1038/nrmicro2858

[10] Lüder CG, Walter W, Beuerle B, Maeurer MJ, Gross U. *Toxoplasma gondii* down-regulates MHC class II gene expression and antigen presentation by murine macrophages via interference with nuclear translocation of STAT1alpha. European Journal of Immunology. 2001;**31**(5):1475–1484

[11] Fukao T, Frucht DM, Yap G, Gadina M, O'shea JJ, Koyasu S. Inducible expression of Stat4 in dendritic cells and macrophages and its critical role in innate and adaptive immune responses. Journal of Immunology. 2001;**166**:4446–4455

[12] Zimmermann S, Murray PJ, Heeg K, Dalpke AH. Induction of suppressor of cytokine signaling-1 by *Toxoplasma gondii* contributes to immune evasion in macrophages by blocking IFN-gamma signaling. Journal of Immunology. 2006;**176**(3):1840–1847

[13] Lang C, Algner M, Beinert N, Gross U, Lüder CG. Diverse mechanisms employed by *Toxoplasma gondii* to inhibit IFN-gamma-induced major histocompatibility complex class II gene expression. Microbes and Infection. 2006;**8**:1994–2005

[14] Howe DK, Sibley LD. *Toxoplasma gondii* comprises three clonal lineages, correlation of parasite genotype with human disease. Journal of Infectious Diseases. 1995;**172**:1561–1566

[15] Dardé ML. Toxoplasma gondii, "new" genotypes and virulence. Parasite. 2008;**15**:366–371

[16] Ajzenberg D, Cogné N, Paris L, Bessieres MH, Thulliez P, Fillisetti D, Pelloux H, Marty P, Dardé ML. Genotype of 86 *Toxoplasma gondii* isolates associated with human congenital toxoplasmosis and correlation with clinical findings. Journal of Infectious Diseases. 2002b;**186**:684–689

[17] Sibley LD, Khan A, Ajioka JW, Rosenthal BM. Genetic diversity of *Toxoplasma gondii* in animals and humans. Philosophical Transactions of the Royal Society B: Biological Sciences. 2009;**364**(1530):2749–2761

[18] Ferreira IMR, Vidal JE, De Mattos CCB, De Mattos LC, Qu D, Su C, Pereira-Chioccola VL. *Toxoplasma gondii* isolates: Multilocus RFLP PCR genotyping from human patients in Sao Paulo State, Brazil identified distinct genotypes. Experimental Parasitology. 2011;**129**:190–195

[19] Sibley LD, Ajioka JW. Population structure of *Toxoplasma gondii*: Clonal expansion driven by infrequent recombination and selective sweeps. Annual Review of Microbiology. 2008;**62**:329–351

[20] Radke JR, et al. Defining the cell cycle for the tachyzoite stage of Toxoplasma gondii. Molecular and Biochemical Parasitology. 2001;**115**:165–175

[21] Barragan A, Sibley LD. Transepithelial migration of *Toxoplasma gondii* is linked to parasite motility and virulence. Journal of Experimental Medicine. 2002;**195**:1625–1633

[22] Ning H-R, Huang S-Y, Wang J-L, Xu Q-M, Zhu X-Q. Genetic diversity of *Toxoplasma gondii* strains from different hosts and geographical regions by sequence analysis of GRA20 gene. The Korean Journal of Parasitology. 2015;**53**(3):345–348. DOI: 10.3347/kjp.2015.53.3.345

[23] Maubon D, Ajzenberg D, Brenier-Pinchart MP, Darde ML, Pelloux H. What are the respective host and parasite contributions to toxoplasmosis? Trends in Parasitology. 2008;**24**:299–303

[24] Khan A, Shaik JS, Behnke M, Wang Q, Dubey JP, Lorenzi HA, Ajioka JW, Rosenthal BM, Sibley LD. NextGen sequencing reveals short double crossovers contribute disproportionately to genetic diversity in Toxoplasma gondii. BMC Genomics. 2014;**15**:1168. DOI: 10.1186/1471-2164-15-1168

[25] Su C, Shwab EK, Zhou P, Zhu XQ, Dubey JP. Moving towards an integrated approach to molecular detection and identification of Toxoplasma gondii. Parasitology. 2010;**137**:1–11

[26] Su C, Khan A, Zhou P, Majumdar D, Ajzenberg D, Darde ML, Zhu XQ, Ajioka JW, Rosenthal BM, Dubey JP, Sibley LD. Globally diverse *Toxoplasma gondii* isolates comprise six major clades originating from a small number of distinct ancestral lineages. Proceedings of the National Academy of Sciences of the United States of America. 2012;**109**:5844–5849

[27] Wang JL, Li TT, Li ZY, Huang SY, Ning HR, Zhu XQ. Rhoptry protein 47 gene sequence: A potential novel genetic marker for population genetic studies of Toxoplasma gondii. Experimental Parasitology. 2015;**154**:1–4. DOI: 10.1016/j.exppara.2015.03.006

[28] Wang S, Cao A, Li X, Zhao Q, Liu Y, Cong H, He S, Zhou H. Sequence variation in superoxide dismutase gene of *Toxoplasma gondii* among various isolates from different hosts and geographical regions. The Korean Journal of Parasitology. 2015;**53**(3):253–258. DOI: 10.3347/kjp.2015.53.3.253

[29] Li ZY, Song HQ, Chen J, Zhu XQ. Sequence diversity in MIC6 gene among *Toxoplasma gondii* isolates from different hosts and geographical locations. The Korean Journal of Parasitology. 2015;**53**(3):341–344. DOI: 10.3347/kjp.2015.53.3.341

[30] Wujcicka W, Wilczyński J, Nowakowska D. SNPs in toll-like receptor (TLR) genes as new genetic alterations associated with congenital toxoplasmosis? The European Journal of Clinical Microbiology & Infectious Diseases. 2013;**32**(4):503–511. DOI: 10.1007/s10096-012-1763-y

[31] Patni S, Wynen LP, Seager AL, Morgan G, White JO, Thornton CA. Expression and activity of toll-like receptors 1-9 in the human term placenta and changes associated with labor at term. Biology of Reproduction. 2009;**80**(2):243–248

[32] Nishimura M, Naito S. Tissue-specific mRNA expression profiles of human toll-like receptors and related genes. The Biological and Pharmaceutical Bulletin. 2005;**28**(5):886–892

[33] Aboussahoud W, Bruce C, Elliott S, Fazeli A. Activation of toll-like receptor 5 decreases the attachment of human trophoblast cells to endometrial cells in vitro. Human Reproduction. 2010;**25**(9):2217–2228. DOI: 10.1093/humrep/deq185 [Epub: July 23, 2010]

[34] Riley JK, Nelson DM. Toll-like receptors in pregnancy disorders and placental dysfunction. Clinical Reviews in Allergy & Immunology. 2010;**39**(3):185–193

[35] Minns LA, Menard LC, Foureau DM, Darche S, Ronet C, et al. TLR9 is required for the gut-associated lymphoid tissue response following oral infection of Toxoplasma gondii. Journal of Immunology. 2006;**176**:7589–7597

[36] Plattner F, Yarovinsky F, Romero S, Didry D, Carlier M, et al. Toxoplasma profilin is essential for host cell invasion and TLR11-dependent induction of an interleukin-12 response. Cell Host & Microbe. 2008;**3**:77–87

[37] Pifer R, Benson A, Sturge CR, Yarovinsky F. UNC93B1 is essential for TLR11 activation and IL-12-dependent host resistance to *Toxoplasma gondii*. Journal of Biological Chemistry. 2011;**286**(5):3307–3314. DOI: 10.1074/jbc.M110.171025

[38] Andrade WA, Souza Mdo C, Ramos-Martinez E, Nagpal K, Dutra MS, Melo MB, Bartholomeu DC, Ghosh S, Golenbock DT, Gazzinelli RT. Combined action of nucleic acid-sensing toll-like receptors and TLR11/TLR12 heterodimers imparts resistance to *Toxoplasma gondii* in mice. Cell Host & Microbe. 2013;**13**(1):42–53. DOI: 10.1016/j.chom.2012.12.003

[39] Wujcicka W, Gaj Z, Wilczyński J, Nowakowska D. Possible role of TLR4 and TLR9 SNPs in protection against congenital toxoplasmosis. The European Journal of Clinical Microbiology & Infectious Diseases. 2015;**34**(10):2121–2129. DOI: 10.1007/s10096-015-2461-3

[40] Wujcicka W, Wilczyński J, Nowakowska D. Do the placental barrier, parasite genotype and toll-like receptor polymorphisms contribute to the course of primary infection with various *Toxoplasma gondii* genotypes in pregnant women? The European Journal of Clinical Microbiology & Infectious Diseases. 2014;**33**(5):703–709

[41] Dutra MS, Béla SR, Peixoto-Rangel AL, Fakiola M, Cruz AG, Gazzinelli A, Quites HF, Bahia-Oliveira LM, Peixe RG, Campos WR, Higino-Rocha AC, Miller NE, Blackwell JM, Antonelli LR, Gazzinelli RT. Association of a NOD2 gene polymorphism and T-helper 17 cells with presumed ocular toxoplasmosis. Journal of Infectious Diseases. 2013;**207**(1):152–163. DOI: 10.1093/infdis/jis640

[42] Witola WH, Mui E, Hargrave A, Liu S, Hypolite M, Montpetit A, et al. NALP1 influences susceptibility to human congenital toxoplasmosis, proinflammatory cytokine response, and fate of Toxoplasma gondii-infected monocytic cells. Infection and Immunity. 2011;**79**:756–766

[43] Shimokawa PT, Targa LS, Yamamoto L, Rodrigues JC, Kanunfre KA, Okay TS. HLA-DQA1/B1 alleles as putative susceptibility markers in congenital toxoplasmosis. Virulence. 2016;**7**(4):456–464. DOI: 10.1080/21505594.2016.1150401

[44] Wallon M, Gaucherand P, Al Kurdi M, Peyron F. Toxoplasma infections in early pregnancy: Consequences and management. Journal de Gynécologie, Obstétrique et Biologie de la Reproduction (Paris). 2002;**31**(5):478–484

[45] Mazzola A, Casuccio A, Romano A, Schimmenti MG, Titone L, Di Carlo P. Diagnostic problems and postnatal follow-up in congenital toxoplasmosis. Minerva Pediatrica. 2007;**59**(3):207–213

[46] Tan CD, Halushka MK, Rodriguez ER. Cardiovascular Pathology. Chapter 17. pp. 679–719

[47] Dubey JP, Beattie CP. Toxoplasmosis of Animals and Man. Boca Raton, FL: CRC Press; 1988

[48] McGovern KE, Wilson EH. Dark side illuminated: Imaging of Toxoplasma gondii through the decades. Parasites & Vectors. 2013;**6**:334. DOI: 10.1186/1756-3305-6-334

[49] Patterson JW. Weedon's Skin Pathology. Chapter 27. pp. 747–755.e4

[50] Matossian RM, Nassar VH, Basmadji A. Direct immunofluorescence in the diagnosis of toxoplasmic lymphadenitis. Journal of Clinical Pathology. 1977;**30**(9):847–850

[51] Kozar Z. Badania nad toksoplazmoza wsrod umyslowo chorych. Bulletin of the State Institute of Marine and Tropical Medicine in Gdansk, Poland. 1953;**5**:146–173. [Summary in English: Studies of toxoplasmosis among the mentally sick. Bulletin of the State Institute of Marine and Tropical Medicine in Gdańsk, Poland. 1953;**5**:142–145]

[52] Ling VJ, Lester D, Mortensen PB, Langenberg PW, Postolache TT. *Toxoplasma gondii* seropositivity and suicide rates in women. Journal of Nervous and Mental Disease. 2011;**199**(7):440–444

[53] Okusaga O, Langenberg P, Sleemi A, et al. *Toxoplasma gondii* antibody titers and history of suicide attempts in patients with schizophrenia. Schizophrenia Research. 2011;**133**(1–3):150–155

[54] Del Grande C, Galli L, Schiavi E, Dell'Osso L, Bruschi F. Is *Toxoplasma gondii* a trigger of bipolar disorder? Pathogens. 2017;**6**(1). pii: E3. DOI: 10.3390/pathogens6010003

[55] Sutterland AL, Fond G, Kuin A, Koeter MW, Lutter R, van Gool T, Yolken R, Szoke A, Leboyer M, de Haan L. Beyond the association. *Toxoplasma gondii* in schizophrenia, bipolar disorder, and addiction: Systematic review and meta-analysis. Acta Psychiatrica Scandinavica. 2015;**132**(3):161–179. DOI: 10.1111/acps.12423. [Review]

[56] Hamdani N, Daban-Huard C, Godin O, Laouamri H, Jamain S, Attiba D, Delavest M, Lépine JP, Le Corvoisier P, Houenou J, Richard JR, Yolken RH, Krishnamoorthy R, Tamouza R, Leboyer M, Dickerson FB. Effects of cumulative Herpesviridae and *Toxoplasma gondii* infections on cognitive function in healthy, bipolar, and schizophrenia subjects. Journal of Clinical Psychiatry. 2017;**78**(1):e18–e27. DOI: 10.4088/JCP.15m10133

[57] Fekadu A, Shibre T, Cleare AJ. Toxoplasmosis as a cause for behaviour disorders—overview of evidence and mechanisms. Folia Parasitologica (Praha). 2010;**57**(2):105–113

[58] Flegr J, Vedralova M. Specificity and nature of the associations of twenty-four neuropsychiatric disorders with contacts with cats and dogs. Schizophrenia Research. 2017. pii: S0920-9964(17)30078-6. DOI: 10.1016/j.schres.2017.02.007

[59] Arias I, Sorlozano A, Villegas E, de Dios Luna J, McKenney K, Cervilla J, Gutierrez B, Gutierrez J. Infectious agents associated with schizophrenia: A meta-analysis. Schizophrenia Research. 2012;**136**(1–3):128–136. DOI: 10.1016/j.schres.2011.10.026. [Review]

[60] Torrey EF, Bartko JJ, Lun ZR, Yolken RH. Antibodies to *Toxoplasma gondii* in patients with schizophrenia: A meta-analysis. Schizophrenia Bulletin. 2007;**33**(3):729–736

[61] Carter CJ. Schizophrenia susceptibility genes directly implicated in the life cycles of pathogens: Cytomegalovirus, Influenza, Herpes simplex, Rubella, and *Toxoplasma gondii*. Schizophrenia Bulletin. 2009;**35**(6):1163–1182. DOI: 10.1093/schbul/sbn054

[62] Torrey EF, Bartko JJ, Yolken RH. *Toxoplasma gondii* and other risk factors for schizophrenia: An update. Schizophrenia Bulletin. 2012;**38**(3):642–647. DOI: 10.1093/schbul/sbs043

[63] da Silva RC, Langoni H. Toxoplasma gondii: Host-parasite interaction and behavior manipulation. Parasitology Research. 2009;**105**(4):893–898

[64] Henriquez SA, Brett R, Alexander J, Pratt J, Roberts CW. Neuropsychiatric disease and *Toxoplasma gondii* infection. Neuroimmunomodulation. 2009;**16**(2):122–133

[65] Petitto JM, McCarthy DB, Rinker CM, Huang Z, Getty T. Modulation of behavioral and neurochemical measures of forebrain dopamine function in mice by species-specific interleukin-2. Journal of Neuroimmunology. 1997;**73**:183–190

[66] Flegr J, Preiss M, Klose J, Havlícek J, Vitáková M, Kodym P. Decreased level of psychobiological factor novelty seeking and lower intelligence in men latently infected with the protozoan parasite *Toxoplasma gondii* Dopamine, a missing link between schizophrenia and toxoplasmosis? Biological Psychology. 2003;**63**(3):253–268

[67] Sawa A, Snyder SH. Schizophrenia: Diverse approaches to a complex disease. Science. 2002;**296**:692

[68] Du J, An R, Chen L, Shen Y, Chen Y, et al. *Toxoplasma gondii* virulence factor ROP18 inhibits the host NF-kappaB pathway by promoting p65 degradation. Journal of Biological Chemistry. 2014;**289**:12578–12592

[69] Bouchut A, Chawla AR, Jeffers V, Hudmon A, Sullivan WJ Jr. Proteome-wide lysine acetylation in cortical astrocytes and alterations that occur during infection with brain parasite *Toxoplasma gondii*. PLoS One. 2015;**10**(3):e0117966. DOI: 10.1371/journal.pone.0117966

[70] Harker KS, Ueno N, Lodoen MB. *Toxoplasma gondii* dissemination: A parasite's journey through the infected host. Parasite Immunology. 2015;**37**(3):141–149. DOI: 10.1111/pim.12163

[71] Cetinkaya Z, Yazar S, Gecici O, Namli MN. Anti-*Toxoplasma gondii* antibodies in patients with schizophrenia—preliminary findings in a Turkish sample. Schizophrenia Bulletin. 2007;**33**(3):789–791

[72] Leweke FM, Gerth CW, Koethe D, et al. Antibodies to infectious agents in individuals with recent onset schizophrenia. European Archives of Psychiatry and Clinical Neuroscience. 2004;**254**:4–8

[73] Yolken RH, Bachmann S, Rouslanova I, et al. Antibodies to *Toxoplasma gondii* in individuals with first-episode schizophrenia. Clinical Infectious Diseases. 2001;**32**:842–844

[74] Esshili A, Thabet S, Jemli A, Trifa F, Mechri A, Zaafrane F, Gaha L, Juckel G, Babba H, Bel Hadj Jrad B. *Toxoplasma gondii* infection in schizophrenia and associated clinical features. Psychiatry Research. 2016;**245**:327–332. DOI: 10.1016/j.psychres.2016.08.056. [Epub: August 22, 2016]

[75] Dickerson F, Boronow J, Stallings C, Origoni A, Yolken R. *Toxoplasma gondii* in individuals with schizophrenia: Association with clinical and demographic factors and with mortality. Schizophrenia Bulletin. 2007;**33**(3):737–740

[76] Alvarado-Esquivel C, Urbina-Álvarez JD, Estrada-Martínez S, Torres-Castorena A, Molotla-de-León G, Liesenfeld O, Dubey JP. *Toxoplasma gondii* infection and schizophrenia: A case control study in a low Toxoplasma seroprevalence Mexican population. Parasitology International. 2011;**60**(2):151–155

[77] Emelia O, Amal RN, Ruzanna ZZ, Shahida H, Azzubair Z, Tan KS, Noor Aadila S, Siti NA, Aisah MY. Seroprevalence of anti-*Toxoplasma gondii* IgG antibody in patients with schizophrenia. Tropical Biomedicine. 2012;**29**(1):151–159

[78] Tamer GS, Dundar D, Yalug I, Caliskan S, Yazar S, Aker A. The schizophrenia and *Toxoplasma gondii* connection: Infectious, immune or both? Advances in Therapy. 2008;**25**(7):703–709. DOI: 10.1007/s12325-008-0063-5

[79] Karabulut N, Bilgiç S, Gürok MG, Karaboğa F. Is there any role of latent toxoplasmosis in schizophrenia disease? Journal of the Chinese Medical Association. 2015;**78**(9):533–537. DOI: 10.1016/j.jcma.2015.06.007. [Epub: July 29, 2015]

[80] Lupi O, Bartlett BL, Haugen RN, Dy LC, Sethi A, Klaus SN, Machado Pinto J, Bravo F, Tyring SK. Tropical dermatology: Tropical diseases caused by protozoa. Journal of the American Academy of Dermatology. 2009;**60**:897–925

[81] Fong MY, Wong KT, Rohela M, Tan LH, Adeeba K, Lee YY, et al. Unusual manifestation of cutaneous toxoplasmosis in a HIV positive patient. Tropical Biomedicine. 2010;**27**(3):447–450

[82] Binazzi M. Profile of cutaneous toxoplasmosis. International Journal of Dermatology. 1986;**25**(6):357–363

[83] Lo Schiavo A, Ruocco E, Brancaccio G, Caccavale S, Ruocco V, Wolf R. Bullous pemphigoid: Etiology, pathogenesis, and inducing factors: Facts and controversies. Clinics in Dermatology. 2013;**31**(4):391–399. DOI: 10.1016/j.clindermatol.2013.01.006

[84] Mawhorter SD, Effron D, Blinkhorn R, Spagnuolo PJ. Cutaneous manifestations of toxoplasmosis. Clinical Infectious Diseases. 1992;**14**(5):1084–1088. [Back to cited text no]

[85] Jeffrey L, Pollock MD. Toxoplasmosis appearing to be dermatomyositis. Archives of Dermatology. 1979;**115**(6):736–737. DOI: 10.1001/archderm.1979.04010060044028

[86] Ivanova K, Glatz K, Zippelius A, Nicolas G, Itin P. Acute toxoplasmosis mimicking melanoma metastases: Review of conditions causing false-positive results on (18)F-FDG PET/CT. Dermatology. 2012;**225**(4):349–353. DOI: 10.1159/000346333. [Review. Annals of Agricultural and Environmental Medicine. 2016;**23**(4):570–575]

[87] Marina S, Broshtilova V, Botev I, Guleva D, Hadzhiivancheva M, Nikolova A, Kazandjieva J. Cutaneous manifestations of toxoplasmosis: A case report. Serbian Journal of Dermatology and Venereology. 2014;**6**(3):113–119

[88] Nandedkar S, Bajpai T, Malukani K, Bhatambare GS. Unusual manifestation of isolated cutaneous toxoplasmosis in an immunocompetent patient. Indian Journal of Dermatopathology and Diagnostic Dermatology. 2015;**2**:18–22

[89] Montoya JG, Liesenfeld O. Toxoplasmosis. Lancet. 2004;**363**:1965–1976

[90] Sroka J, Wójcik-Fatla A, Zając V, Sawczyn A, Cisak E, Karamon J, Dutkiewicz J, Bojar I. Comparison of the efficiency of two commercial kits—ELFA and Western blot in estimating the phase of *Toxoplasma gondii* infection in pregnant women. Annals of Agricultural and Environmental Medicine. 2016;**23**(4):570–575. DOI: 10.5604/12321966.1226848

[91] Abdoli A, Dalimi A, Soltanghoraee H, Ghaffarifar F. Molecular detection and genotypic characterization of *Toxoplasma gondii* in paraffin-embedded fetoplacental tissues of women with recurrent spontaneous abortion. International Journal of Fertility & Sterility. 2017;**10**(4):327–336

[92] Chu JQ, Jing KP, Gao X, Li P, Huang R, Niu YR, Yan SQ, Kong JC, Yu CY, Shi G, Fan YM, Lee YH, Zhou Y, Quan JH. *Toxoplasma gondii* induces autophagy and apoptosis in human umbilical cord mesenchymal stem cells via downregulation of Mcl-1. Cell Cycle. 2017:1–10. DOI: 10.1080/15384101.2017.1281484

[93] Mumcuoglu I, Toyran A, Cetin F, Coskun FA, Baran I, Aksu N, Aksoy A. Evaluation of the toxoplasmosis seroprevalence in pregnant women and creating a diagnostic algorithm. Mikrobiyoloji Bülten. 2014;**48**(2):283–291

[94] Asgari Q, Fekri M, Monabati A, Kalantary M, Mohammadpour I, Motazedian MH, Sarkari B. Molecular genotyping of *Toxoplasma gondii* in human spontaneous aborted fetuses in Shiraz, Southern Iran. Iranian Journal of Public Health. 2013;**42**(6):620–625

[95] Holec-Gąsior L. *Toxoplasma gondii* recombinant antigens as tools for serodiagnosis of human toxoplasmosis—the current status of studies. Clinical and Vaccine Immunology. 2013;**20**:1343–1351

[96] Tanyuksel M, Guney C, Araz E, Saracli MA, Doganci L. Performance of the immunoglobulin G avidity and enzyme immunoassay IgG/IgM screening tests for differentiation of the clinical spectrum of toxoplasmosis. Journal of Microbiology. 2004;**42**(3):211–215

[97] Liesenfeld O, Montoya JG, Kinney S, Press C, Remington JS Effect of testing for IgG avidity in the diagnosis of *Toxoplasma gondii* infection in pregnant women: Experience in a US reference laboratory. Journal of Infectious Diseases. 2001;**183**(8):1248–1253

[98] Iqbal J, Khalid N. Detection of acute *Toxoplasma gondii* infection in early pregnancy by IgG avidity and PCR analysis. Journal of Medical Microbiology. 2007;**56**(Pt 11):1495–1499

[99] de Oliveira Azevedo CT, do Brasil PE, Guida L, Lopes Moreira ME. Performance of polymerase chain reaction analysis of the amniotic fluid of pregnant women for diagnosis

of congenital toxoplasmosis: A systematic review and meta-analysis. PLoS One. 2016;**11**(4):e0149938. DOI: 10.1371/journal.pone.0149938. [eCollection 2016]

[100] Armengol C, Cassaing S, Roques-Malecaze C, Chauvin P, Iriart X, Berry A, Fillaux J. Time before anti-Toxoplasma IgG seroconversion detection by 7 commercial assays in French pregnant women. Diagnostic Microbiology and Infectious Disease. 2017;**87**(2):103–107. DOI: 10.1016/j.diagmicrobio.2016.10.020

[101] Pomares C, Zhang B, Arulkumar S, Gonfrier G, Marty P, Zhao S, Cheng S, Tang M, Dai H, Montoya JG. Validation of IgG, IgM multiplex plasmonic gold platform in French clinical cohorts for the serodiagnosis and follow-up of *Toxoplasma gondii* infection. Diagnostic Microbiology and Infectious Disease. 2017;**87**(3):213–218. DOI: 10.1016/j.diagmicrobio.2016.09.001

[102] Mahmoudi S, Mamishi S, Suo X, Keshavarz H. Early detection of *Toxoplasma gondii* infection by using a interferon gamma release assay: A review. Experimental Parasitology. 2017;**172**:39–43. DOI: 10.1016/j.exppara.2016.12.008

[103] Mohammadpour N, Saki J, Rafiei A, Khodadadi A, Tavalla M, Cheraghian B. Design of indigenous ELISA using tachyzoites from the RH strain of *Toxoplasma gondii* and comparison with commercial kits in Ahvaz, Southwest of Iran, 2015. Jundishapur Journal of Microbiology. 2016;**9**(10):e36666

[104] Robert-Gangneux F, Brenier-Pinchart MP, Yera H, Belaz S, Varlet-Marie E, Bastien P, Molecular Biology Study Group of the French National Reference Center for Toxoplasmosis. Evaluation of the Toxoplasma ELITe MGB® real-time PCR assay for the diagnosis of toxoplasmosis. Journal of Clinical Microbiology. 2017. pii: JCM.02379-16. DOI: 10.1128/JCM.02379-16. [Epub ahead of print]

[105] Gencer M, Cevizci S, Saçar S, Vural A, Güngör ANÇ, Uysal A, Hacıvelioğlu SÖ, Çelik M, Duru E, Coşar E. Çanakkale Onsekiz Mart Üniversitesi Tıp Fakültesi Hastanesi Obstetri Polikliniğine Müracaat Eden Gebelerde Anti-Toxoplasma gondii Antikorlarının Dağılımı ve Risk Faktörlerinin İrdelenmesi. Türkiye Parazitoloji Dergisi. 2014;**38**(2):76–80

[106] Cevizci S, Bakar C. Halk sağlığı bakışıyla Toxoplasma gondii. Türkiye Halk Sağlığı Dergisi. 2013;**11**(1):45–58

[107] Cevizci S, Babaoğlu ÜT, Öyekçin DG. *Toxoplasma gondii*, Ruh Sağlığı ve Şizofreni. TAF Preventive Medicine Bulletin. 2013;**12**(2):199–208. DOI: 10.5455/pmb.1-1337514352

[108] Cevizci S, Celik M, Akcali A, Öyekçin DG, Şahin O, Bakar C. Seroprevalence of anti-Toxoplasma gondii and anti-Borrelia species antibodies in patients with schizophrenia: A case-control study from Western Turkey. World Journal of Biological Psychiatry. 2015;**16**(4):230–236. DOI: 10.3109/15622975.2015.1012224

# 7

# Microparticle Vaccines Against *Toxoplasma gondii*

Chung-Da Yang

**Abstract**

Significant information indicates that future investigations on *Toxoplasma* vaccine development have to include adjuvants for enhancing protective immunity against *Toxoplasma gondii*. Especially, safe and effective adjuvants capable of fulfilling Th1-dependent cell-mediated immunity appear to be more likely to be allowed to use for anti *Toxoplasma* vaccine development. Recently, biodegradable and biocompatible polymers, such as poly (lactide-co-glycolide) (PLG) polymers, have been utilized as safe and efficacious adjuvants to encapsulate antigens for producing long-term release microparticle-based vaccines. PLG microencapsulation allows the sustained release of antigens and facilitates antigen uptake via antigen-presenting cells (APCs) to favorably generate Th1 cell-mediated immunity, which is required for the prevention of *T. gondii* infection. In our recent work, recombinant surface antigens (rSAGs), including rSAG1, rSAG2, and rSAG1/2, have been, respectively, encapsulated with the PLG polymer for production of PLG-encapsulated rSAG1 (PLG-rSAG1), PLG-encapsulated rSAG2 (PLG-rSAG2), or PLG-encapsulated rSAG1/2 (PLG-rSAG1/2) microparticles. This chapter describes adjuvant effect of PLG microparticles, controlled release of PLG microparticles, PLG microparticles-immune system interaction, *Toxoplasma* SAG-loaded PLG microparticles, protective immunity by *Toxoplasma* SAG-loaded PLG microparticles, and future prospects. PLG microparticle vaccines would be advantageous for their application in the development of long-lasting vaccines against *T. gondii* for future use in humans and animals.

**Keywords:** adjuvants, poly(lactide-co-glycolide) (PLG), antigen-presenting cells (APCs), PLG-rSAG1 microparticles, PLG-rSAG2 microparticles, PLG-rSAG1/2 microparticles

## 1. Introduction

*Toxoplasma gondii* is an intracellular protozoan parasite that uses felines as final hosts and various endothermic animals, including humans, as intermediate hosts [1]. Toxoplasmosis is of major clinical and veterinary importance. The infection in domestic animals such as sheep or pigs usually generates adverse economic impact due to the induction of severe abortion and neonatal loss [2]. In addition, toxoplasmosis in pregnant women may result in severe congenital fetal disorders, including hydrocephaly, blindness, and mental retardation [3]. Toxoplasmosis in immunocompromised individuals such as AIDS patients often develops lethal toxoplasmic encephalitis as an important opportunistic infection [4]. Although prophylactic anti-*Toxoplasma* vaccines have been studied for a long time, only one commercial attenuated vaccine (Toxovax) has been licensed for use in sheep [5]. Most inactivated and recombinant vaccines developed in the past have produced only little to moderate protective efficacy against infections with a lethal challenge dose of the virulent strain of *T. gondii* [6].

Numerous earlier studies have demonstrated that cell-mediated immunity is considered as the 'appropriate' immune response in the prevention of *T. gondii* infection [7]. Therefore, potent adjuvants that can improve cell-mediated immunity have to include in *Toxoplasma* vaccine development in the future. In addition, gamma interferon (IFN-$\gamma$), one of Th1-type cytokines, mainly produced by CD4$^+$ Th1 cells is able to subsequently stimulate CD8$^+$ Tc cells to convert into cytotoxic effector cells for preventing acute and chronic *T. gondii* infection [6–8]. Thus, effective protection against *T. gondii* infection is critically dependent on the IFN-$\gamma$-associated Th1 cell-mediated immunity. Therefore, effective vaccines formulated with potent adjuvants that are promised to induce an IFN-$\gamma$-associated Th1 cell-mediated immune response seem more likely to be approved for use.

Most modern vaccines based on subunits of pathogens, such as purified proteins, are likely to be less immunogenic than traditional vaccine antigens and are often unable to initiate a strong immune response [9]. These subunit vaccines require effective adjuvants to aid them to elicit strong protective immune responses [10, 11]. Therefore, one of the current important issues in vaccinology is the urgent need for the development of new or improved adjuvants to enhance the immunogenicity or effectiveness of vaccines [9, 10, 12]. Different adjuvants capable of improving immunity and protection have been described in numerous studies [9, 10, 12]. However, the safety concern of an adjuvant is still a crucial issue to limit adjuvant development [13].

Adjuvants are special substances used in combination with an antigen to generate a more robust immune response than the antigen alone [11, 14, 15]. This broad definition encompasses a very wide range of materials for adjuvant development. Actually, adjuvants can be broadly separated into two classes, vaccine delivery systems and immunostimulatory agents, based on their main mechanisms of action [11]. Vaccine delivery systems are generally particulate, such as emulsions [16], micro/nano particles [17], iscoms, and liposomes [18], and their main function is to deliver antigens into antigen-presenting cells (APCs) [11]. In contrast, immunostimulatory agents are predominantly derived from pathogens and often represent pathogen-associated molecular patterns (PAMP), such as lipopolysaccharides (LPS) [19], monophosphoryl Lipid A (MPL-A) [20], and CpG oligodeoxynucleotides (CpG-ODN) [21], which activate cells of the innate immune system to induce the following acquired immune response [11].

This chapter will focus predominantly on microparticle adjuvant, especially poly(lactide-co-glycolide) (PLG) polymer, to be used in tachyzoite surface antigen (SAG)-based subunit vaccines against *T. gondii*, the etiological agent of toxoplasmosis. In our recent work, recombinant SAGs (rSAGs), including rSAG1, rSAG2, and rSAG1/2, have been, respectively, encapsulated with the PLG polymer for production of PLG-encapsulated rSAG1 (PLG-rSAG1) [22], PLG-encapsulated rSAG2 (PLG-rSAG2) [23], or PLG-encapsulated rSAG1/2 (PLG-rSAG1/2) microparticles [24]. This chapter describes adjuvant effect of PLG microparticles, controlled release of PLG microparticles, PLG microparticles-immune system interaction, *Toxoplasma* SAG-loaded PLG microparticles, protective immunity by *Toxoplasma* SAG-loaded PLG microparticles, and future prospects. The capability of these PLG microparticle vaccines to control the stable release of antigenic rSAG1 and effectively induce and extend protective immunity would be advantageous for their application in the development of long-lasting vaccines against *T. gondii* for future use in humans and animals.

## 2. Adjuvants effects of PLG microparticles

Microparticles, one of the vaccine delivery systems, derived from different biodegradable and biocompatible polymers, including poly(lactide-co-glycolide), alginate, starch, and other carbohydrate polymers, can be designed as safe carriers for proteins or drugs to perform the main function of delivery systems [25]. Particularly, PLG polymers approved by the US Food and Drug Administration (FDA) have been extensively used as sutures [26] and drug carriers [27] for many years. Different forms of PLG polymers can be generated according to the ratio of lactide to glycolide used for the polymerization [28]. In the recent 10 years, PLG polymers have further become safe and potent adjuvants or delivery systems to encapsulate vaccine antigens for the development of controlled release microparticle vaccines [29]. The PLG microparticles are biodegradable through hydrolysis to break down into the biocompatible metabolites, lactic and glycolic acids, which produce little inflammatory activity and are excreted from the body via natural metabolic pathways [28]. PLG polymers provide a number of practical advantages in acting as vaccine adjuvants or delivery systems following PLG encapsulation. The PLG microencapsulation protects antigens from unfavorable degradation [30], allows the sustained and extended release of antigens for a long period [31], and enhances antigen uptake by APCs, such as macrophages and dendritic cells, in specific lymphoid regions [32]. These adjuvant effects strengthen antigen immunogenicity to favorably generate strong specific immunity, especially cell-mediated immunity [29], which is urgently required for eliminating intracellular pathogens, such as *T. gondii*.

## 3. Microparticles-immune system interaction

Earlier significant studies have shown that potent cell-mediated immunity induced by PLG microparticles following vaccination is likely to be due to the uptake of PLG microparticles into APCs and the effective delivery of microparticle-containing APCs to specific lymphoid compartments [25, 32, 33]. The size of PLG microparticles used for animal vaccination is a crucial parameter in facilitating the uptake of APCs [32]. Particles smaller than 10 μm in diameter are appropriate for direct uptake by APCs, such as macrophages and dendritic cells [25, 32].

The proper size range thus can stimulate APCs to facilitate the microparticle uptake. Following the uptake of microparticles, the APCs containing microparticles then migrate to other lymphoid compartments [25], such as the spleen and mesenteric lymph nodes, where they effectively present antigenic epitopes to T lymphocytes, especially Th1 and Tc, thereby inducing strong specific cell-mediated immunity [32, 33]. In other words, facilitation of uptake and delivery of PLG microparticles by APCs can lead to more effective antigen processing and presentation to T lymphocytes capable of inducting cell-mediated immune responses [25, 32–34]. Significant earlier studies have further demonstrated that the APCs containing microparticles can travel to specialized mucosal lymphoid compartments, including mucosal-associated lymphoid tissues (MALTs), the inductive sites for stimulating potent immunity following intranasal or oral vaccination [35, 36]. Thus, PLG-encapsulated antigens can be designed as effective mucosal vaccines that have potential to stimulate mucosal systems, such as intestinal and vaginal tracks via intranasal or oral administration [36].

## 4. Controlled release of PLG microparticles

The capability of PLG microparticles to regulate the extended release rate of PLG-encapsulated antigens can lead to long-term immunity in microparticle-vaccinated animals [29, 37]. Various studies have demonstrated that PLG microparticles may perform pulsed and/or slow release of encapsulated antigens to promote effective immune responses [38]. The sustained and extended antigen release appears to substantially enhance and prolong antigen-specific immunity for achieving long-term protection [29, 31]. The antigen release from PLG microparticles is controlled by the degradation rate of PLG copolymer, which is largely due to the ratio of lactide to glycolide of PLG polymer, the molecular weight, and hydrophilicity of PLG polymer as well as the characteristics of PLG microparticles such as the morphology, size, and encapsulation efficiency [38]. The sustained antigen release of antigen-loaded PLG microparticles have been applied in the development of various potent microparticle vaccines [29, 31]. In addition, antigen-loaded PLG microparticles capable of sustaining release of an antigen also show potential for being designed as a single-dose vaccine without the need for booster doses [37, 39]. However, as some sophisticated events, including enhancement of protein load in PLG microparticles as well as optimization and stabilization of protein release are involved in the design of a single-dose vaccine [40], the feasibility needs to be assessed in future studies.

## 5. Encapsulation methods

The microparticles based on biodegradable PLG polymers can be prepared by number of methods, such as spray drying, double emulsion, and phase separation-coacervation [30]. However, the most widely used technique for preparation of protein-loaded microparticles is the double emulsion method [30].

The protein is encapsulated in 50:50 poly(lactide-co-glycolide) microparticles using the double emulsion method as described previously [41, 42], with minor modifications [22–24]. In the process, PLG polymer is first dissolved in an organic solvent. The organic solvent dichloromethane is mainly used to dissolve PLG polymer. Protein in aqueous solvent is then emulsified with nonmiscible organic solution of PLG polymer by high speed homogenization or sonication to produce a water/oil emulsion. The resulting emulsion is further transferred to a solution of polyvinyl alcohol, which is used as a stabilizer. Again homogenization or intensive stirring is necessary to generate a double emulsion of water/oil/water. The water/oil/water emulsion is then stirred for 18 h at room temperature (RT) and pressurized to promote solvent evaporation and microparticle formation in a laboratory fume hood. Solvent extraction can also be undertaken yielding microparticles containing protein. The microparticles are collected by centrifugation and washed with distilled water to remove nonentrapped protein.

Based on previous studies, proteins used for PLG encapsulation can be scaled down by using the water/oil/water double emulsion method [30]. In addition, this method also results in high microparticle yields and encapsulation efficiencies [30]. However, there is still a potential concern of antigen denaturation due to organic solvent exposure during the encapsulation process [41, 42], although numerous proteins have been successfully entrapped in PLG microparticles without loss of structural integrity, immunogenicity, or bioactivity [25, 30]. Especially, antigenicity retention following the process of double emulsion method is a critical event to subsequently initiate effective immunity by vaccinating antigen-loaded microparticles [30].

## 6. Preparation of *Toxoplasma* SAG-loaded microparticles

Development efforts of subunit vaccines against *T. gondii* in our laboratory have been focused mainly on the major immunodominant SAGs of tachyzoites [22–24, 43, 44], the rapidly multiplying stage during the acute phase infection. Furthermore, SAG1 and SAG2 proteins have been identified as two major tachyzoite SAGs in the previous study [45]. These two proteins are involved in the process of host cell invasion [46] and can induce anti *Toxoplasma* immune responses [6]. Therefore, both SAG1 and SAG2 can be considered as potential candidate antigens for *Toxoplasma* vaccine development. SAG1 gene, SAG2 gene, and a hybrid gene consisting of SAG1 and SAG2 sequences had been, respectively, cloned in our previous work to produce recombinant SAG1 (rSAG1) protein [22, 43], recombinant SAG2 (rSAG2) protein [23, 43], and a recombinant chimeric protein, rSAG1/2 [24, 43]. Further animal studies in mice demonstrated that rSAG1, rSAG2, or rSAG1/2 emulsified with an oil adjuvant, Vet L-10, induced partial protection against a lethal subcutaneous challenge of *T. gondii* tachyzoites [43]. If alternative effective adjuvants, such as the PLG polymer are used to make these recombinant proteins more immunogenic, more protective immunity against *T. gondii* may be achieved in animals.

In our recent work, rSAG1, rSAG2, or rSAG1/2 was then, respectively, encapsulated with the PLG polymer by using the double emulsion method for production of PLG-encapsulated rSAG1 (PLG-rSAG1) [22], PLG-encapsulated rSAG2 (PLG-rSAG2) [23], or PLG-encapsulated rSAG1/2 (PLG-rSAG1/2) microparticles [24]. Some microparticle characteristics, such as size (diameter), microparticle morphology, protein entrapment, and *in vitro* release were analyzed after PLG encapsulation (**Tables 1** and **2**). The morphological studies based on scanning electron microscopy showed that these microparticles are uniform population of spherical particles with a smooth surface. In addition, particle sizes of all three PLG microparticles in diameter were smaller than 10 μm (**Table 1**). Thus, the three PLG microparticles have an appropriate feature for direct uptake by APCs, such as macrophages and dendritic cells.

More importantly, the release of rSAG1, rSAG2, or rSAG1/2 from PLG microparticles was also analyzed (**Table 2**). We found that the *in vitro* cumulative release of rSAG1, rSAG2, and rSAG1/2 from PLG microparticles suspended in phosphate buffered saline (PBS) could be, respectively, sustained for 35, 33, and 56 days with three distinct phases consisting of an initial burst release, a very slow release, and a final rapid release (**Table 2**). Actually, based on previous critical investigations, such three-phase fluctuation in antigen release from PLG microparticles is due to the initial rapid diffusion of coated antigen on the PLG microparticle surface, the very slow and gradual diffusion of encapsulated antigen, and the final rapid diffusion of antigen because of the PLG microparticle degradation [47–49]. Furthermore, in the triphasic antigen release profile, both initial and final rapid release of entrapped antigen, respectively, look like priming and boosting doses usually employed in a conventional immunization procedure [49]. Thus, vaccination with a single dose of PLG-rSAG microparticles that are able to fulfill the triphasic rSAG release may be thought of as treating with two doses of rSAG protein. However, further improvements such as enhancement of protein load in PLG microparticles, as well as, optimization and stabilization of protein release are needed to evaluate the feasibility [40]. On the other hand, Western blotting assay with use of mouse monoclonal antibodies specific to tachyzoite SAGs demonstrated that released rSAG proteins from PLG microparticles still retained the original SAG antigenicity during the release from PLG microparticles [22–24]. These data indicate that both the encapsulation procedure and release from microparticles in our previous work are not detrimental to the antigenicity of

| Microparticle | Mean particle size (μm) | Entrapment efficiency (%) | Reference |
|---|---|---|---|
| PLG-rSAG1 | 4.25–6.58 | 69–81 | [22] |
| PLG-rSAG2 | 2.14–3.63 | 74–80 | [23] |
| PLG-rSAG1/2 | 1.27–1.65 | 72–83 | [24] |

**Table 1.** Particle size and entrapment efficiency of PLG-rSAG microparticles.

| Microparticle | Release protein | Release period | Release profile | Reference |
|---|---|---|---|---|
| PLG-rSAG1 | 87.8% rSAG1 | 35 days | Three phases | [22] |
| PLG-rSAG2 | 88.3% rSAG2 | 33 days | Three phases | [23] |
| PLG-rSAG1/2 | 88.5% rSAG1/2 | 56 days | Three phases | [24] |

**Table 2.** Release of rSAG from PLG microparticles.

rSAG. Thus, rSAG proteins have been successfully encapsulated with PLG polymers by the double emulsion method and the resulting PLG-rSAG microparticles not only properly preserved the SAG's antigenicity, but also sustained the controlled, stable release of the antigenic rSAG proteins from PLG microparticles. Based on these data, therefore, released rSAG proteins from PLG microparticles have the potential to induce anti SAG immune responses.

## 7. Protective immunity by *Toxoplasma* SAG-loaded microparticles

Although different adjuvants capable of improving immune responses and protection against *T. gondii* have been studied [6, 50], the biodegradable and biocompatible PLG polymers are so far seldom used as potent adjuvants for *Toxoplasma* vaccine development. Stanley and his coauthors first employed the double emulsion method to produce PLG-encapsulated microparticle vaccine against *T. gondii* [51]. In the same study, the PLG microparticle vaccine containing a tachyzoite extract plus a mucosal adjuvant, cholera toxin, failed to provide protection in sheep [51]. The unexpected protection in sheep indicates that more effort is therefore needed to improve not only the stability of encapsulated *Toxoplasma* antigens but also the immune responses and protection they induce in animals.

On the other hand, the adjuvant effects of the PLG encapsulation had been exercised to, respectively, prepare PLG-rSAG1, PLG-rSAG2, and PLG-rSAG1/2 microparticles in our three previous studies [22–24]. The ability of these PLG-rSAG microparticles to trigger protective immunity against *T. gondii* was subsequently evaluated in BALB/c mice by vaccination through the intraperitoneal route. Results showed that both PLG-rSAG1 and PLG-rSAG1/2 microparticles effectively induced not only significant long-lasting (10 weeks) specific humoral and cell-mediated immune responses, accompanied by secretion of a large amount of IFN-γ, but also high protection (80% for PLG-rSAG1 microparticles and 83% for PLG-rSAG1/2 microparticles) against *T. gondii* tachyzoite infection [22, 24]. However, PLG-rSAG2 microparticles could induce sustained (10 weeks) lymphocyte proliferation and IFN-γ production [23]. Furthermore, after a lethal subcutaneous challenge of $1 \times 10^4$ *T. gondii* tachyzoites (RH strain), PLG-rSAG2 microparticles also improved anti *Toxoplasma* protection (87%) [23], which is higher, though not statistically significant, than either 80% of PLG-rSAG1 microparticles [22] or 83% of PLG-rSAG1/2 microparticles [24].

As *T. gondii* is an obligate intracellular parasite, protective immunity to *T. gondii* is largely mediated by Th1 cell-mediated immunity [6, 7]. Previous studies have shown that induction of both lymphocyte proliferation and IFN-γ production (one of Th1-type cytokines) positively correlates with protective Th1 cell-mediated immunity against *T. gondii* [43, 44, 51]. In addition, IFN-γ has been demonstrated to be a critical mediator that has to be secreted for as long as possible in order to maintain anti *Toxoplasma* immunity [52, 53]. We found that sustained lymphocyte proliferation and significant IFN-γ production readily detected in mice immunized with PLG-rSAG microparticles in our previous studies [22–24]. These findings indicate that immunization with PLG-rSAG microparticles really elicits the IFN-γ-associated Th1 cell-mediated immunity, which is the expected response that we aimed to induce in mice.

Based on previous studies, PLG microparticles appear to favorably facilitate a size-dependent interaction with APCs, such as macrophages and dendritic cells [32–34]. The particles, like PLG-rSAG microparticles prepared in our previous studies (**Table 1**), smaller than 10 μm in diameter are directly taken by APCs [32]. Based on our previous results, the proper size range thus could stimulate peritoneal macrophages to facilitate the uptake of these PLG-rSAG microparticles administered in the mouse peritoneal cavity [22–24]. Therefore, the microparticle-containing macrophages in the peritoneal cavity then traveled to other lymphoid compartments, including the spleen, and effectively presented SAG epitopes to Th1 and Tc; thereby, inducing strong SAG-specific Th1 cell-mediated immunity to protect mice from the tachyzoite challenge. Our previous studies [22–24] and those recorded by others [32–34] have shown that facilitation of uptake and delivery of PLG-rSAG microparticles by macrophages can lead to more effective antigen processing and presentation to T lymphocytes capable of inducting cell-mediated immunity. Thus, the high survival rates in mice have demonstrated that PLG-rSAG microparticles effectively elicit protective Th1 cell-mediated immunity to remove tachyzoite-infected cells for limiting parasite dissemination during the experimental tachyzoite challenge [7].

In addition to Th1-dependent cell-mediated immunity, in our previous studies, high titers of anti *Toxoplasma* IgG in mouse sera elicited by PLG-rSAG microparticles have indicated that systemic humoral immunity mediated by Th2 may participate in the prevention of *T. gondii* infection [54, 55]. However, further measurements by the dye test are still needed to assay these antibodies to elucidate their functional lytic activities. Therefore, peritoneal vaccination of mice with PLG-rSAG microparticles may generate mixed Th1/Th2 immunity against *T. gondii*.

## 8. Conclusions and future prospects

PLG polymers are the primary candidates for the development of microparticle vaccines [25]. The rSAG proteins (rSAG1, rSAG2, and rSAG1/2) prepared in our laboratory have been successfully encapsulated with PLG polymers to generate PLG-rSAG microparticles capable of sustaining long-term stable release of antigenic rSAG proteins. Moreover, following peritoneal immunization in mice, PLG-rSAG microparticles induce not only long-term (10 weeks) SAG-specific humoral and cell-mediated immune responses, but also high protection against a lethal challenge of *T. gondii* tachyzoites [22–24]. Our studies provide a valuable basis for developing long-lasting vaccines against *T. gondii* for future use in humans and animals. Our experimental data indicate that the encapsulation procedure we used for production of PLG-rSAG microparticles is feasible at the laboratory level. However, this procedure have never been used to try mass production of PLG-rSAG microparticles. More effort is therefore needed to evaluate the optimized encapsulation conditions used to fulfill the need for mass production [40].

The PLG-rSAG microparticles we prepared previously could allow the sustained and extended release of rSAG proteins over a long period. Such long-term release of rSAG proteins could repeatedly stimulate the immune effector cells to maintain enhanced immunity following immunization with PLG-rSAG microparticles [29, 37]. However, the triphasic rSAG release detected in the cumulative release assay we carried out in the previous studies was done *in vitro* in PBS and; therefore, may not completely reflect *in vivo* release in mice [22–24]. Further studies are therefore needed to confirm the critical effect of triphasic rSAG release on *in vivo* anti *Toxoplasma* immune responses.

One adjuvant effect acted by PLG microparticle vaccines is to facilitate antigen uptake via APCs [25, 32, 33]. Different APCs populated in various administrating routes are able to perform the uptake of antigen-loaded PLG microparticles and then process and present the epitopes of PLG-encapsulated antigen on the major histocompatibility (MHC) molecules [32]. Therefore, different routes of delivery of antigen-loaded PLG microparticles give rise to different vaccine efficacy in animals [32]. The mouse protective immunity induced by intraperitoneally administered PLG-rSAG microparticles protected mice from a lethal subcutaneous challenge of *T. gondii* tachyzoites. However, such intraperitoneal administration of the microparticle vaccine appears to be inappropriate for use in large animals such as sheep or swine. In order to corroborate the conclusions drawn from the mouse model, more studies are needed to evaluate the proper route for administration of PLG-rSAG microparticles in target animals. In addition, due to the natural infection initiated by ingesting oocysts released in cat feces or consuming meat from infected animals containing the long-lived tissue cysts, future experiments will also be necessary to assess whether mucosal administration (oral or nasal route) of PLG-rSAG microparticles protects these animals from an oral challenge of oocysts or tissue cysts of *T. gondii*.

## Author details

Chung-Da Yang

Address all correspondence to: cdyang@mail.npust.edu.tw

Graduate Institute of Animal Vaccine Technology, College of Veterinary Medicine, National Pingtung University of Science and Technology, Pingtung, Taiwan

## References

[1] Hill D, Dubey JP. *Toxoplasma gondii*: Transmission, diagnosis and prevention. Clinical Microbiology and Infection. 2002;**8**(10):634-640. DOI: http://dx.doi.org/10.1046/j.1469-0691.2002.00485.x

[2] Dubey JP. The history of *Toxoplasma gondii*–the first 100 years. The Journal of Eukaryotic Microbiology. 2008;**55**(6):467-475. DOI: 10.1111/j.1550-7408.2008.00345.x

[3] Kravetz JD, Federman DG. Toxoplasmosis in pregnancy. American Journal of Medicine. 2005;**118**(3):212-216. DOI: S0002-9343(04)00700-4 [pii]

[4] Contini C. Clinical and diagnostic management of toxoplasmosis in the immunocompromised patient. Parassitologia. 2008;**50**(1–2):45-50.

[5] Buxton D. Toxoplasmosis: The first commercial vaccine. Parasitology Today. 1993;**9**(9): 335-337. DOI: 0169-4758(93)90236-9 [pii]

[6] Jongert E, Roberts CW, Gargano N, Forster-Waldl E, Petersen E. Vaccines against *Toxoplasma gondii*: Challenges and opportunities. Memórias do Instituto Oswaldo Cruz. 2009;**104**(2):252-266. DOI: http://dx.doi.org/10.1590/S0074-02762009000200019

[7] Jongert E, Lemiere A, Van Ginderachter J, De Craeye S, Huygen K, D'Souza S. Functional characterization of in vivo effector CD4(+) and CD8(+) T cell responses in acute toxoplasmosis: An interplay of IFN-gamma and cytolytic T cells. Vaccine. 2010;**28**(13):2556-2564. DOI: 10.1016/j.vaccine.2010.01.031

[8] Innes EA, Bartley PM, Maley S, Katzer F, Buxton D. Veterinary vaccines against *Toxoplasma gondii*. Memórias do Instituto Oswaldo Cruz. 2009;**104**(2):246-251. DOI: http://dx.doi.org/10.1590/S0074-02762009000200018

[9] Nascimento IP, Leite LC. Recombinant vaccines and the development of new vaccine strategies. Brazilian Journal of Medical and Biological Research. 2012;**45**(12):1102-1111.

[10] Schijns VE, Lavelle EC. Trends in vaccine adjuvants. Expert Review of Vaccines. 2011;**10**(4):539-550. DOI: 10.1586/erv.11.21

[11] Spickler AR, Roth JA. Adjuvants in veterinary vaccines: Modes of action and adverse effects. Journal of Veterinary Internal Medicine. 2003;**17**(3):273-281. DOI: 10.1111/j.1939-1676.2003.tb02448.x

[12] Wilson-Welder JH, Torres MP, Kipper MJ, Mallapragada SK, Wannemuehler MJ, Narasimhan B. Vaccine adjuvants: Current challenges and future approaches. Journal of Pharmaceutical Sciences. 2009;**98**(4):1278-1316. DOI: 10.1002/jps.21523

[13] Tomljenovic L, Shaw CA. Aluminum vaccine adjuvants: Are they safe? Current Medicinal Chemistry. 2011;**18**(17):2630-2637. DOI: 10.2174/092986711795933740

[14] O'Hagan DT, MacKichan ML, Singh M. Recent developments in adjuvants for vaccines against infectious diseases. Biomolecular Engineering. 2001;**18**(3):69-85. DOI: S1389-0344(01)00101-0 [pii]

[15] Singh M, O'Hagan DT. Recent advances in veterinary vaccine adjuvants. International Journal of Parasitology. 2003;**33**(5–6):469-478. DOI: S0020751903000535 [pii]

[16] Schijns VE, Strioga M, Ascarateil S. Oil-based emulsion vaccine adjuvants. Current Protocols in Immunology. 2014;**106**(2):181-187. DOI: 10.1002/0471142735.im0218s106

[17] Malyala P, Singh M. Micro/nanoparticle adjuvants: Preparation and formulation with antigens. Methods in Molecular Biology. 2010;**626**:91-101. DOI: 10.1007/978-1-60761-585-9_7

[18] Kersten GF, Crommelin DJ. Liposomes and ISCOMs. Vaccine. 2003;**21**(9–10):915-920. DOI: http://dx.doi.org/10.1016/S0264-410X(02)00540-6

[19] Thompson BS, Chilton PM, Ward JR, Evans JT, Mitchell TC. The low-toxicity versions of LPS, MPL adjuvant and RC529, are efficient adjuvants for CD4+ T cells. Journal of Leukocyte Biology. 2005;**78**(6):1273-1280. DOI: 10.1189/jlb.0305172

[20] Kaur T, Thakur A, Kaur S. Protective immunity using MPL-A and autoclaved *Leishmania donovani* as adjuvants along with a cocktail vaccine in murine model of visceral leishmaniasis. Journal of Parasitic Diseases. 2013;**37**(2):231-239. DOI: 10.1007/s12639-012-0171-7

[21] Rothenfusser S, Tuma E, Wagner M, Endres S, Hartmann G. Recent advances in immunostimulatory CpG oligonucleotides. Current Opinion in Molecular Therapeutics. 2003;**5**(2):98-106.

[22] Chuang SC, Ko JC, Chen CP, Du JT, Yang CD. Induction of long-lasting protective immunity against *Toxoplasma gondii* in BALB/c mice by recombinant surface antigen 1 protein encapsulated in poly (lactide-co-glycolide) microparticles. Parasites & Vectors. 2013;**6**:34. DOI: 10.1186/1756-3305-6-34

[23] Chuang SC, Yang CD. Sustained release of recombinant surface antigen 2 (rSAG2) from poly(lactide-co-glycolide) microparticles extends protective cell-mediated immunity against *Toxoplasma gondii* in mice. Parasitology. 2014;**141**(12):1657-1666. DOI: 10.1017/S0031182014000997

[24] Chuang SC, Ko JC, Chen CP, Du JT, Yang CD. Encapsulation of chimeric protein rSAG1/2 into poly(lactide-co-glycolide) microparticles induces long-term protective immunity against *Toxoplasma gondii* in mice. Experimental Parasitology. 2013;**134**(4):430-437. DOI: 10.1016/j.exppara.2013.04.002

[25] Heegaard PM, Dedieu L, Johnson N, Le Potier MF, Mockey M, Mutinelli F, Vahlenkamp T, Vascellari M, Sorensen NS. Adjuvants and delivery systems in veterinary vaccinology: Current state and future developments. Archives of Virology. 2011;**156**(2):183-202. DOI: 10.1007/s00705-010-0863-1

[26] Ulery BD, Nair LS, Laurencin CT. Biomedical applications of biodegradable polymers. Journal of Polymer Science Part B: Polymer Physics. 2011;**49**(12):832-864. DOI: 10.1002/polb.22259

[27] Tiwari G, Tiwari R, Sriwastawa B, Bhati L, Pandey S, Pandey P, Bannerjee SK. Drug delivery systems: An updated review. International Journal of Pharmaceutical Investigation. 2012;**2**(1):2-11. DOI: 10.4103/2230-973X.96920

[28] Eldridge JH, Staas JK, Meulbroek JA, McGhee JR, Tice TR, Gilley RM. Biodegradable microspheres as a vaccine delivery system. Molecular Immunology. 1991;**28**(3):287-294. DOI: http://dx.doi.org/10.1016/0161-5890(91)90076-V

[29] Jain S, O'Hagan DT, Singh M. The long-term potential of biodegradable poly(lactide-co-glycolide) microparticles as the next-generation vaccine adjuvant. Expert Review of Vaccines. 2011;**10**(12):1731-1742. DOI: 10.1586/erv.11.126

[30] Sinha VR, Trehan A. Biodegradable microspheres for protein delivery. Journal of Controlled Release. 2003;**90**(3):261-280. DOI: http://dx.doi.org/10.1016/S0168-3659(03)00194-9

[31] Lim TY, Poh CK, Wang W. Poly (lactic-co-glycolic acid) as a controlled release delivery device. Journal of Materials Science. Materials in Medicine. 2009;**20**(8):1669-1675. DOI: 10.1007/s10856-009-3727-z

[32] Newman KD, Elamanchili P, Kwon GS, Samuel J. Uptake of poly(D,L-lactic-co-glycolic acid) microspheres by antigen-presenting cells *in vivo*. Journal of Biomedial Materials Research. 2002;**60**(3):480-486. DOI: 10.1002/jbm.10019

[33] Men Y, Audran R, Thomasin C, Eberl G, Demotz S, Merkle HP, Gander B, Corradin G. MHC class I- and class II-restricted processing and presentation of microencapsulated antigens. Vaccine. 1999;**17**(9–10):1047-1056. DOI: http://dx.doi.org/10.1016/S0264-410X(98)00321-1

[34] Luzardo-Alvarez A, Blarer N, Peter K, Romero JF, Reymond C, Corradin G, Gander B. Biodegradable microspheres alone do not stimulate murine macrophages in vitro, but prolong antigen presentation by macrophages *in vitro* and stimulate a solid immune response in mice. Journal of Controlled Release. 2005;**109**(1–3):62-76. DOI: 10.1016/j.jconrel.2005.09.015

[35] Vajdy M, O'Hagan DT. Microparticles for intranasal immunization. Advanced Drug Delivery Reviews. 2001;**51**(1–3):127-141. DOI: http://dx.doi.org/10.1016/S0169-409X(01)00167-3

[36] McNeela EA, Lavelle EC. Recent advances in microparticle and nanoparticle delivery vehicles for mucosal vaccination. Current Topics in Microbiology and Immunology. 2012;**354**:75-99. DOI: 10.1007/82_2011_140

[37] Gupta RK, Singh M, O'Hagan DT. Poly(lactide-co-glycolide) microparticles for the development of single-dose controlled-release vaccines. Advanced Drug Delivery Reviews. 1998;**32**(3):225-246. DOI: http://dx.doi.org/10.1016/S0169-409X(98)00012-X

[38] Raman C, Berkland C, Kim K, Pack DW. Modeling small-molecule release from PLG microspheres: Effects of polymer degradation and nonuniform drug distribution. Journal of Controlled Release. 2005;**103**(1):149-158. DOI: http://dx.doi.org/10.1016/j.jconrel.2004.11.012

[39] He XW, Wang F, Jiang L, Li J, Liu SK, Xiao ZY, Jin XQ, Zhang YN, He Y, Li K et al. Induction of mucosal and systemic immune response by single-dose oral immunization with biodegradable microparticles containing DNA encoding HBsAg. Journal of General Virology. 2005;**86**(Pt 3):601-610. DOI: 10.1099/vir.0.80575-0

[40] Ye M, Kim S, Park K. Issues in long-term protein delivery using biodegradable microparticles. Journal of Controlled Release. 2010;**146**(2):241-260. DOI: 10.1016/j.jconrel.2010.05.011

[41] Jeffery H, Davis SS, O'Hagan DT. The preparation and characterization of poly (lactide-co-glycolide) microparticles. II. The entrapment of a model protein using

a (water-in-oil)-in-water emulsion solvent evaporation technique. Pharmaceutical Research. 1993;**10**(3):362-368. DOI: 10.1023/A:1018980020506

[42] Ghaderi R, Carlfors J. Biological activity of lysozyme after entrapment in poly(d,l-lactide-co-glycolide)-microspheres. Pharmaceutical Research. 1997;**14**(11):1556-1562. DOI: 10.1023/A:1012122200381

[43] Yang CD, Chang GN, Chao D. Protective immunity against *Toxoplasma gondii* in mice induced by a chimeric protein rSAG1/2. Parasitology Research. 2004;**92**(1):58-64. DOI: 10.1007/s00436-003-0992-5

[44] Yang CD, Chang GN, Chao D. Protective immunity against *Toxoplasma gondii* in mice induced by the SAG2 internal image of anti-idiotype antibody. Parasitology Research. 2003;**91**(6):452-457. DOI: 10.1007/s00436-003-1006-3

[45] Couvreur G, Sadak A, Fortier B, Dubremetz JF. Surface antigens of *Toxoplasma gondii*. Parasitology. 1988;**97**(Pt 1):1-10. DOI: https://doi.org/10.1017/S0031182000066695

[46] Grimwood J, Smith JE. *Toxoplasma gondii*: The role of parasite surface and secreted proteins in host cell invasion. International Journal of Parasitology. 1996;**26**(2):169-173. DOI: 0020-7519(95)00103-4 [pii]

[47] Kavanagh OV, Earley B, Murray M, Foster CJ, Adair BM. Antigen-specific IgA and IgG responses in calves inoculated intranasally with ovalbumin encapsulated in poly(DL-lactide-co-glycolide) microspheres. Vaccine. 2003;**21**(27–30):4472-4480. DOI: http://dx.doi.org/10.1016/S0264-410X(03)00432-8

[48] Sturesson C, Carlfors J. Incorporation of protein in PLG-microspheres with retention of bioactivity. Journal of Controlled Release. 2000;**67**(2–3):171-178. DOI: S0168365900002054 [pii]

[49] Uchida M, Natsume H, Kishino T, Seki T, Ogihara M, Juni K, Kimura M, Morimoto Y. Immunization by particle bombardment of antigen-loaded poly-(DL-lactide-co-glycolide) microspheres in mice. Vaccine. 2006;**24**(12):2120-2130. DOI: 10.1016/j.vaccine.2005.11.027

[50] Lim SS, Othman RY. Recent advances in *Toxoplasma gondii* immunotherapeutics. Korean Journal of Parasitology. 2014;**52**(6):581-593. DOI: 10.3347/kjp.2014.52.6.581

[51] Stanley AC, Buxton D, Innes EA, Huntley JF. Intranasal immunisation with *Toxoplasma gondii* tachyzoite antigen encapsulated into PLG microspheres induces humoral and cell-mediated immunity in sheep. Vaccine. 2004;**22**(29-30):3929-3941. DOI: 10.1016/j.vaccine.2004.04.022

[52] Subauste CS, Remington JS. Immunity to *Toxoplasma gondii*. Current Opinion in Immunology. 1993;**5**(4):532-537. DOI: http://dx.doi.org/10.1016/0952-7915(93)90034-P

[53] Casciotti L, Ely KH, Williams ME, Khan IA. CD8(+)-T-cell immunity against *Toxoplasma gondii* can be induced but not maintained in mice lacking conventional CD4(+) T cells. Infection and Immunity. 2002;**70**(2):434-443. DOI: 10.1128/IAI.70.2.434–443.2002

[54] Johnson LL, Sayles PC. Deficient humoral responses underlie susceptibility to *Toxoplasma gondii* in CD4-deficient mice. Infection and Immunity. 2002;**70**(1):185-191. DOI: 10.1128/IAI.70.1.185–191.2002

[55] Kang H, Remington JS, Suzuki Y. Decreased resistance of B cell-deficient mice to infection with *Toxoplasma gondii* despite unimpaired expression of IFN-gamma, TNF-alpha, and inducible nitric oxide synthase. The Journal of Immunology. 2000;**164**(5):2629-2634. DOI: ji_v164n5p2629 [pii]

# 8

# *Toxoplasma gondii* Tissue Cyst: Cyst Wall Incorporation Activity and Matrix Cytoskeleton Proteins Paving the Way to Nutrient Acquisition

Mariana Acquarone,
Marialice da F. Ferreira-da-Silva,
Erick V. Guimarães and Helene S. Barbosa

**Abstract**

*Toxoplasma gondii* is an intracellular parasite that causes chronic infection by the development of bradyzoites housed in tissue cysts, preferably in the muscles and central nervous system. The composition and the function of the cyst wall are still not fully understood. Are *T. gondii* cysts able to incorporate nutrients through its wall? If so, how would these nutrients be traversed to cross the cyst matrix to reach the bradyzoite forms? Herein, we tested the uptake capacity of the Toxoplasma tissue cyst wall by employing some fluid-phase endocytosis tracers as peroxidase (HRP) and bovine serum albumin (BSA). Fluorescence images revealed these molecules on the cyst wall as well as in the cyst matrix. The subcellular localization of the tracer was confirmed by ultrastructural analysis showing numerous labeled vesicles and tubules distributed within the cyst matrix in close association with intracystic bradyzoite membrane, suggesting the cyst wall as a route of nutrient uptake. Furthermore, we confirmed the presence of cytoskeleton proteins, such as tubulin, actin, and myosin, in the tissue cyst matrix that may explain the nutrient input mechanism through the cyst wall. A better understanding of the nutrient acquisition process by the cyst might potentially contribute to the development of new therapeutic targets against chronic toxoplasmosis.

**Keywords:** *Toxoplasma gondii*, tissue cysts, endocytosis, macromolecules, cytoskeleton

## 1. Introduction

Toxoplasmosis is a worldwide human protozoan infection caused by an intracellular protozoan, *Toxoplasma gondii.* Characterized by the presence of slow replicative bradyzoites surrounded by a thick wall, the tissue cysts have a striking predilection for infecting the central nervous system and skeletal muscle cells of the host [1]. It is widely accepted that the chronic phase of the disease in an immunologically competent person is normally asymptomatic and self-resolving. However, *T. gondii* has been associated with an increase in the incidence of many relevant psychiatric disorders. This relates to the fact that the brain is an immune-privileged site for lifelong existence of *T. gondii* tissue cysts [2]. Although the current pharmacological treatments have been ineffective against the cyst form, it is possible that the tissue cyst wall acts as a biological barrier preventing the interaction of drugs with intracystic bradyzoites [3].

Despite the clinical relevance of chronic toxoplasmosis, the biology of the cyst wall as yet has not been completely elucidated [4–9]. A 116-kDa glycoprotein termed CST1 [7] and two lectins, *Dolichos biflorus* and succinylated wheat-germ agglutinin, that bind specifically to the cyst wall, were identified, and it was suggested that chitin probably represents an important component of the cyst wall [10]. There are few evidences of the composition of the cyst matrix. Parmley et al. [11] described a cyst matrix antigen named MAG1, which was also found inside the parasitophorous vacuole matrix, forming a filamentous-like protein material.

Our previous ultrastructural analysis demonstrated that the cyst wall displays endocytic activity through the engulfing of negatively charged molecules in the cystic wall [3]. These molecules are incorporated by tubules and vesicles formed from the membrane that delimits the cyst wall and localized in the granular region and posteriorly in the cyst matrix. Within the cyst, the presence of vesicles containing the tracer in close contact to the bradyzoite membrane or in its neighborhood suggests that it could be one of the incorporated molecule pathways from the host cell cytoplasm to intracystic parasites [8]. The current knowledge of mechanisms involved in the process of nutrient uptake by this parasite still presents many gaps, restricted to few reports [12, 13]. As an obligate intracellular parasite, *T. gondii* actively invades and replicates in a wide variety of nucleated vertebrate cells where it resides in a parasitophorous vacuole. The ultrastructural analysis also demonstrated that *T. gondii* is able to invade host cell nuclei, and this invasion could reflect an alternative parasite route for immune evasion or may be a nutrient source when scarce in the host cell cytoplasm [14]. The vacuole membrane is the interface between the host and parasite, playing a role in the nutrient acquisition from the host cell by the parasite. The physiological significance of the endocytosis in the *T. gondii* lifestyle with tachyzoite forms is in the incipient stages of elucidation [15, 16], as the basic mechanisms delineating endocytosis in tachyzoites, bradyzoites, and tissue cysts are still poorly understood [17].

In all eukaryotes, endocytosis and intracellular vesicle traffic are events mediated by several proteins including a complex cytoskeleton network. Cytoskeleton proteins are indispensable components of a number of vital parasite structures and functions, like cell division, membrane and cytoplasmic architectures, parasite gliding motility (glideosome), and host-cell invasion [18–20]. Besides conventional cytoskeleton elements, many components of *T. gondii* are novel proteins. Two examples are Actin-Like Protein 1 (ALP1), which plays a role during cell division [21], and a protein called TgSIP, a structural cytoskeleton component of the parasite inner membrane complex [22].

Herein, the putative mechanisms employed by *T. gondii* cysts involved in nutrient incorporation and the cytoskeletal protein network in the tissue cysts were investigated, which could explain the endocytic activity of the tissue cyst wall and vesicle traffic in the cyst matrix. The endocytosis process and the cytoskeleton network are crucial to *T. gondii* replication, motility, invasion, and maintenance, indicative as excellent drug targets for antiparasitic therapies.

## 2. Experimental design

### 2.1. Parasites

Mice infected with ME-49 strain *T. gondii* and maintained for 4–8 weeks in C57BL/6 were euthanized and the brain cysts isolated as described [23]. License CEUA LW 50/14 from Fundação Oswaldo Cruz Committee of Ethics for Use of Animals was authorized.

### 2.2. Endocytosis assays

Cysts were incubated with bovine serum albumin (BSA) labeled with fluorescein isothiocyanate (BSA-FITC), a fluid phase endocytic tracer, for 2 or 3 h at 37°C and processed for analysis in a confocal laser scanning microscopy FV300/BX51 Olympus and differential interference contrast (DIC) microscopy. Serial optical sections of each cyst incubated with BSA-FITC were converted into a volume performing 3D reconstruction. Additionally, the ultrastructural analysis was performed with two fluid phase endocytic tracers, BSA and peroxidase (HRP), both conjugated with colloidal gold (Au) particles.

### 2.3. Identification of cytoskeleton proteins

Brain cryosections of *T. gondii*-infected mice as well as *ex vivo*-isolated tissue cysts (pre-fixed with 4% PFA) were processed for immunolabeling. Briefly, the samples were incubated with polyclonal primary antibodies (anti-actin 1:500, anti-tubulin 1:200, anti-myosin 1:200, and microtubule-associated proteins (MAPs) 1:200), followed by incubation in CY3-conjugated secondary antibody (goat anti-rabbit IgG, 1:1000) and processed for fluorescence microscopy analysis. Control samples were processed omitting primary antibodies. Brains of uninfected animals were the controls for the experiment.

## 3. Results

### 3.1. *T. gondii* is able to incorporate macromolecules through the tissue cyst wall

*T. gondii* tissue cysts incubated for 2 or 3 h with BSA-FITC at 37°C were analyzed by DIC and confocal microscopy, **Figure 1A–C** and **D–F**, respectively. The BSA-FITC presented a strong

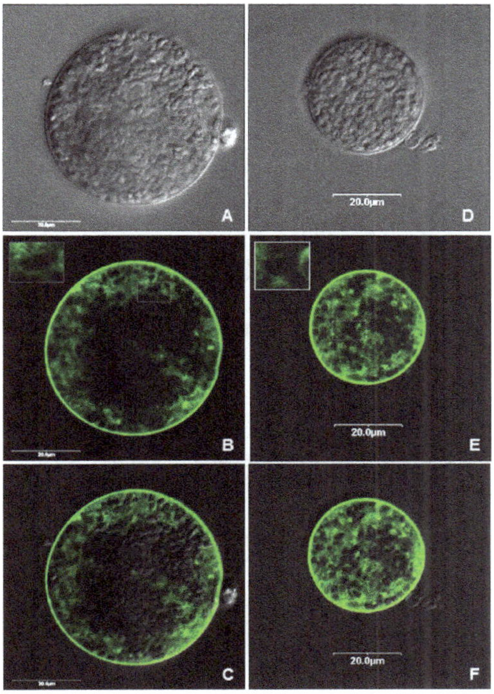


**Figure 1.** Confocal microscopy of *Toxoplasma* cyst incubated with BSA-FITC. (A–C) *Toxoplasma gondii* tissue cyst incubated at 37°C for 2 h and (D–F) 3 h with BSA-FITC. (A and D) Interferential microscopy (DIC) showing the cyst wall and numerous parasites inside the cyst. (B and E) Cyst fluorescence microscopy after 2 and 3 h of BSA-FITC incubation showing the tracer in the matrix, fulfilling the free spaces between the bradyzoites and throughout the cyst wall. (C and F) Overlay of fluorescence and DIC images showing the matrix and cyst wall labeled with BSA-FITC. Note that the cysts incubated for 3 h presented higher tracer incorporation. Scale bars: 20 μm.

labeling throughout the cyst wall and also located in the cyst matrix between the intracyst bradyzoites (**Figure 1B**, **C**, **E**, and **F**). These features were reinforced by merge obtained from DIC and fluorescence images (**Figure 1C** and **F**). The incorporation of BSA-FITC by tissue cysts was time dependent (**Figure 1C** and **F**). During the 3D reconstruction performance of a whole cyst from a set of 351 serial sections of 0.3 μm thickness, cyst wall transparency was strategically maintained in order to permit the visualization of the intracystic tracer (Video 1, supplementary material).

### 3.2. Ultrastructural analysis confirmed distinct molecule incorporation through the cyst wall

In order to examine whether the predicted protein labeling was in fact throughout the cyst wall, an ultrastructural analysis was conducted, incubating cysts with electron dense tracers, such as BSA-Au and HRP-Au. The incubation for 30 min at 4°C with BSA-Au revealed the marker at the surface as well as within invaginations of the cyst wall (**Figure 2A**). The internalization of BSA-Au occurred after 2 or 4 h of incubation at 37°C. Colloidal gold particles could be found within small vesicles and tubules localized at the granular region independent of the time of BSA-Au incubation (**Figure 2B** and **C**).

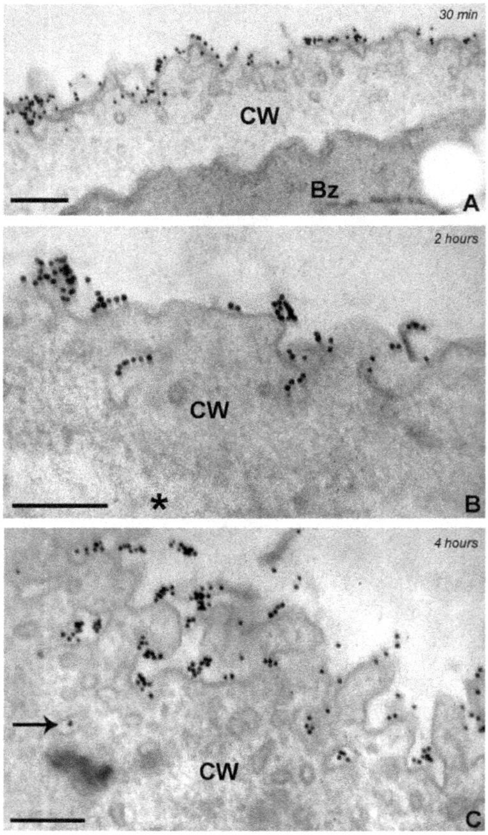


**Figure 2.** Transmission electron microscopy of *Toxoplasma gondii* cysts incubated with BSA-Au. (A) Tissue cyst presents many BSA-Au particles on cyst wall membrane after incubation for 30 min at 4°C. (B) Tissue cysts incubated for 2 h at 37°C displaying gold particles lining the cyst wall membrane and within the cyst membrane invaginations. (C) Tissue cysts incubated for 4 h at 37°C present BSA-Au particles in the uncoated vesicles and within tubules full of particles (arrow). Scale bars: 0.2 μm.

Similar results were obtained with HRP-Au by incubation of tissue cysts for 30 min at 4°C (**Figure 3A**). When the temperature was elevated to 37°C, the HRP-Au particles were observed within uncoated vesicles and tubules localized in the granular region of the cyst (**Figure 3B** and **C**).

### 3.3. Tissue cysts display a cytoskeleton network both in vivo and ex vivo

Aiming to reveal the cytoskeletal proteins in *T. gondii* tissue cysts, immunofluorescence assays were carried out with different polyclonal antibodies. Anti-myosin demonstrated the protein in

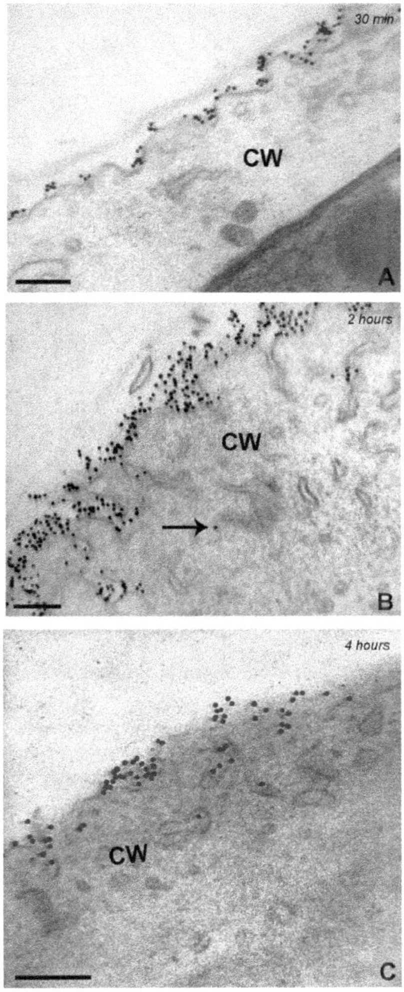


**Figure 3.** Transmission electron microscopy of *Toxoplasma* cyst incubated with Au-HRP. (A) Tissue cyst incubated for 18 h at 37°C with HRP-Au displaying gold particles lining the cyst membrane (arrow) and within the cyst membrane invaginations (large arrow). Scale bar: 0.2 μm. (B) Cysts present different regions of their surface with the distribution of HRP-Au (arrows) lining the cyst wall followed by spaces without any labeling. Absence of the marker in the cyst interior. Scale bar: 0.5 μm.

the cyst matrix as a diffuse staining and on the tissue cyst wall as intense heterogeneous fluorescent dots (**Figure 4A–C**). Brain cryosections from C57BL/6 mice chronically infected with *T. gondii* were incubated with the anti-myosin antibody, revealing that the distribution in tissue cysts *in vivo* followed the same pattern as *in vitro* (**Figure 4D** and E). For positive control, bradyzoites were incubated with the same antibody, and the myosin was localized mainly at the anterior pole (conoid region) or diffused through the parasite plasma membrane and cytosol (**Figure 4F**).

DIC microscopy (**Figure 5A**) and the immunofluorescence with the anti-tubulin antibody revealed a homogeneous labeling along the cyst wall in an area correspondent to the

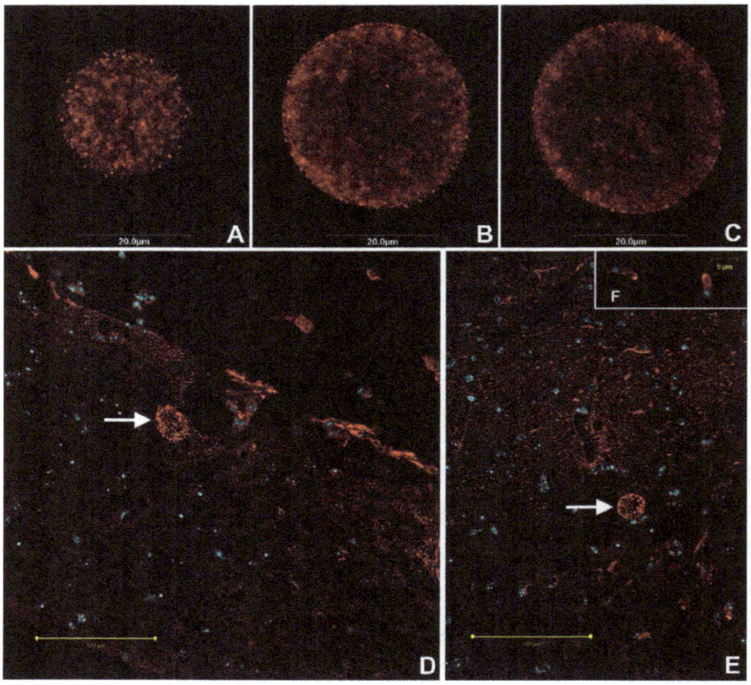

Figure 4. Immunofluorescence for detection of myosin in *T. gondii* tissue cysts. (A–C) Different confocal sections of the same isolated tissue cyst show that myosin was located along the tissue cyst wall with a dotted distribution, and the labeling was seen inside parasites as well. Scale bars: 20 μm. (D) Cryosection of a chronically infected brain showed that *in vivo* the tissue cyst wall had the same myosin distribution pattern as *in vitro*. (E) Different brain area labeled for myosin. Scale bars: 100 μm. (F) Positive control of myosin staining in *T. gondii* bradyzoites confirms the localization of the protein at the anterior pole and associated with the plasma membrane, similarly as described for tachyzoites. Scale bar: 5 μm.

granular region (**Figure 5B**). This intense wall labeling was better visualized in the merged figure (**Figure 5C**). Different virtual confocal sections of the same cyst disclosed the presence of tubulin inside bradyzoites (**Figure 5D–I**). In *T. gondii* chronically infected brains, the pattern of tubulin distribution was the same as in isolated tissue cysts (**Figure 6A**). In bradyzoites, tubulin was strongly labeled in the region corresponding to the subpellicular microtubules (**Figure 6B**), conferring the typical elongated shape of the parasite and the apical polarity of apicomplexan phylum. Microtubule-associated proteins (MAPs) form bridges linking with themselves and other structures. Tissue cysts in infected brain cryosections incubated with the anti-MAPs antibody colocalize with tubulin distribution (**Figure 6C** and **D**).

The most intense fluorescence labeling was for actin detection in *T. gondii* tissue cysts with homogeneous distribution along the cyst wall of isolated cysts (**Figure 7A**), presenting the same pattern of labeling as in the infected brain cryosections (**Figure 7B**). The revelation of actin inside the cyst (**Figure 7A**) suggested the detection of bradyzoites. To confirm this distribution, isolated bradyzoites were incubated with the same antibody, the labeling apparent on the conoid and extending below the apical region of the parasite body (**Figure 7C**).

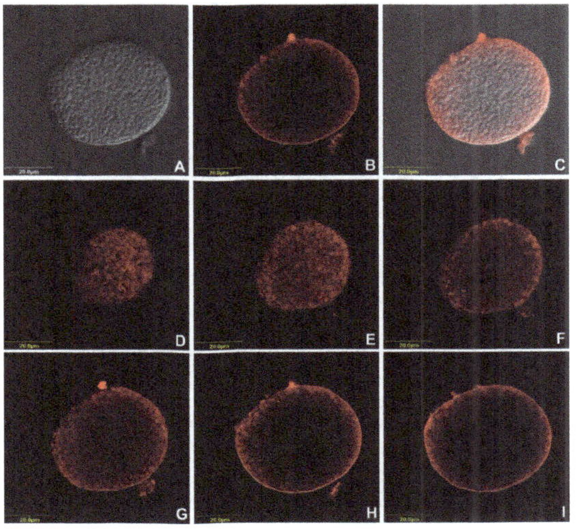


**Figure 5.** Immunofluorescence for detection of tubulin in *T. gondii* tissue cysts. (A) DIC microscopy, (B) fluorescence, and (C) a merge of figures A and B of an isolated tissue cyst labeling for tubulin detection showed an intense and homogeneous staining around the tissue cyst wall as well as parasite staining. (D–I) Different confocal sections of the same isolated tissue cyst confirm this distribution. Scale bars: 20 μm.

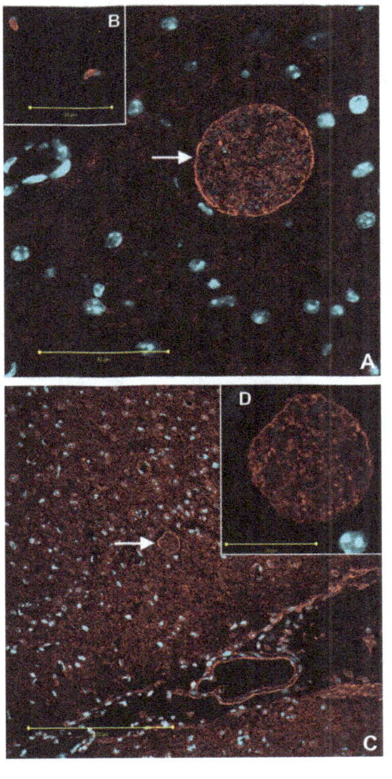


**Figure 6.** Immunofluorescence for detection of tubulin and microtubule-associated proteins (MAPs) in *T. gondii* tissue cysts. (A and B) Cryosections of chronically infected brains showed that, as *in vitro, in vivo* staining for tubulin and MAPs was intense and homogeneous around the tissue cyst wall. Scales bars 50 and 200 μm, respectively. (A′) Positive control for tubulin staining in bradyzoites of *T. gondii* revealed the population of subpellicular microtubules of the parasite. Scale bars: 20 μm. (B′) Detail of tissue cyst in cryosection. Scale bars: 20 μm.

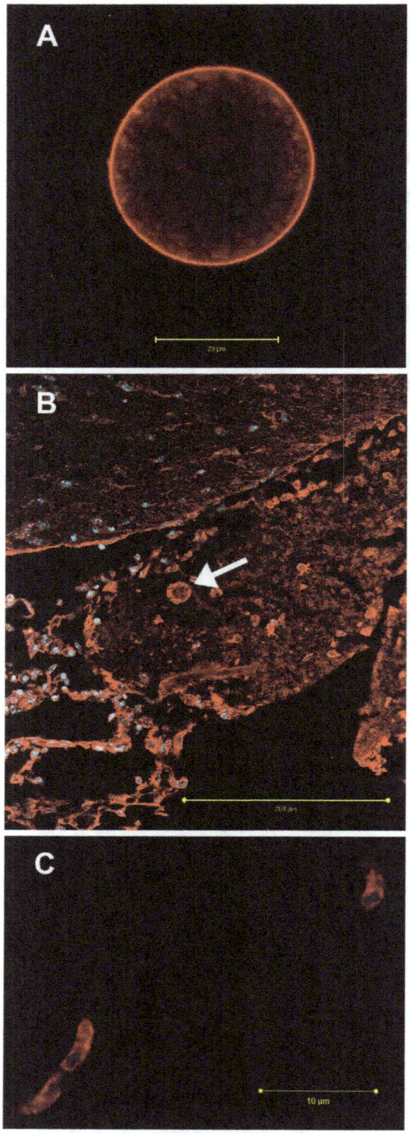


**Figure 7.** Immunofluorescence for detection of actin in *T. gondii* tissue cysts. (A) In isolated tissue cysts, actin detection was more intense than tubulin but still homogeneous around the tissue cyst wall. Scale bars: 20 µm. (B) In cryosections of chronically infected brains, the staining was the same as *in vitro*. Scale bars: 200 µm. (C) In positive control, anti-actin antibody labeled bradyzoites in the apical region and appeared as a diffuse staining in the parasite cytosol. DAPI stained both the cell and parasite nuclei (in blue). Scale bar: 10 µm.

## 3.4. Ultrastructural localization of cytoskeleton proteins through the cyst matrix

The detection by ultrastructural immunocytochemical of actin and tubulin proteins in tissue cysts revealed many gold particles distributed along the granular region and dispersed in the cyst matrix of tissue cysts (**Figure 8A**). In bradyzoites, some particles were located in the

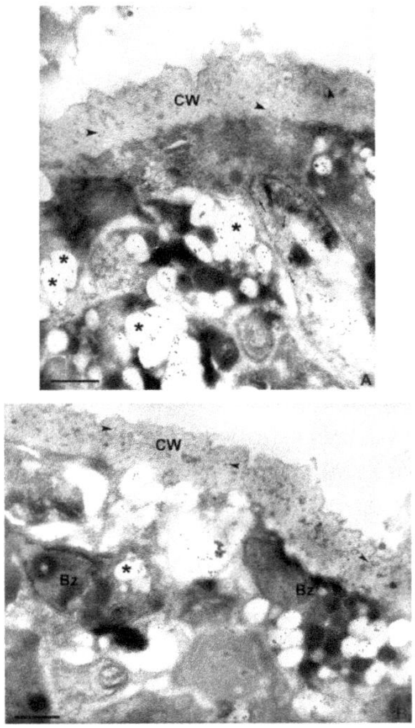


**Figure 8.** Transmission electron micrographs (TEM) of *T. gondii* tissue cyst labeled for actin by immunogold assays. (A) In tissue cyst, many gold particles were distributed along the granular region (arrowhead) and in the matrix (circle). In bradyzoites, some particles were located in the cytoplasm (arrows), most of them inside amylopectin granules (asterisk). (B) In bradyzoites, the gold particles were seen along the cyst granular region (arrowhead) and in clusters in the parasite cytoplasm (circle). Cyst wall (CW) and bradyzoites (Bz). Scale bars: 0.5 μm.

cytoplasm, most of them inside amylopectin granules, along the cyst granular region (arrowhead) and in clusters in the parasite cytoplasm (**Figure 8B**). The immunogold reaction for tubulin identified some gold particles on the cyst wall membrane along the granular region and in the matrix (**Figure 9A**). In bradyzoites, tubulin gold particles were detected mainly inside and around the amylopectin granules as well as in the cytoplasm and membrane (**Figure 9B**).

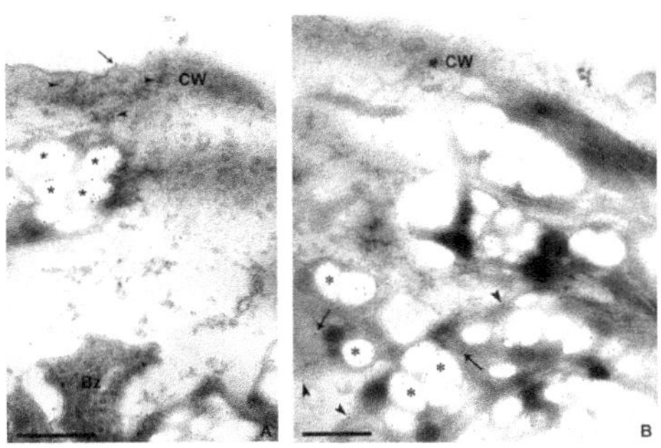


**Figure 9.** Transmission electron micrographs (TEM) of *T. gondii* tissue cyst labeled for tubulin by immunogold staining. (A) In the tissue cyst, gold particles are seen on the cyst wall membrane (arrows) along the granular region (arrowheads). In the bradyzoites, gold particles were present mainly inside and around the amylopectin granules (asterisk). (B) Bradyzoites cytoplasm (arrow) and membrane (arrowhead) showed some gold particles. Cyst wall (CW) and bradyzoites (Bz). Scale bars: 0.5 μm.

## 4. Discussion

This study reveals the ability of the *T. gondii* cyst wall to incorporate macromolecules *in vitro* as well as the presence of cytoskeleton elements in tissue cysts. A critical question in the lifelong persistence of host *Toxoplasma* cysts is how these intracellular parasites are able to survive for long periods within the cyst. The nutrients required by bradyzoites surrounded by the cyst wall may be necessary for its maintenance, multiplication, and amylopectin granule synthesis [23, 24]. The cyst wall, due to its limiting, highly invaginated membrane, provides an enhancement of the cyst surface area, affording the traffic of material between the parasite intracyst and the host cell cytosol [25–27]. Our results show that the *T. gondii* cyst wall is able to incorporate fluids and macromolecules from the external environment via the formation of vesicles and tubules, corroborating findings [8], when there is endocytic activity of the cystic wall, a dynamic process that occurs in *ex-vivo* cysts. These properties might be an alternative method for parasite survival, remaining enclosed within cysts for a long period of time or, as proposed, for the entire life of the infected host [28, 29]. These data point to the endocytosis, described for mammalian cells [30, 31] as well as the endocytic pathway of other pathogenic protozoa [32], as a mechanism of tissue cysts during intracellular development for nutrient acquisition from the host cell.

The exposure of Toxoplasma cysts to BSA-FITC for 2 or 3 h exhibited for the first time, the incorporation dynamics of this endocytic marker located at and attached initially to the cyst wall and afterward, the transit within vesicles toward the cyst matrix. Ultrastructural images from cysts incubated with the two different fluid-phase endocytic tracers (BSA-Au and HRP-Au) demonstrated that they were capable to associate with the cystic wall and be internalized via vesicle and tubules. The incubation of tracers and cysts at 37°C for periods 1–4 h displayed a heterogeneous labeling with formation of clusters on the cyst wall. Guimarães et al. [8] obtained similar images after cyst incubation with cationized ferritin. This labeling type may be due to the motility of cyst wall components or even the presence of different surface micro domains. Some images suggested fusion between the vesicles originating from invagination of the cyst wall with the parasite membrane. However, we have been unable to visualize vesicles discharging the marker or the marker inside the parasite. The present results corroborate previous data of our group with cationized ferritin showing vesicles and tubules containing particles in close contact with the membrane bradyzoite intracystics [8]. The previous data added together with those presented in this work suggest an active process of membrane fusion involved in the bradyzoite macromolecule uptake. It could be one of the pathways for parasite nutrient acquisition through the molecules available in the host cell cytoplasm (see **Scheme 1**, supplementary material). Moreover, we believe that the tubules and vesicles between the filaments of the cyst wall play a key role in delivering internalized molecules from the cyst wall to the intracellular bradyzoites and vice versa.

This cyst wall property opens new perspectives to the investigation of cytoskeletal element involvement in the process of nutrient incorporation by *T. gondii* tissue cysts. Thus, research was initiated concerning the molecular motors that move vesicles and tubules along actin filaments or microtubules, which might mediate the movement from the wall to the matrix cyst. Immunofluorescence of infected brain cryosections and isolated tissue cysts revealed that the tissue cyst wall and matrix are surrounded by a network of cytoskeleton proteins containing at least actin, tubulin, and myosin. Previously, our group demonstrated that the cyst wall is

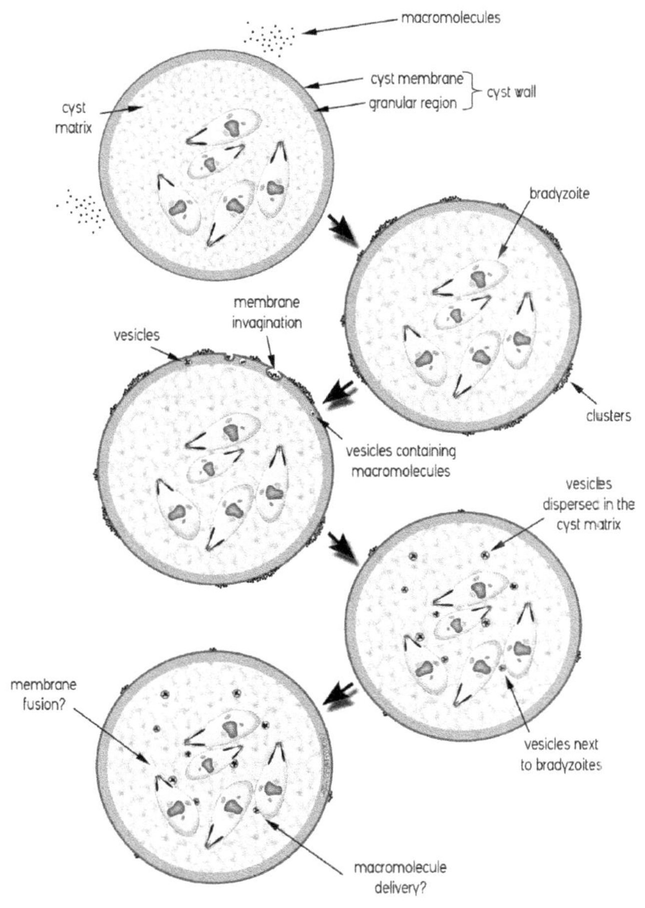


**Scheme 1.** *Toxoplasma* cyst endocytosis. Schematic representation illustrating macromolecules endocytosis by *Toxoplasma* cyst showing each step of this process: (**A**) *Toxoplasma* cyst exposed to macromolecules; (**B**) binding of macromolecules on the cyst wall and cluster formation; (**C–E**) macromolecule incorporation through the cyst membrane invagination followed by the formation of vesicles which migrate from the granular region toward the cyst matrix where they were visualized next to bradyzoites.

formed by negatively charged molecules, and that these molecules are incorporated in the matrix through an endocytic process, involving tubules and vesicles formed from the membrane delimiting the cyst wall [8]. Additionally, we verified that these vesicles and tubules were at different locals of the cyst wall, intimating that they are certainly moving from the outer membrane of the cyst toward the bottom of the cyst wall. Moreover, some vesicles were seen in the matrix very close to the bradyzoite plasma membrane.

Until now, there has been no evidence of the fusion of these vesicles with the parasite membrane. However, we suggest that it might be an important pathway for host cell nutrient acquisition. Nutrient required for bradyzoites is extremely important, as the parasite is confined inside the tissue for long periods and can persist throughout the life of the host [1]. Di Cristina et al. [33] observed that fluorescence molecules, such as D-luciferin, have access to bradyzoites within intact cysts both *in vitro* and *in vivo*. Lemgruber et al. [9] described that the tissue cyst wall incorporation is dependent upon the molecular weight of the tracers. Our data are therefore consistent with both of these studies.

In this way, our interest was to explain how these molecules are incorporated by the cyst wall and also how they can move within the cyst matrix considering that the cyst is not one cell but a structure that maintains various parasites in its interior. The endocytic activity of the cyst wall requires a stimulus induced by molecular signaling which involves cytoskeleton proteins as described for eukaryotic cells. Both actin and tubulin contribute to intracellular vesicle trafficking and endocytic activity in a series of dynamic events in the endomembrane system. The strong positive staining of tubulin and actin, revealed with polyclonal mammalian antibodies throughout the cyst matrix, indicated the presence of a cytoskeleton network within the cyst. Further investigation would be needed to evaluate the origin of these proteins. Eukaryotic cells exhibit tubulin dimers that can be easily altered by posttranslational modifications that differentially mark distinct microtubule subpopulations [34, 35]. Each microtubule subpopulation is organized for specific functions, such as the mitotic spindle, tracks for vesicular transport plus the basal body, and associated flagellar axoneme. In *T. gondii*, there are at least five discrete tubulin-based structures including the conoid, cortical microtubules, intraconoid microtubules, and centrioles, as well as a spindle in replicating parasites [19]. Studies may be required to confirm whether or not tissue cyst matrix cytoskeleton proteins originate from the parasite or from mammalian host cells during the parasitophorous vacuole formation.

Numerous protozoan parasites have the ability to form the cyst stage that normally allows them to survive under adverse environmental conditions. Chávez-Munguía et al. [36] showed that during the encystation process of *Entamoeba invadens*, the cyst wall components are concentrated and transported in specific vesicle, which contain a fibrillar material. This material is then deposited on the parasite plasma membrane through the aperture of the vesicles. Vesicles with a similar appearance may also be present in the cytoplasm of *E. invadens* mature cysts and in the parasite *Acanthamoeba castellanii*. Benchimol [37] also described this structural mechanism involved in the deposition and transport of material to the *Giardia lamblia* pseudocyst wall. After releasing their contents, the membranes may reseal to form empty vesicles, which may be endocytosed by the parasite and/or remain as empty vesicles. Hausen et al. [38] suggested that *G. lamblia* cysts treated with the benzimidazole derivative drug Albendazole, which binds to α-β-tubulin heterodimers of assembling microtubules, link to cyst tubulin, strongly interfering in the excystation process of the parasite. The demonstration of actin, tubulin, and myosin in the composition of the *T. gondii* cyst wall and their distribution in the cyst matrix, as shown here, by immunofluorescence in the *ex-vivo* and *in vivo* systems, is a potential key to the understanding of the incorporation and traffic of molecules by the *T. gondii* cyst wall.

Actin is a highly conserved microfilament protein that plays an important role for gliding motility and in *T. gondii* tachyzoites host cell invasion [39]. By indirect immunofluorescence, actin has been reported to be primarily concentrated in the anterior third of the tachyzoite and in a diffuse staining pattern throughout the cytoplasm [40, 41], our immunofluorescence for actin in the bradyzoite stage revealing the same staining pattern. We also considered that the strong fluorescence staining along the cyst wall could be a false positive and may be caused by adsorptions of the antibody. This hypothesis was discarded when an infected brain was sectioned, and the cyst stain pattern was the same as for intact isolated tissue cysts.

In conclusion, *T. gondii* cyst wall endocytic activity has been demonstrated to provide insight in the parasite cell biology. The relationship of the cyst wall dynamics and cytoskeleton elements maintained in *ex-vivo* cysts corroborate the hypothesis that the cyst wall incorporates and circulates molecules, which could guarantee the parasite survival and persistence during *T. gondii* host infection. In addition, this data potentially provides prospects for new strategies and drug design for toxoplasmosis treatment.

**Funding**

Our work was supported by grants from Conselho Nacional de Desenvolvimento Científico e Tecnológico (CNPq), Fundação Carlos Chagas Filho de Amparo à Pesquisa do Estado do Rio de Janeiro (FAPERJ), Fundação Oswaldo Cruz (Programa Estratégico de Apoio à Pesquisa em Saúde—PAPES IV e VI), Pronex—Programa de Apoio a Núcleos de Excelência—CNPq/FAPERJ, and Instituto Oswaldo Cruz/Fiocruz. MFFS is currently supported by the Re-entry grant of the University of Cologne.

## Acknowledgements

The authors thank Carlos Bizarro, Genilton Vieira, Bruno Ávila for all the image management and Dr. Maurício Paiva for the scheme designed in this work. We are grateful to Sandra Maria for technical support. English review and revision by Mitchell Raymond Lishon, native of Chicago, Illinois, USA—UCLA 1969.

## Author details

Mariana Acquarone[1†], Marialice da F. Ferreira-da-Silva[2†], Erick V. Guimarães[3] and Helene S. Barbosa[3*]

*Address all correspondence to: helene@ioc.fiocruz.br

1 Laboratory Frontiers in Neurosciences, Institute of Biomedical Sciences, Federal University of Rio de Janeiro, RJ, Brazil

2 Institute for Medical Microbiology, Immunology and Hygiene, CECAD, University of Cologne, Cologne, Germany

3 Laboratory of Structural Biology, Oswaldo Cruz Institute, Oswaldo Cruz Foundation, Rio de Janeiro, RJ, Brazil

† These authors contributed equally.

## References


[1] Weiss LM, Dubey JP. Toxoplasmosis: A history of clinical observation. International Journal for Parasitology. 2009;**39**:895–901. DOI: 10.1016/j.ijpara.2009.02.004

[2] Xiao J, Yolken RH. Strain hypothesis of *Toxoplasma gondii* infection on the outcome of human diseases. Acta Physiologica (Oxford). 2015;**213**:828–845. DOI: 10.1111/apha.12458

[3] Neville AJ, Zach SJ, Wang X, Larson JJ, Judge AK, Davis LA, Vennerstrom JL, Davis PH. Clinically available medicines demonstrating anti-toxoplasma activity. Antimicrobial Agents and Chemotherapy. 2015;**59**:7161–7169. DOI: 10.1128/AAC.02009-15

[4] Sethi KK, Rahman A, Pelster B, Brandis H. Search for the presence of lectin-binding sites on *Toxoplasma gondii*. Journal of Parasitology. 1977;**63**:1076–1080

[5] Meingassner JG, Matthaei C, Teutsch HF, Sasse D. Histochemistry of the carbohydrate metabolism in cysts of *Toxoplasma gondii*. Zeitschrift fur Parasitenkunde. 1977;**51**:219–228

[6] Derouin F, Beauvais B, Lariviere M, Guillot J. Binding of fluorescein-labelled lectins on trophozoites and cysts of 3 strains of *Toxoplasma gondii*. Comptes Rendus Des Seances De La Societe De Biologie Et De Ses Filiales. 1981;**175**:761–768

[7] Zhang YW, Halonen SK, Ma YF, Wittner M, Weiss LM. Initial characterization of CST1, a *Toxoplasma gondii* cyst wall glycoprotein. Infection and Immunity. 2001;**69**:501–507

[8] Guimarães EV, Acquarone M, de Carvalho L, Barbosa HS. Anionic sites on *Toxoplasma gondii* tissue cyst wall: Expression, uptake and characterization. Micron. 2007;**38**:651–658

[9] Lemgruber L, Lupetti P, Martins-Duarte ES, De Souza W, Vommaro RC. The organization of the wall filaments and characterization of the matrix structures of *Toxoplasma gondii* cyst form. Cellular Microbiology. 2011;**13**:1920–1932. DOI: 10.1111/j.1462-5822.2011.01681.x

[10] Boothroyd JC, Black M, Bonnefoy S, Hehl A, Knoll LJ, Manger ID, Ortega-Barria E, Tomavo S. Genetic and biochemical analysis of development in *Toxoplasma gondii*. Philosophical Transactions of the Royal Society of London. Series B: Biological Sciences. 1997;**352**:1347–1354

[11] Parmley SF, Yang S, Harth G, Sibley LD, Sucharczuk A, Remington JS. Molecular characterization of a 65-kilodalton *Toxoplasma gondii* antigen expressed abundantly in the matrix of tissue cysts. Molecular and Biochemical Parasitology. 1994;**66**:283–296

[12] Saliba KJ, Kirk K. Nutrient acquisition by intracellular apicomplexan parasites: Staying in for dinner. International Journal for Parasitology. 2001;**31**:1321–1330

[13] Ortíz-Estrada G, Luna-Castro S, Piña-Vázquez C, Samaniego-Barrón L, León-Sicairos N, Serrano-Luna J, de la Garza M. Iron-saturated lactoferrin and pathogenic protozoa: Could this protein be an iron source for their parasitic style of life? Future Microbiology. 2012;**7**:149–164. DOI: 10.2217/fmb.11.140

[14] Barbosa HS, Ferreira-Silva MF, Guimarães EV, Carvalho L, Rodrigues RM. Absence of vacuolar membrane involving *Toxoplasma gondii* during its intranuclear localization. Journal of Parasitology. 2005;**91**:182–184

[15] Coppens I, Sinai AP, Joiner KA. *Toxoplasma gondii* exploits host low-density lipoprotein receptor-mediated endocytosis for cholesterol acquisition. Journal of Cell Biology. 2000;**149**:167–180

[16] Robibaro B, Hoppe HC, Yang M, Coppens I, Ngô HM, Stedman TT, Paprotka K, Joiner KA. Endocytosis in different lifestyles of protozoan parasitism: Role in nutrient uptake with special reference to *Toxoplasma gondii*. International Journal for Parasitology. 2001;**12**:1343–1353

[17] Polonais V, Soldati-Favre D. Versatility in the acquisition of energy and carbon sources by the Apicomplexa. Biology of the Cell. 2010;**102**:435–445. DOI: 10.1042/BC20100005

[18] Jacot D, Daher W, Soldati-Favre D. *Toxoplasma gondii* myosin F, an essential motor for centrosomes positioning and apicoplast inheritance. EMBO Journal. 2013;**32**:1702–1716. DOI: 10.1038/emboj.2013.113

[19] Morrissette N. Targeting toxoplasma tubules: Tubulin, microtubules, and associated proteins in a human pathogen. Eukaryotic Cell. 2015;**14**:2–12. DOI: 10.1128/EC.00225-14

[20] Kumpula EP, Kursula I. Towards a molecular understanding of the apicomplexan actin motor: On a road to novel targets for malaria remedies? Acta Crystallographica Section F-Structural Biology and Crystallization Communications. 2015;**71**:500–513. DOI: 10.1107/S2053230X1500391X

[21] Gordon JL, Buguliskis JS, Buske PJ, Sibley LD. Actin-like protein 1 (ALP1) is a component of dynamic, high molecular weight complexes in *Toxoplasma gondii*. Cytoskeleton (Hoboken). 2010;**67**:23–31. DOI: 10.1002/cm.20414

[22] Lentini G, Kong-Hap M, El Hajj H, Francia M, Claudet C, Striepen B, Dubremetz JF, Lebrun M. Identification and characterization of Toxoplasma SIP, a conserved apicomplexan cytoskeleton protein involved in maintaining the shape, motility and virulence of the parasite. Cellular Microbiology. 2015;**17**:62–78. DOI: 10.1111/cmi.12337

[23] Guimarães EV, de Carvalho L, Barbosa HS. An alternative technique to reveal polysaccharides in *Toxoplasma gondii* tissue cysts. Memórias do Instituto Oswaldo Cruz. 2003;**98**:915–917

[24] Dzierszinski F, Nishi M, Ouko L, Roos DS. Dynamics of *Toxoplasma gondii* differentiation. Eukaryotic Cell. 2004;**3**:992–1003

[25] Jones TC, Bienz KA, Erb P. In vitro cultivation of *Toxoplasma gondii* cysts in astrocytes in the presence of gamma interferon. Infection and Immunity. 1986;**51**:147–156

[26] Ferguson DJ, Hutchison WM. An ultrastructural study of the early development and tissue cyst formation of *Toxoplasma gondii* in the brains of mice. Parasitology Research. 1987;**73**:483–491

[27] Nichols BA, Chiappino ML, Pavesio CE. Endocytosis at the micropore of *Toxoplasma gondii*. Parasitology Research. 1994;**80**:91–98

[28] Tenter AM, Heckeroth AR, Weiss LM. *Toxoplasma gondii*: From animals to humans. International Journal for Parasitology. 2000;**30**:1217–1258

[29] Rougier S, Montoya JG, Peyron F. Lifelong persistence of toxoplasma cysts: A questionable dogma? Trends in Parasitology. 2017;**33**:93–101. DOI: 10.1016/j.pt.2016.10.007

[30] Mukherjee S, Ghosh RN, Maxfield FR. Endocytosis. Physiological Reviews. 1997;**77**: 759–803

[31] Vega-Cabrera LA, Pardo-López L. Membrane remodeling and organization: Elements common to prokaryotes and eukaryotes. IUBMB Life. 2017;**69**:55–62. DOI: 10.1002/iub.1604

[32] de Souza W, Sant'Anna C, Cunha-e-Silva NL. Electron microscopy and cytochemistry analysis of the endocytic pathway of pathogenic protozoa. Progress in Histochemistry and Cytochemistry. 2009;**44**:67–124. DOI: 10.1016/j.proghi.2009.01.001

[33] Di Cristina M, Marocco D, Galizi R, Proietti C, Spaccapelo R, Crisanti A. Temporal and spatial distribution of *Toxoplasma gondii* differentiation into bradyzoites and tissue cyst formation in vivo. Infection and Immunity. 2008;**76**:3491–3501. DOI: 10.1128/IAI.00254-08

[34] Verhey KJ, Gaertig J. The tubulin code. Cell Cycle. 2007;**6**:2152–2160

[35] Wloga D, Gaertig J. Post-translational modifications of microtubules. Journal of Cell Science. 2010;**123**:3447–3455. DOI: 10.1242/jcs.063727

[36] Chávez-Munguía B, Cristóbal-Ramos AR, González-Robles A, Tsutsumi V, Martínez-Palomo A. Ultrastructural study of *Entamoeba invadens* encystation and excystation. Journal of Submicroscopic Cytology and Pathology. 2003;**35**:235–243

[37] Benchimol M. The release of secretory vesicle in encysting *Giardia lamblia*. FEMS Microbiology Letters. 2004;**235**:81–87

[38] Hausen MA, de Oliveira RP, Gadelha AP, Campanati L, de Carvalho JJ, de Carvalho L, Barbosa HS. *Giardia lamblia*: A report of drug effects under cell differentiation. Parasitology Research. 2009;**105**:789–796. DOI: 10.1007/s00436-009-1463-4

[39] Blader IJ, Coleman BI, Chen CT, Gubbels MJ. Lytic cycle of *Toxoplasma gondii*: 15 years later. Annual Review of Microbiology. 2015;**69**:463–485. DOI: 10.1146/annurev-micro-091014-104100

[40] Cintra WM, Silva-Filho FC, De Souza W. The surface charge of *Toxoplasma gondii*: A cytochemical and electrophoretic study. Journal of Submicroscopic Cytology. 1986;**18**:773–781

[41] Endo T, Yagita K, Yasuda T, Nakamura T. Detection and localization of actin in *Toxoplasma gondii*. Parasitology Research. 1988;**75**:102–106

# 9

# *Toxoplasma gondii* in Meat for Human Consumption – A Brief Review of the Most Described Strategies for its Detection and Quantification

G.F. Dzib Paredes, A. Ortega-Pacheco, J.A. Rosado-Aguilar, K.Y. Acosta-Viana, E. Guzmán -Marín and M. Jiménez-Coello

**Abstract**

Toxoplasmosis is a parasitic zoonotic disease widely distributed worldwide and is caused by the intracellular parasite *Toxoplasma gondii*. The definitive host of *T. gondii* is the domestic cat and the entire cat family, in which the sexu-al stages of the parasite develop. *T. gondii* can also infect a wide range of inter-mediate hosts, affecting most warm-blooded animals including humans. In humans, toxoplasmosis is usually asymptomatic in healthy individuals, but can develop lymphadenopathy and nonspecific symptomatology or even be fatal in infants with congenital toxoplasmosis and in immunocompromised pa-tients. Transmission to humans is mainly through food, especially by eating undercooked meat or meat contaminated with tissue cysts. This has led to vari-ous public health organizations worldwide monitoring programs on *T. gondii* in animals intended for human consumption, especially in meat samples. One of the techniques employed in the laboratory is that based on the polymerase chain reaction and some of its variants, which have proven to be valuable tools for the detection of *T. gondii* in tissues for human consumption and many other types of biological samples. The development of different strategies for the mo-lecular detection of *T. gondii* has led to the identification and quantification methodologies varying widely among laboratories. Therefore, this chapter re-views the main methods of extraction, purification, detection and quantifica-tion of *T. gondii* DNA in tissue samples from different species destined for human consumption.

**Keywords:** *T. gondii*, meat, DNA quantification, parasite load, zoonosis

## 1. Introduction

Toxoplasmosis is a zoonotic disease widely distributed throughout the world and is caused by the intracellular parasite *Toxoplasma gondii*. The definitive host of the parasite is the domestic cat and the entire cat family, in which the parasite reproduces sexually. *T. gondii* can also infect a wide range of intermediate hosts, affecting most warm-blooded animals [1].

In humans, toxoplasmosis is usually asymptomatic in healthy individuals, but can develop lymphadenopathy and nonspecific symptomatology or even be fatal in infants with congenital toxoplasmosis (CT) and in immunocompromised patients (such as people with AIDS), in persons with problems in bone marrow and recipient patients of transplanted organs) [2].

*Toxoplasmosis* transmission to humans is mainly through food and from exposure to different stages of *T. gondii,* particularly by ingestion of sporulated oocysts found in the environment and contaminated water and food, or by ingestion of tissue cysts or tachyzoites contained in meat and products derived from the meat of various animals, [1,3,4].

The consumption of undercooked, raw or cured meat is a major mode of transmission of *Toxoplasmosis* to humans, especially in cases of CT, which has been attributed to 30% to 60% of cases of infection during pregnancy [5]. This has led to various public health organizations worldwide monitoring programs introduced on *T. gondii* in animals intended for human consumption, mainly in meat samples [6].

## 2. Occurrence of toxoplasmosis

*T. gondii* is a parasite that is widely distributed around the world, showing a higher incidence in tropical areas and a decrease when the latitude increases [7]. The estimated prevalence in the human population varies widely in different geographical areas, between different cities within the same city and between different ethnic groups even when they live in the same area [6,8]. In humans, toxoplasmosis is considered the third leading cause of death among food-borne diseases [7].

As well in humans, *T. gondii* is widely distributed worldwide. Parasite presence has been described in several animal species (wild, companion and production animals). However, food-producing animals may represent a real risk for transmission of the disease to humans, either directly or through farming [9]. Several serological assays have been performed in free-ranging chickens, because the information provided is usually used as an index of environmental contamination with oocysts [10]. Prevalence rates in these animals in Central and South America ranges from 40 to 60% [11],and other reports from India describe prevalence rates from 20 to 40% [12,13]; in Egypt there are rates reported around 40% [10,14] and in China, 30.36% [15]. Pigs and sheep are also commonly infected. Pigs are very susceptible to become experimentally infected and show high prevalence rates in some regions of the United States, as well in warm and tropical countries [16–21]. Prevalence rates of *T. gondii* in sheep are also widely distributed. For example in the United States, there has been described prevalence rate in range of 27 to 73 %; Uruguay, Argentina, Chile, Mexico and the United Kingdom showed prevalence rates of around 30%, but there are some countries with higher rates such as Ivory Coast, France and Turkey, where prevalence rates of 68, 89 and 95.7%, respectively, have been reported [22]. Cattle and buffaloes are not considered as probably sources of significant infection [22] as cows are relatively resistant to experimental infection [24].

In general, the occurrence infection by *T. gondii* in animals varies depending on weather conditions, geographical area, type of species, either productive or wild, as well as the age of the animals, the type of farming system (extensive, semi-extensive, intensive), the management and the existence of health programs [22,25,26]. Also, there have been described many factors that have an important impact on foodborne transmission of *T. gondii* to humans, such as the type of management and production of livestock, hygienic standards of slaughterhouses, food processing and technology, the density of cats or wild felines in the area and climate change, which may influence the sporulation of oocysts in the environment (i.e., temperature, humidity, wind) [6].

## 3. Clinical signs in animals and humans

### 3.1. Toxoplasmosis in humans

The clinical spectrum of the disease varies widely and depends primarily on the immune status of the host and *Toxoplasma* lineage to which a person was exposed. In humans, toxoplasmosis may manifest basically in five ways: asymptomatic, acute infection, congenital, ocular and the immunocompromised patient. In immunocompetent persons toxoplasmosis is usually asymptomatic or develops mild symptoms that go unnoticed in 80–90% of cases [27]. The usual clinical manifestations, trend to be laterocervical lymphadenopathy which is often treated, less frequently supraclavicular nodes, occipital, inguinal, mediastinal lymph node or any other chain are affected; patients with lymphadenopathy also have other symptoms such as fever, malaise, arthralgia, asthenia, night sweats, sore throat or maculopapular rash, no itching, which usually spares the palms and soles. The clinical picture of acute toxoplasmosis is usually benign and self-limiting; in <1 month, progression to the severe form is rare in immunocompetent hosts [27–30]. In immunocompromised subjects, acute toxoplasmosis usually occurs widely where the main sites of spread are the central nervous system, eyes, heart, liver and lungs, with preference in the tissues where the immune response is limited, causing injuries. In immunocompromised patients, such as AIDS patients with very low CD4 counts, patients under immunosuppression to prevent or treat transplant rejection and fetuses, a reactivation of an earlier infection, rather than a newly acquired one, is common. In these individuals the parasite can induce besides encephalitis and retinochoroiditis, carditis, pneumonia, and meningitis, among other manifestations [31]. Ocular toxoplasmosis is produced in most cases by breaking tissue cysts that are congenitally acquired; however, it can occur in acquired infections too. It manifests as uveitis or retinochoroiditis with exudate and decreased vision; the lesion can be observed by fundus evaluation. The ocular presentation is commonly characterized by necrotic lesions destroying retinal architecture, sometimes engaging and choroid (retinochoroiditis) [28,30]. CT is the most significant complication of active infection. When the infection is acquired during pregnancy, either by reactivation of latent-phase bradyzoites or by a primary infection, the parasites migrate to the placenta and from there to the fetus. The severity of the disease depends on the stage of pregnancy when the parasites cross the placenta. At the beginning of pregnancy, fetal infection is rare, but when it happens, it triggers severe injury or death of the fetus. As the pregnancy progresses, congenital infection is most common, but the damage tends to be lower [29,32]. When the disease occurs in utero, there may be consequences observed at birth. Most congenital infections are asymptomatic, although in some cases the child is born with acute illness, where cases of hydrocephalus, eye damage and visceral can be found. In other cases, the disease develops after birth or become dormant for a long time [29,32].

### 3.2. Toxoplasmosis in animals

Natural infection in non-pregnant animals usually elapses without symptoms, but primary infection during pregnancy can cause embryonic death, abortion, birth weak or clinically normal but infected animals. Globally, *T. gondii* is the cause of 11–14% of the abortions that occur in sheep and goats [33]. In cattle, by contrast, *T. gondii* infection is not considered a common cause of abortion and presented asymptomatic. *T. gondii* in dogs is considered an opportunistic pathogen and infection is usually subclinical, but under certain conditions clinical signs are present, predominantly respiratory and neuromuscular manifestations (Dubey, 2010). Cats even as definitive hosts usually enrolled asymptomatic infection, even during removal of oocysts; however, sometimes clinical signs are present, primarily associated with respiratory type interstitial pneumonia, dyspnea, lethargy and anorexia, ocular signs (uveitis, retinochoroiditis) or neuromuscular signs [34]. In cats it has also been described as intrauterine infection; thus, infected animals generally have more severe signs: encephalitis, hepatitis, ascites, respiratory signs and perinatal death or weaning [35]. In the pigs, the disease usually attends in subclinical and can be seen in some cases of weak animals born or stillborn; in adult animals weight loss, anorexia and fever have been observed, which usually disappear by the third week after infection regardless of variant of *T. gondii*. Pigs are considered an important source of infection for humans because of the high parasite loads encountered in their tissues compared to other productive animals [22,35].

## 4. Economic impact of toxoplasmosis

The real economic impact of toxoplasmosis is difficult to estimate, because in most immunocompetent individuals, the infection goes unnoticed or has claimed clinical presentation to other diseases [22,29]. However, it is estimated that the economic impact should be very high due to the loss of one or more days of work in mild cases, treatment and care needs, sick children, especially those with mental retardation and blindness, loss of quality lifestyle and the costs of hospitalization in severe cases and the cost of monitoring pregnant women and treatment during pregnancy who are *T. gondii* positive [26,36,37].

In United States,, despite the low incidence, the economic impact of CT is high due to the severity of the infection, associated complications, treatment and social costs. CT costs have been estimated as $ 1.26 million per case and were mainly attributed to drug costs, annual losses of productivity, special education and health care costs [38]. On the other hand, in the United States, some 3,000 babies are born every year with CT and the annual cost of treating this disease is between US$ 31 and US$ 40 million [39]. The total economic impact of CT just in the United States has been estimated as over $ 7.7 billion per year, which makes it the second most important infection to humans after foodborne salmonellosis [40]. In the United Kingdom, the annual economic impact is estimated $ 12 million [26].

In most productive animals, toxoplasmosis occurs asymptomatically; however, in animal production, toxoplasmosis is considered as an economically important disease of livestock, especially sheep and goats, where it can cause early embryonic death and resorption, fetal death and mummification, abortion, stillbirth and neonatal death [41].

Regarding economic impact of infection with *T. gondii* in productive species, just in the United Kingdom, economic losses were estimated to be between 15 and 20%, from scanning to sale, but on some farms losses can reach over 30% [42]. This is often a result of a disease outbreak of *T. gondii* abortion. Other authors had mentioned that cost of *Toxoplasma* in the UK flock was estimated to be £12 million [43]. These estimates included loss of production, cost of treatment, control and monitoring but did not include the costs associated with human health. As a matter of fact, the economic losses caused by *T. gondii* infection in sheep are difficult to estimate because the disease occurs sporadically. Moreover, only a small number of the lambs aborted are subjected to diagnosis [43]. In addition, the material sent for diagnosis, besides being potentially inadequate, might also be examined erroneously and, finally, serological testing lacks specificity [45].

In pigs, the infection with *T. gondii* also use to be asymptomatic, but in some cases, the active infection or parasitemia reactivation could impact over reproductive parameters (abortions or weak stillborns), mainly when is present in concomitance with other viral agents such as parvovirus [46] or circovirus.

## 5. Molecular biology techniques for *T. gondii* detection

The diagnosis of toxoplasmosis is usually based on the detection of antibodies by ELISA serology, agglutination assays or other methods such as Western blot immuno- or Sabin-Feldman [47] staining. However, there are times when serological or with any of the aforementioned detection methods are not possible; in these cases the techniques of molecular biology have been helpful in the diagnosis of *T. gondii*, especially the PCR technique, which has proved to be a valuable tool [2,48].

Currently different strategies for molecular diagnosis of *T. gondii* have been developed; this has meant that various methodologies are reported (both for the extraction of nucleic acids and for the detection of different amplification targets) and brings about a large variation between results from different laboratories [49]. So the aim of this chapter is to review the main methods of extraction, purification, detection and quantification of DNA from *T. gondii* in different species intended for human consumption.

### 5.1. DNA extraction methods

The extraction and purification of nucleic acids is the first stage of most molecular biological studies; extraction methods allow to obtain nucleic acids from various sources and then perform specific analysis by polymerase chain reaction (PCR) or its variants [49]. The quality and purity of the nucleic acids are two of the most important elements of such analysis since contaminants can interfere by inhibiting the amplification process in which PCR [50] rests. This makes clear that the importance of the process of sample preparation and DNA extraction methodology used, to have significant impact on the sensitivity of the test [50,51].

To extract the nucleic acids of the biological material, samples must be homogenized, causing cell lysis, proteins be removed by incubation with a protease and finally nucleic acids should be separated from other cellular components [50]. The ideal lysis procedure, which usually consists of a balancing techniques, must be strong enough to break the complex starting material (a fabric, for example), but gentle enough to preserve the nucleic acids. The lysis process is generally performed by physical or chemical processes, which break the bonds between the cells to facilitate interaction with lysis solutions that help release the genetic material [50, 51]. Among the conventional methods for extracting genetic material from T. *gondii* in tissue include the following procedures previous to DNA extraction.

#### *5.1.1. Mechanical homogenization with liquid nitrogen*

This process involves macerating the sample with liquid nitrogen using a mortar to obtain a fine powder. The nitrogen immediately can freeze the sample to prevent crystals formation, thus avoiding the breakdown of cell structures and the start of DNA degradation process by the action of DNase [51].

#### *5.1.2. Chemical homogenization*

In the chemical homogenization, the samples are maintained in solution at high temperatures in the presence of proteases, detergents and chaotropic agents to break the bonds between the cells or can even pierce the cell membrane. In fibrous tissue it is recommended that you cut into small pieces to facilitate their decomposition. Before starting this type of homogenization it is necessary to have information about the right amount of tissue; for rapid and complete homogenization, it is necessary to ensure the recovery of DNA and prevent degradation [51].

#### *5.1.3. Pepsin digestion*

Pepsin digestion is a method developed by Jacos et al. in 1960 and is modified by Dubey (1998) for retrieving from *T. gondii* from 50 g of muscle tissue (Dubey, 2010). The method is based on the digestion process by which the parasite is released from tissue cysts to invade its host. In this method, the homogenization of muscle tissue occurs by digestion with porcine pepsin solution, HCl, NaCl and distilled water at 37°C for 1 hour. Subsequently, a series of centrifugations allow the parasites to concentrate and be more likely to find their genetic material when purification is performed. At the end of centrifugation the product has to be buffered with bicarbonate to prevent degradation of the nucleic acids contained in the homogenate [22].

Pepsin requires acidic pH for activation; it breaks the bonds between tyrosine and phenylalanine partially degraded proteins. Pepsin polypeptides of different sizes and some amino acids are obtained without degrading completely, so this procedure is commonly followed by the enzymatic action of another protease [52].

#### *5.1.4. Proteinase K*

Proteinase K is most often used because it is the widest-spectrum (degrades all proteins) protease and it is often used with buffers containing SDS and EDTA [50]. Proteinase K is a protease obtained from the fungus saprophyte *Tritirachium album* and is particularly suitable for digestion in a short time. Proteinase k acts on the carboxyl group of amino acids and is highly stable in a wide range of temperatures and pH values, having its greatest activity at elevated temperatures [53].

### 5.2. DNA purification methods

The DNA purification methods can be classified into two major branches: traditional protocols and by commercial kits [51].

#### *5.2.1. Conventional protocols*

They were developed in the 1950s; organic solvents used to separate proteins and DNA, once suspended in the aqueous phase by ethanol precipitation isolate [51]. In the case of *T. gondii*, more purification methodology used in the traditional methods is performed by phenol/chloroform.

#### *5.2.2. Phenol/chloroform*

The phenol/chloroform purification is a method of liquid-liquid organic extraction consisting of separate mixtures of molecules, which is based on the difference in solubility of individual molecules in two different liquids [52,53]. The nucleic acid extraction with phenol/chloroform involves adding equal volumes of phenol/chloroform aqueous cell lysate or tissue homogenate, mixing the two phases and allowing to separate by centrifugation (Alejos et al., 2014). The phenol/chloroform method ensures the separation of liquids in two phases (organic and aqueous lower than), because chloroform is miscible with phenol due to its higher density (1.47 g/cm3) phenol [54,55].

Nucleic acids are soluble in the upper aqueous phase because of their negatively charged phosphate backbone, while proteins and lipids are separated in the organic phase [55]. Phenol causes precipitation of proteins and polymers (including carbohydrates) that are contained in the interface between the two phases (often as a white supernatant); in the case of lipids, these

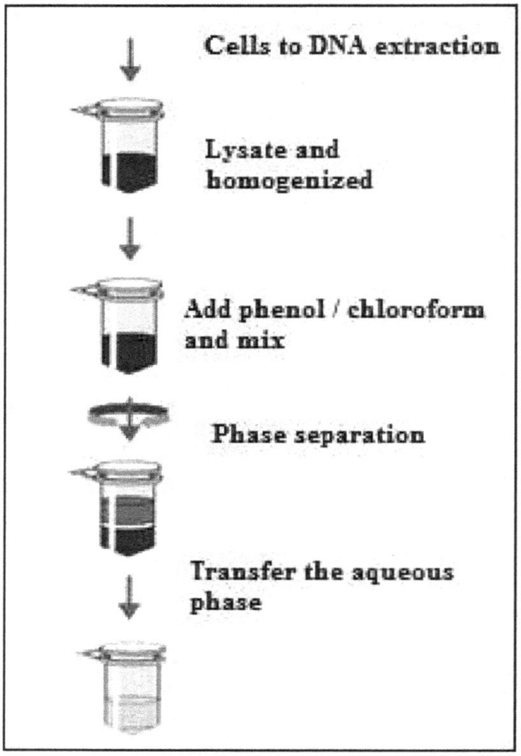


**Figure 1.** DNA purification with phenol/chloroform [55].

are dissolved in the lower organic phase. The separation between the aqueous and organic phase by centrifugation allows isolation of the DNA in the aqueous phase (Karp, 2009; Soma, 2010). Subsequently the DNA is recovered from the aqueous phase with ethanol and is insoluble, causing centrifugation to precipitate it [51].

### 5.3. DNA extraction using commercial kits

From the 1990s were introduced to market commercial purification kits; these kits commonly used membranes or inorganic matrices to which the DNA will bind to specific conditions (Karp, 2009). Often these arrays are stacked into small columns in centrifuge tubes so that the binding steps, washing and elution can be performed efficiently by applying a centrifugal force. Some of the advantages of using commercial kits are to increase efficiency of DNA recovery, to obtain inhibitor-free extract and to decrease the time spent for purification {51,54]

The purification procedure with commercial kits can be summarized in three steps: 1) homogenization of tissues to facilitate the selective attachment of DNA to the matrix; 2) washing to remove DNA contaminants and 3) recovering the DNA from the matrix using an eluting buffer [51].

### 5.3.1. *Silica matrix*

This method is based in selectively adsorption/desorption of nucleic acids and it has proven more efficient for the recovery of pure DNA beside biological samples (i.e., blood, tissue). Silica extraction methods produce increased DNA yield while efficiently removing PCR inhibitors; those protocols usually include a small-scale silica-based spin column. The selective adsorption/desorption occurs when, by the action of ethanol, the DNA loses its humectant layer, exposing its phosphate groups and thereby facilitating the adsorption of the molecule to the positively charged membrane. Lipids and proteins are not related to the membrane and are removed using the wash solution and a cycle of centrifugation, while the genetic material remained is bound to the matrix [51].

### 5.3.2. *Magnetic beads*

Extraction methodology using magnetic beads or a magnet that attracts magnet to separate the beads from solutions in which they are suspended is applicable. In this case, the lysis buffer solution at acidic pH, which allows to positively charge the beads, favoring DNA binding [51,53], is added.

The methodology for the extraction and purification of DNA from *T. gondii* in tissue with magnetic beads was described by Opsteegh et al. [56]. Tissue homogenization is carried out in a bag filter Stomacher400 containing a lysis buffer (100 mM Tris HCl pH 8.0, 5 mM EDTA pH 8.0, 0.2% SDS, 200mMNaCl and 40mg/L Proteinase k), by reaction using 2.5 mL of lysis buffer per gram of sample for 2 minutes at high speed. The homogenate is placed in incubation at 55°C overnight and, after the incubation, the extract obtained is homogenized again for 1 minute; 50 mL of the homogenate is transferred to a 50-mL tube and is centrifuged at 3500 g × 45 min; 12 mL of the supernatant (crude extract) is collected for use in the purification of the genetic material of *T. gondii*.

The first step in the purification process based on magnetic beads is the removal of free biotin in the sample because this method is based on the target binding sequence labeled with biotin to the magnetic beads that are coated with streptavidin (protein high affinity for biotin). To remove free biotin from the sample streptavidin sepharose should be added to allow the biotin precipitation and to form a pellet by centrifuging and 10 mL of the supernatant are finally used for purification process [56,57].

To mark the sequences of interest with biotin is needed the addition of specific primers that are marked with this molecule [57]. The bonding occurs during hybridization, so it is first necessary to denature the sample nucleic acids by heating at 95°C for 15 min and then lower the temperature to allow hybridization; if the proposed protocol is by Opsteegh et al. [56]. the hybridization temperature is 55°C for 45 min. Once labeled primers are hybridized to the target sequence, we proceed to introduce the magnetic beads in the sample and proceed to incubate at room temperature for 60 minutes to allow binding sequences labeled with magnetic beads. They are separated from the beads using a magnet and then the DNA of the beads was recovered by washing with buffer B & W (Binding & Washing) provided in the kit extraction and finally the DNA recovered is resuspended in distilled water. Magnetic capture process is presented in Figure 2.

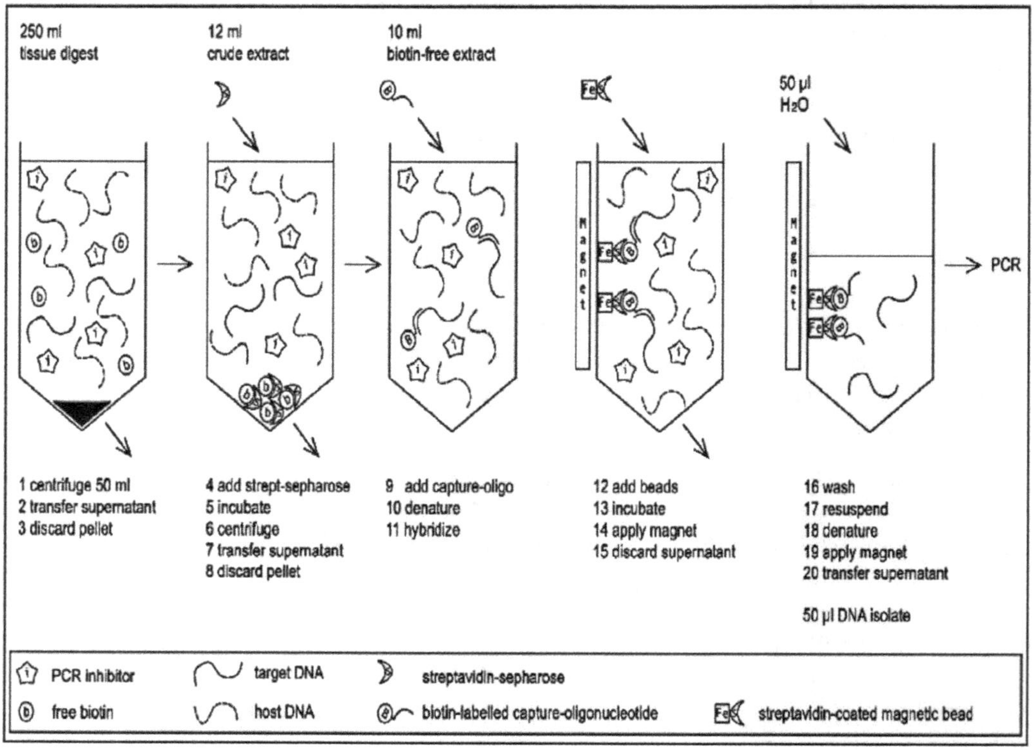


**Figure 2.** DNA purification from tissue employing magnetic beads [56].

Today there are also cases that implement business purification methods with organic solvents. Usually these methods are based on the phenol/chloroform by adding guanidine or any other part that improves the extraction and purification of nucleic acids. Examples of these traditional methods are converted to commercial kits extraction and extraction with TRIzol® DNAzol® [58,59]. These commercial kits based home methods are usually cheaper than commercial kits based on inorganic matrices, although purification performance is very similar in some cases, there is a risk of contamination of samples with phenol and inhibition of amplification in the PCR process [60]. Another important factor to consider is security, since this type of extraction involves the use of corrosive and irritant substances and therefore requires some experience to handle; accidental contact with the reagents that can burn skin and vapors inhalation could cause damage to the respiratory system, in both cases, medical assistance is required. Table 1 presents the main commercial kits used for the extraction and purification of DNA from *T. gondii*.

| Commercial kit | Fundamental | Column material | Amount of recovered DNA | Reference |
|---|---|---|---|---|
| Universal Genomic DNA Extraction Kit (TaKaRa, USA) | Absorption/ desorption | Silica | 10μg (2–30 mg of tissue) | [61]. |
| Easy-DNA®Kit (Invitrogen) | Organic extraction | N/A | 150μg (50 mg of tissue) 5–10 ng/μL blood | [62]. |
| High Pure PCR Template Preparation Kit (Roche Diagnostics, Mannheim Germany) | Absorption/ desorption | Glass fiber filter | 3–9 μg (200–300 μL blood) 25–50 mg of tissue (variable amount recovered depending the tissue tested) | [6]. [63]. |
| QIAamp DNA Mini Kit (QIAGEN, Valencia, CA) | Absorption/ desorption | Silica | 4–12μg (200μL blood) 25–45μg (25mg of cardiac tissue) | [21,47,64–68]. |
| TRIzol® LS Reagent (Invitrogen, Paisley, the United Kingdom) (Fenol-Cloroformo) | Organic liquid-liquid extraction | N/A | 2–3μg (for each mg of sample) | [69]. |
| Phenol-Chloroform | Organic liquid-liquid extraction | N/A | --- | [70–76] |
| NucleoSpin Tissue Kit (Macherey Nagel, Czech Republic) | absorption/ desorption | Silica | 20–35μg (25mg of tissue) | [77]. |
| Biotin labeled capture oligonucleotides and Streptavidin labeled magnetic beads (Invitrogen) | magnetic capture | Magnetic beads | Recovered DNA from 5–100pb | [5,47,56] |
| NucliSens easy MAG system (BIOMERIEUX) | magnetic capture | Magnetic Silica | --- | [49,78,79] |
| Genomic Prep Blood DNA isolation kit (Amersham Pharmacia Biotech, the United Kingdom) | absorption/ desorption | Silica | Recovered DNA from 100–200 kb | |
| DNAzol® (Life technologies) | organic extraction | N/A | 3–5μg/mg from tissue | [80]. |
| Qiaquick y PCR purification kit (QIAGEN, Valencia) | absorption/ desorption | Silica | 10 μg DNA recovered from 100pb–10kb | [81,82] |
| DNeasy Blood & Tissue Kit (QIAGEN) | absorption/ desorption | Silica | 10–30ug (25mg of tissue) | [83,84] |

**Table 1.** Leading commercial kits used for DNA extraction and purification from different tissues for *T. gondii* detection

## 6. Methods for molecular detection of *T. gondii* in meat for consumption

The presence of *T. gondii* in biological samples can be diagnosed by molecular techniques aimed at detecting its genetic material [74,85] (Switaj et al., 2005; Garcia et al., 2006). A specific fragment of the parasite genome can be amplified by PCR to visualize on a polyacrylamide or agarose gel, to stain, to sequence directly in real time. The sensitivity and specificity of PCR-based techniques rely on an appropriate method of purification of genetic material from the samples, the characteristics of the DNA sequences chosen for amplification and the parameters of the amplification reaction [50,85]. Various amplification methods for *T. gondii* will be explained below.

### 6.1. Conventional PCR (endpoint)

The PCR is a molecular biology technique developed by Dr. Kary B. Mullis in 1985 [54,86]. The impact of his discovery was such that Dr. Mullis received the Nobel Prize for Chemistry in 1993 (Welch, 2012). PCR is a technique "*in vitro*" used to amplify enzymatically a specific region of DNA located between two regions of DNA whose sequence is known [86]. PCR simulates what happens during cell replication taking advantage of features of the chemical structure and semiconservative DNA replication [50].

DNA is a polymer formed from two complementary strands anti-parallel, each chain consists of nucleotide units which in turn are comprised of a nitrogenous base (adenine = A, guanine = G, cytokine = C and thymine = T) attached to sugar deoxyribose and a triphosphate group [50,87]. To replicate the DNA separates its two complementary strands, serving each mold or template for the "de novo synthesis" of its complementary strand, the specificity of pairing of the nitrogenated bases (TA, CG) to obtain two identical DNA molecules, each consisting of an original and a new chain. The enzyme that performs this process is called DNA polymerase [54,87]. PCR synthesis of new DNA strands is performed by mixing: containing DNA or fragments to be amplified; polymerase; primers (DNA fragment of 15 to 30 nucleotides flanking the region to be amplified and to provide the free 3 'end to initiate transcription); deoxynucleotides (dNTPs); magnesium chloride (MgCl2) or other cofactor necessary to work polymerase [86]. Generally, the PCR begins with denaturation or separation of the double helix of DNA by heating the sample at a temperature between 94 and 96°C to break the hydrogen bonds that bind them, so as each string is a template for synthesis A new complementary strand of DNA [88].

Once separated the chains of DNA primers (initiators or primers) are aligned in complementary-specific sites of the single strands in the region to be amplified; for this to happen it is necessary to lower the temperature between 40 and 60°C, allowing binding (hybridization or alignment) of the primers. Finally, a new strand is synthesized in the 5′ to 3′ for which the temperature is increased, generally at 72°C, which is the optimum temperature to work Taq polymerase [89]. These three stages — 1) denaturation, 2) hybridization and 3) elongation of DNA — are repeated successively in each new cycle and amplified the region of interest of the two complementary strands [86] simultaneously. The essential equipment for the process to take place is the thermal cycler, which has a heating pad where each reaction is placed and where temperature changes are accurate and can be pre-programmed in three stages by several cycles [50, 86].

Detecting the PCR product is usually accomplished by electrophoresis. Separation matrices (agarose, polyacrylamide) at various concentrations are used depending on the size of the amplification product and the resolution desired. The posterior viewing can be done with ethidium bromide with a UV lamp, silver staining, fluorescence or radioactivity light. The sizes of the PCR products are determined by comparing them with markers containing DNA fragments of known size, which are run in a gel with PCR products.

### 6.2. Nested PCR

Nested PCR (nested) consists of two successive processes of amplification, using the product of the first amplification as template for the second [2]. In the second amplification primers used should be different from the first amplification and are targeted to amplify a smaller fraction contained within the product of the first PCR [90]. This methodology increases both the sensitivity and specificity of the test. Furthermore, the risk of contamination increases significantly due to the increased amount of amplification products and work steps involved [91]. In this type of test validation it is always recommended by both negative and positive controls, ensuring that the positive controls are highly diluted to avoid contamination of the samples [90].

### 6.3. PCR-LAMP

This is a variant of PCR developed for parasites of the phylum Apicomplexa, among which is *T. gondii*. The amplification method LAMP (Loop-mediated isothermal amplification) is based on a displacement auto cyclic reaction chain using a set of four oligonucleotides (primers) which recognize six sequences within the genomic DNA target region and form a loop structured amplicon, the polymerase that performs this function is Bst polymerase having activity displacement [92,93].

### 6.4. Real-time PCR (qPCR)

Real-time PCR is a technique used to quantify specific nucleic acid sequences in a sample of interest. The assay is based on generating a fluorescent signal that is directly proportional to the amount of target DNA. Real-time PCR is able to monitor the fluorescence emission that occurs during the reaction progress, so is said to be in real time [94]. Among the major fluorophores used for determination of *T. gondii* load are as follows:

#### *6.4.1. SYBR Green™*

It is an intercalator that binds to dsDNA resulting fluorescence increased with increasing the amount of PCR product. An important aspect to consider is that the SYBR Green™ can also join primer dimers and nonspecific amplification products, resulting in an overestimation of the concentration of target DNA. The detection of DNA of *T. gondii* using SYBR Green it could be useful mainly during experimental infections. It has been used for monitoring parasitemia loads in animal models, however for clinical diagnosis or monitoring any other natural infection (i.e., in animals for consumption) the performance it is not enough sensitive to detect the presence of low amount of the target in the sample.

*6.4.2. TaqMan™*

TaqMan probes are hydrolysis probes which allow increase the specificity of quantitative PCR. They have attached a reporter (a fluorophore) and a quencher. When both (fluorophore and the quencher) are in proximity, the reporter emits no signal, however, when the probe hybridizes to the sequence of interest during PCR, the endonuclease activity of Taq polymerase to short photochromic other reporter probe, allowing emission of a fluorescent signal. The reporter fluorescent signal is cumulative in each of the subsequent cycles [79].

## 7. Determination of parasite load in meat by qPCR

### 7.1. Absolute quantification

Absolute quantitation is a quantization strategy based on comparison of the test samples against a standard curve created from a template of known concentration (Sivaganesan et al., 2010). This template of known concentration is used to make serial dilutions and generate a curve from the CT values (threshold cycle) obtained for each concentration. The curve can interpolate directly the CT values of the test samples and get your concentration by the equation $Q=10\left(\frac{CT-b}{m}\right)$ where: Q = amount shown, CT = amplification cycle, b = insertion axis "and" m = gradient of the line. In traditional protocols creating absolute quantification standard curve in each qPCR experiment conducted it suggested, however, can also be employed master calibration curve generated from multiple experiments qPCR [95]. The absolute quantification method is conceptually easy, however, requires a reliable source as a template of known concentration.

### 7.2. Relative quantification

Such quantification measures changes in the basal state of a gene of interest versus constant gene expression that acts as a control. The difference lies in the absolute quantification that are not part of a known amount of DNA, but an endogenous housekeeping gene control or reference "housekeeping". Because the absolute amount of internal standard is unknown, can be determined only relative changes of the gene of interest with reference to the endogenous gene. Some of the most commonly used reference genes include glyceraldehyde 3-phosphate dehydrogenase (GAPDH), β-actin, hypoxanthine guanine phosphoribosyl transferase (HPRT) and 18S ribosomal RNA.

The advantage of using mass units and normalizing the experimental design is that it is conceptually simple, but requires accurate quantitation of starting material to be used as a normalizer. There are some methods and models to determine the amount of DNA that are based on comparison of the CT values using the efficiency of PCR reaction as a correction factor. However, there is also a model that does not require the reaction efficiency of accessing a correction factor, assuming 100% efficiency in the PCR reaction in real time, both study gene as reference gene, this Method 2 is delta-delta CT (2-ΔΔCT) (Vinuesa, 2009; Aguilera et al, 2014.). Method 2-ΔΔCT expresses the ratio obtained from the relationship between the CT values of the sample and control values CT. Assay validation is made by serial dilution problem for both the endogenous gene to gene. ΔCt values (CT gen – CT endogenous) are obtained. These are plotted on the "y" axis versus the logarithm of the concentration in each of the dilutions in the "x" axis. The slope of the line should be less than or equal to 0.1 so that the method is valid [69]. Table 2 shows the most commonly used primers for the detection by different variants of PCR and also are listed the ones used to estimate the parasite load of *T. gondii* in tissues.

| **Amplification target** | **primers** | **Sequence 5′–3′** | **Amplicon size** | **Reference** |
|---|---|---|---|---|
| **PCR endpoint** | | | | |
| 529pb Repeat Element (*RE*) | Toxo4 | CGCTGCAGGGAGGAAGACGAAAGTTG | 529pb | [52,74,75] |
| | Toxo5 | CGCTGCAGACACAGTGCATCTCGGATT | | |
| Gen B1 | Tg1 | AAAAATGTGGGAATGAAAGAG | 469pb | [3,21,64] |
| | Tg2 | ACGAATCAACGGAACTGTAAT | | |
| Gen B1 | F | AGCCTCTCTCTTCAAGCAGCGTA | 300pb | [71,83] |
| | R | TCGGAGAGAGAAGTTCGTCGCAT | | |
| **Nested PCR** | | | | |
| Gen B1 | S1 | TGTTCTGTCCTATCGCAACG | 580 pb | [49] |
| | AS1 | ACGGATGCAGTTCCTTTCTG | 530pb | |
| | S2 | TCTTCCCAGACGTGGATTTC | | |
| | AS2 | CTCGACAATACGCTGCTTGA | | |
| Gen GRA6 | GRA6-F1x | ATTTGTGTTTCCGAGCAGGT | 546pb | [76] |
| | GRA6-R1 | GCACCTTCGCTTGTGGTT | 351pb | |
| | GRA6-F1 | TTTCCGAGCAGGTGACCT | | |
| | GRA6-R1x | TCGCCGAAGAGTTGACATAG | | |
| Gen B1 | B1F1 | TCAAGCAGCGTATTGTCGAG | 194pb | [96] |
| | B1R1 | CCGCAGCGACTTCTATCTCT | | |
| | B1F2 | GGAACTGCATCCGTTCATGAG | | |
| | B1R2 | TCTTTAAAGCGTTCGTGGTC | | |
| 529 pb *RE* | REF1 | TGACTCGGGCCCAGCTGCGT-3′ | 164pb | [93,95] |
| | RER1 | CTCCTCCCTTCGTCCAAGCCTCC-3′ | | |
| | REF2 | AGGGACAGAAGTCGAAGGGG-3′ | | |
| | RER2 | GCAGCCAAGCCGGAAACATC-3′ | | |
| PCR LAMP | | | | |
| 529bp *RE* | F3 | ACGAGAGTCGGAGAGGGA | 202pb | [93, 96] |
| | B3 | TGGATTCCTCTCCTACCCCT | | |
| | FIP (F1 c-F2) | GGATCGCATTCCGGTGTCTCTTAAGATGTTTCCGGCT | | |
| | BIP (B1c-B2) | TGGC | | |

| Amplification target | primers | Sequence 5′–3′ | Amplicon size | Reference |
|---|---|---|---|---|
| | | GACGACGCTTTCCTCGTGGTCAAGCCTCCGACTCTGT CT | | |
| 529bp *RE* | F3<br>B3<br>FIP<br>BIP<br>LF<br>LB | CCACAGAAGGGACAGAAGTC<br>TCCGGTGTCTCTTTTTCCAC<br>TCCTCACCCTCGCCTTCATCTAGGACTACAGACGCGA<br>TGC<br>TGGTTGGGAAGCGACGAGAGTTCCAGGAAAAGCAG<br>CCAAG<br>TCCAAGACGGCTGGAGGAG<br>CGGAGAGGGAGAAGATGTTTCC | 202pb | [96,97] |
| Gen B1 | BIP<br>FIP<br>F3<br>B3 | TCGCAACGGAGTTCTTCCCAGTTTTGGCCTGATATTA<br>CGACGGAC<br>TGACGCCTTTAGCACATCTGGT<br>TTTTGATGCTCAAAGTCGACCGC<br>GGGAGCAAGAGTTGGGACTA<br>CAGACAGCGAACAGAACAGA | 212 pb | [96] |
| **qPCR** | | | | |
| Gen B1 | SYBR Green™ | BE-F: CTCCTTCGTCCGTCGTAATATC<br>BE-R: TGGTGTACTGCGAAAATGAATC | 451pb | [47] |
| SAG 1 | SYBR Green™ | F: CTGATGTCGTTCTTGCGATGTGGC<br>R: GTGAAGTG-GTTCTCCGTCGGTGT | 128pb | [61] |
| Gen B1 | SYBR Green™ | F: CGTCCGTCGTAATATCAG<br>R: GACTTCATGGGACGATATG | 98pb | [47] |
| 529pb *RE* | TaqMan™ | F: CACAGAAGGGACAGAAGT<br>R: TCGCCTTCATCTACAGTC<br>RE probe: (JOE[e])-CTCTCCTCCAAGACGGCTGG-(TAMRA[f]) | 94pb | [47,63,69] |
| Gen B1 | TaqMan™ | GENE_B1_TG-TX2F: CTAGTATCGTGCGGCAATGTG<br>GENE_B1_TG-TX2R: GGCAGCGTCTCTTCCTCTTTT<br>GENE_B1_TG-TX2M1: 6-FAM)-CCACCTCGCCTCTTGG-(NFQ-MGB) | 62 pb | [79] |
| Gen B1 | TaqMan™ | BE-F: CCCCACAAGACGGCTGABE-R: TGGTGTACTGCGAAAATGAATC<br>TaqMan probe: (6-FAM)-CATTTGCAAAACAGCGGCAGCGTCT-(DQ) | 248pb | [47] |
| 529pb *RE* | TaqMan™ | TOX-9F: AGGAGAGATA TCAGGACTGT AG<br>TOX-11R: GCGTCGTCTC GTCTAGATCG<br>TOX-TP1: (6-FAM)-CCGGCTTGGC TGCTTTTCCT-(BHQ1) | 524pb | [5,47,56,77] |

**Table 2.** Amplification targets, primers and probes used in the diagnosis and quantification of *T. gondii* in meat.

Although there are several methods for the diagnosis of toxoplasmosis, the present work focused on the most used by researchers working with *T. gondii* in animal tissue samples. In this aspect the molecular, especially the PCR technique and its variants, has been a major technique for diagnosing the presence and in some cases abundance of the parasite in the tissues of the various productive species that are commonly consumed tool.

The sensitivity of PCR techniques is influenced by several factors, among which are tissue type, sample handling, the process employed in the extraction and purification of nucleic acids and the type of card selected amplification. All these factors cause variation sensitivity in these tests of about 20% to over 80% in some cases. Variations of the PCR most commonly used for the diagnosis of toxoplasmosis are conventional PCR, LAMP-PCR, nested PCR and real time PCR, considered as the most sensitive nested PCR and PCR techniques in real time, can detect the presence of nucleic acids of *T. gondii* from a single parasite in the sample.

The techniques of DNA extraction and purification significantly affect the development of PCR techniques; the presence of contaminants may inhibit the amplification process. Nowadays, there are different methodologies used for DNA extraction and also, there is a wide variety of commercial options available to perform the procedures, however, even almost all of them have been designed to obtain as much amount of DNA as possible from any specimen while minimizing manual handling and co-extraction of PCR inhibitors. Methodologies based in small-scale silica-based spin column, has proven more efficient for the recovery of pure DNA in comparison with phenol/chloroform extraction, because they have showed several disadvantages besides being unable to remove potential PCR inhibitors efficiently.

The sensitivity of PCR assays depends heavily on the number of copies of the target sequence; in the case of *T. gondii* although various cards amplification as is the case of SAG1, SAG2, SAG3 and GRA6 genes, most widely used are those which are directed to highly repetitive genes as gene B1 is repeated 35 times in the genome of *T. gondii* or repeated 529pb fraction, which is repeated 200 to 300 times in the parasite genome. Although the B1 gene is considered to be the gene of choice for the diagnosis, repeated fraction 529pb has begun to have a greater impact due to it being repeated more times increases the sensitivity of PCR testing. This trend toward the use of these cards amplification is observed in most variants of the PCR.

An important aspect for the selection of the PCR technique used in the diagnosis of toxoplasmosis has been the cost involved, the techniques of real-time PCR are usually much more expensive due to the use of probes and specialized equipment for reading the results, so this type of quantitative PCR are mainly used for research.

It is important to consider that molecular methods allow us to estimate whether the presence (when we use some variants as endpoint PCR or nested PCR) or quantity (by qPCR) parasite DNA in the evaluated sample. However, these findings do not allow for determination whether the parasites are viable and capable of producing infection.

Tissues that tend to have higher parasite loads are often brain, heart and spleen, but it is feasible to detect the presence of the parasite in other tissues intended for human consumption. Loading and distribution of parasites depends on biotype and density involved in the environment, as well as the animal's age and the type of production system. Due to this high variability, it is important to determine which tissues have higher loads and biotypes which are involved in order to avoid risks of transmission to consumers of meat from different regions and emphasize the importance of giving proper management to meat products (such as cooking or freeze) to reduce the risk of acquiring infection by eating them.

## 8. Conclusion and recommendation

Toxoplasmosis is a zoonotic disease transmitted by common foods; the occurrence of cysts of *T. gondii* in meat for human consumption represents a potential health risk, especially if the meat is consumed raw or cooked at lower temperatures of 67°C. In this sense the existence of accurate and reliable diagnostic tests is essential for the detection, monitoring and control of infections in intermediate hosts and to minimize the risk of infection in humans.

For the diagnosis of infection in tissue samples from naturally infected animals intended for consumption, it is desirable to use the technique Taqman qPCR probes since it is a more sensitive alternative to the same qPCR detection when used with SYBR Green dye. The format for performance this technique (qPCR with a Taqman probe) is versatile, allowing to evaluate both few samples (in a research environment for example) and in environments where it is required to test a greater number of specimens in a short time period (i.e., specialized laboratories for monitoring food safety), and increasingly, inputs for this procedure are more affordable.

## Author details

G.F. Dzib Paredes[1], A. Ortega-Pacheco[2], J.A. Rosado-Aguilar[2], K.Y. Acosta-Viana[3], E. Guzmán -Marín[3] and M. Jiménez-Coello[1*]

*Address all correspondence to: mjcoello@correo.uady.mx

1 Institutional Postgraduate Agricultural Science and Resource Management, CCBA/UADY, Mérida, Yucatán, México

2 Department of Animal Health and Preventive Medicine, CCBA/UADY, Merida, Yucatan, Mexico

3 Laboratory of Cell Biology, CIR, Dr. Hideyo Noguchi, CA Biomedicine of Infectious and Parasitic Diseases, Autonomous University of Yucatan, Mérida, Yucatán, México

## References

[1] Muñiz - Hernandez, S. & Mondragon -Flores, R. (2009). *Toxoplasma gondii* one murderer reemerging pathogen. Department of Biochemistry. CINVESTAV (CINVESTAV) IPN. Mexico DF. REB. 28 (2): 52-58

[2] Calderaro, A., Piccolo, G., Gorrini, C., Peruzzi, S., Zerbini, L., Bommezzadri, S., Dettori, G. & Chezzi, C. (2006). Comparison between two real-time PCR assays and a nested-PCR for the detection of *Toxoplasma gondii.* Acta Biomedica. 77:75–80.

[3] Rahdar, M., Samarbaf-Zadeh, A.R. & Arab, L. (2012). Evaluating the prevalence of *Toxoplasma gondii* in meat and products in Ahvaz by PCR method. Jundishapur Journal of Microbiology. 5(4):570–573. DOI: 10.5812/jjm.4280.

[4] Hill, D.E. & Dubey, J.P. (2013). *Toxoplasma gondii* prevalence in farm animals in the United States. [Review]. International Journal for Parasitology. 43(2):107–113.

[5] Juránková, J., Opsteegh, M., Neumayerová, H., Kovarcik, K., Frencová, A., Baláz, V., Volf, J. & Koudela, B. (2013b). Quantification of *Toxoplasma gondii* in tissue samples of experimentally infected goats by magnetic capture and real-time PCR. Veterinary Parasitology. 193:95–99.

[6] Tenter A.M. (2009). *Toxoplasma gondii* in animals used for human consumption. Memórias do Instituto Oswaldo Cruz. 104(2):364–369.

[7] Khalil, M., Petr, K., Marek, M., & Intisar, E.L.R. (2012). Socio-economical risk factors associated with *Toxoplasma gondii* infection in rural women at childbearing age in Sudan. Open Access Scientific Reports. 1:488. DOI: 10.4172/scientificreports.488.

[8] USDA (2011). Food Safety information. Available at: www.fsis.usda.gov/wps/wcm/connect/aa9f4a55-2e6f-45a3-8953-d9e986bde1b9/Parasites_Food_Safety_SP.pdf?MOD=AJPERES.

[9] Cenci-Goga, B.T., Rossitto, P.V., Sechi, P., McCrindle, C.M.E. & Cullorm J.S. (2011). *Toxoplasma* in animals, food, and humans: an old parasite of new concern. Foodborne Pathogens and Disease. 8:751–762.

[10] Dubey, J.P., Graham, D.H., Dahl, E., Sreekumar, C., Lehmann, T., Davis, M.F. & Morishita, T.Y. (2003). *Toxoplasma gondii* isolates from free-ranging chickens from the United States. Journal of Parasitology. 89:1060–1062.

[11] Sibley, L.D., Khan A., Ajioka, J.W. & Rosenthal, B.M. (2009). Genetic diversity of *Toxoplasma gondii* in animals and humans. Philosophical transactions of the Royal Society of London. Series B, Biological sciences Royal Society. 364(1530):2749–2761.

[12] Devada, K., Anandan, R. & Dubey, J.P. (1998). Serologic prevalence to *Toxoplasma gondii* in chickens in Madras, India. Journal of Parasitology. 84:621–622.

[13] Sreekumar, C., Graham, D.H., Dahl, E., Lehmann, T., Raman, M., Bhalerao, D.P., Vianna, M.C.B. & Dubey, J.P. (2003). Genotyping of *Toxoplasma gondii* isolates from chickens from India. Veterinary Parasitology. 118:187–194.

[14] El-Massry, A., Mahdy, O.A., El-Ghaysh, A. & Dubey, J. P. (2000). Prevalence of *Toxoplasma gondii* antibodies in sera of turkeys, chickens, and ducks from Egypt. Journal of Parasitology. 86:627–628.

[15] Franco-Hernandez, E.N., Acosta, A., Cortés-Vecino, J. & Gómez-Marín, J.E. (2016). Survey for *Toxoplasma gondii* by PCR detection in meat for human consumption in Colombia. Parasitology Research. 115:691–695.

[16] Zhao, G., Shen, B., Xie, Q., Xu, L X., Yan, R.F., Song, X.K., Hassan, I.A. & Li, X.R. (2012). Detection of *Toxoplasma gondii* in free-range chickens in China based on circulating antigens and antibodies. Veterinary Parasitology. 185:72–77.

[17] Onyiche, T.E. & Ademola, I.O. (2015). Seroprevalence of anti-*Toxoplasma gondii* antibodies in cattle and pigs in Ibadan, Nigeria. Journal of Parasitic Diseases. 39(2):309–314.

[18] Bacci, C., Vismarra, A., Mangia, C., Bonardi, S., Bruini, I., Genchi, M., Kramer, L. & Brindani, F. (2015). Detection of *Toxoplasma gondii* in free-range, organic pigs in Italy using serological and molecular methods. International Journal of Food Microbiology. 202:54–56.

[19] Cademartori, B.G., Santos, L.M., Oliveira, F.C., Quevedo, P., Oliveira, P.A., Ramos, T.S., Rocha, A.S., Ruas, J.L. & Farias, N.A. (2014). Isolation and pathogenicity of *Toxoplasma gondii* in naturally infected (rustic farm) pigs in Southern Brazil. Veterinary Parasitology. 203: 207–211.

[20] Alvarado-Esquivel, C., Romero-Salas, D., García-Vázquez, Z., Crivelli-Diaz, M., Barrientos-Morales, M., Lopez-de-Buen, L. & Dubey, J.P. (2014). Seroprevalence and correlates of *Toxoplasma gondii* infection in domestic pigs in Veracruz State, Mexico. Tropical Animal Health and Production. 46(4):705–709.

[21] Ortega-Pacheco, A., Acosta-Viana, K.Y., Guzmán-Marín, E., Segura-Correa, J.C., Álvarez-Fleites, M. & Jiménez-Coello, M. (2013). Prevalence and risk factors of *Toxoplasma gondii* in fattening pigs farm from Yucatán, México. Research article, BioMed Research International. 2013, e231497.

[22] Dubey, J.P. (2010). Toxoplasmosis of animals and humans (second edition). CRC Press, USA.

[23] Tenter, A.M., Heckeroth, A.R. & Weiss, L.M. (2000). *Toxoplasma gondii*: from animals to humans. International Journal for Parasitology. 30:1217–1258.

[24] Dubey, J.P. & Thulliez, P. (1993). Persistence of tissue cysts in edible tissues of cattle fed *Toxoplasma gondii* oocysts. American Journal of Veterinary Research. 54:270–273.

[25] National Institute of Safety and Health at Work (INSHT). (2014). *Toxoplasma gondii,* sheet Available at: http://www.insht.es/RiesgosBiologicos/Contenidos/Fichas%20de%20agentes%20biologicos/Fichas/Parasitos/Toxoplasma%20gondii.pdf.

[26] Kijlstra, A. & Jongert, E. (2008a). Control of the risk of human toxoplasmosis transmitted by meat. International Journal for Parasitology. 38(12):1359–1370, DOI: 10.1016/j.ijpara.2008.06.002.

[27] Ribera-Pascuet, E. (2013). Toxoplasmosis medicina interna (2ª ed.). J. Rodés, 1:1849–1852.

[28] Montoya, J.G. & Lisenfeld, O. (2004). Toxoplasmosis. The LANCET. 363:1965–1976.

[29] Restrepo, M. (2007). Toxoplasmosis: zoonosis parasitaria. Rev. CES Medicine. 21(1): 41–48.

[30] Uribarren-Berrueta, T. (2013). Toxoplasmosis - Resources Parasitology - Department of Microbiology and Parasitology - UNAM. Available at http://www.facmed.unam.mx/deptos/microbiologia/parasitologia/toxoplasmosis.html.

[31] Vallochi, A.L., Goldberg, A.C., Falcai, A., Ramasawmy, R., Kalil, J., Silveira, C., Belfort, R. & Rizzo, L.V. (2008). Molecular markers of susceptibility to ocular toxoplasmosis, host and guest behaving badly. Clinical Ophthalmology. 2:837–48.

[32] Paternina - Vivero, C. (2004). Management Guide toxoplasmosis in pregnancy. District Health Secretariat of Bogotá, Bogotana Association of Obstetrics and Gynecology (Asbog).Available at http://www.saludcapital.gov.co/DDS/Publicaciones/GUIA%202.%20%20MANEJO%20DE%20TOXOPLASMOSIS%20EN%20EL%20EMBARAZO.pdf.

[33] Buxton, D., Maley, S.W., Wright, S.E., Rodger, S., Bartley, P. & Innes, E.A. (2007). *Toxoplasma gondii* and ovine toxoplasmosis: new aspects of an old story. Veterinary Parasitology. 149:25–28.

[34] Hartmann, K., Addie, D., Belák, S., Boucraut-Baralon, C., Egberink, H., Frymus, T., Gruffydd-Jones, T., Hosie, M.J., Lloret, A., Lutz, H., Marsilio, F., Möstl, K., Pennisi, M.G., Radford, A,D., Thiry, E., Truyen, U. & Horzinek, M.C. (2013). *Toxoplasma gondii* infection in cats:ABCD guidelines on prevention and management. Journal of Feline Medicine and Surgery. 15(7):631–637.

[35] Basso, W.U. & Venturini, M. C. (2009). Zoonosis issues IV. Chapter 39. " Toxoplasmosis in domestic and wild animals raised in captivity : epidemiological and diagnostic aspects ". Ed. Association Zoonoses Argentina. Available at: http://www.veterinariargentina.com/revista/2009/05/la-toxoplasmosis-en-los-animales-domesticos-y-silvestres-criados-en-cautiverio-aspectos-epidemiologicos-y-diagnostico/.

[36] Jones, J.L., Kruszon-Moran, D., Rivera, H.N., Price, C. & Wilkins, P.P. (2014). *Toxoplasma gondii* seroprevalence in the United States 2009-2010 and comparison with the

past two decades. American Journal of Tropical Medicine and Hygiene. 90:1135–1139.

[37] Hill, D. & Dubey, J.P. (2002). *Toxoplasma gondii*: transmission, diagnosis and prevention. Clinical Microbiology and Infection. 8:634–640.

[38] Roberts,,F. & McLeod, R. (1999). Pathogenesis of toxoplasmic retinochoroiditis. Parasitology Today. 15:51–57.

[39] Acha, P.N. & Szyfres, B. (2003). Zoonoses and communicable diseases common to man and animals. Parasitic Zoonoses (Vol. 3). Pan American Health Org.

[40] Buzby, J.C. & Roberts, T. (1996). ERS updates U.S. foodborne disease costs for seven pathogens. Food Reveiw. 19(3):20-25.

[41] Abu-Dalbou, M.A., Ababneh, M.M., Giadinis, N.D. & Lafi, S.Q. (2010). Ovine and caprine toxoplasmosis (*Toxoplasma gondii*). Iranian Journal of Veterinary Science and Technology. 2(2):61–76.

[42] Vickers, M. & Wright, N. (2013). Economic Impact of Health and Welfare Issues in Beef Cattle and Sheep in England. Available at http://www.eblex.org.uk/wp/wp-content/uploads/2013/04/Economic-Impact-of-Health-Welfare-Final-Rpt-170413.pdf

[43] Bennett, R. & Ijpelaar, J. (2003). Economic assessment of livestock diseases in Great Britain. Final report to Defra; ZZ0102 University of Reading.

[44] da Silva, A.F., Brandão, F.Z., Oliveira, F.C.R. & Ferreira, A.M.R. (2013). *Toxoplasma gondii* in the sheep industry: a global overview and the situation in Brazil. Revista Brasileira de Ciência Veterinária. 20:456. Available at http://www.uff.br/rbcv/ojs/index.php/rbcv/article/view/456/pdf_1.

[45] Dubey, J.P. (2009) Toxoplasmosis in sheep The last 20 years. Veterinary Parasitology. 163:1–14.

[46] Basso, W., Handke, M., Sydler, T., Borel, N., Grimm, F., Sidler, X. & Deplazes, P. (2015). Involvement of *Toxoplasma gondii* in reproductive disorders in Swiss pig farms. Parasitology International. 64(2):157–160.

[47] Edvinsson, B., Jalal, S., Nord, C.E., Pedersen, B.S. & Evengard, B. (2004). DNA extraction and PCR assays for detection of *Toxoplasma gondii*. APMIS. 112:342–348.

[48] Juránková, J., Basso, W., Neumayerová, H., Baláz, V., Jánová, E., Silder, X., Deplazes, P. & Koudela, B. (2013a). Brain is the predilection site of *Toxoplasma gondii* in experimentally inoculated pigs as revealed by magnetic capture and real-time PCR. Food Microbiology. 38:167–170.

[49] Alfonso, Y., Fraga, J., Cox, R., Bandera, F., Pomier, O., Fonseca, C., Ginorio, D., Torres, G. & Capo, V. (2008). Comparison of four DNA extraction methods from cerebrospinal fluid for the detection of *Toxoplasma gondii* by polymerase chain reaction in AIDS patients. Diagnostics and Medical Technology. 14(3):MT1-6.

[50] Somma, M. & Querci, M. (2010). Analysis of the presence of genetically modified organisms in food samples, Session No. 6 : polymerase chain reaction (PCR). World Health Organization. 84-108. Available at http://gmo-crl.jrc.ec.europa.eu/capacity-building/manuals/Manual%20ES/User%20Manual%20ES%20full.pdf

[51] Alejos-Velásquez, L.P., Aragón-Martínez, M.C. & Cornejo-Romero, A. (2014). DNA extraction and purification. Molecular tools applied in ecology : theoretical and practical aspects 1st edition. Secretariat of Environment and Natural Resources (SEMARNAT), National Institute of Ecology and Climate Change. (INECC), Iztapalapa Metropolitan Autonomous University (UAM -I)

[52] Mataix-Verdú, J. & Victoria-Muñoz, E.M. (2008). Manual de Fisiologia. Sistema Digestivo. Editorial Universidad de Granada.

[53] Pearson, H. & Stirling, D. (2003). DNA Extraction from Tissue. In: PCR Protocols. Bartlett, J., Stirling, D. 2nd Edition. Humana press. 33–34

[54] Karp, G. (2009). Biología celular y molecular, conceptos y experimentos 5ª ed. McGrawHill. 763–765.

[55] Zumbo, P. (2012). Phenol-chloroform extraction protocol. Weill Cornell Medical College, Department of physiology & biophysics. Available at: http://physiology.med.cornell.edu/faculty/mason/lab/zumbo/files/PHENOL-CHLOROFORM.pdf.

[56] Opsteegh, M., Langelaar, M., Sprong, H., Hartog, L., De-Craeye, S., Bokken, G., Ajzenberg, D., Kijlstra, A. & Giessen, J.V.D. (2010). Direct detection and genotyping of *Toxoplasma gondii* in meat samples using magnetic capture and PCR. International Journal of Food Microbiology. 139:193–201.

[57] FIBAO. (2014). Hybrid selection method target sequences for massively parallel sequencing.Available at: http://medmol.es/tecnicas/93/.

[58] Life technologies. (2010a). DNAzol® Reagent, for isolation of genomic DNA from solid and liquid samples. Available at: https://www.lifetechnologies.com/order/catalog/product/10503027.

[59] Life technologies. (2010b). TRIzol® LS Reagent. Available at: http://www.lifetechnologies.com/order/catalog/product/10296010.

[60] Stirling, D. (2003). Quality Control in PCR. In: PCR Protocols. Bartlett, J., Stirling, D. 2nd Edition. Humana press. 21–23.

[61] Yu, H., Huang, B., Zhuo, X., Chen, X. & Du, A. (2013). Evaluation of real-time PCR assay based on the single-copy SAG1 gene for the detection of *Toxoplasma gondii*. Short communication, Veterinary Parasitology. 197:670–673.

[62] Bezerra, R.A., Carvalho, F.S., Guimarães, L.A., Rocha, D.S., Silva, F.L., Wenceslau, A.A. & Albuquerque, G.R. (2012). Comparison of methods for detection of *Toxoplasma gondii* in tissues of naturally exposed pigs. Parasitology Research. 110:509–514.

[63] Gutierrez, J., O′ Donovan, J., Williams, E., Proctor, A., Brady, C., Marques, P.X., Worrall, S., Nally, J.E., McErloy, M., Bassett, H., Sammin, D., Buxton, D., Maley, S. & Markey, B.K. (2010). Detection and quantification of *Toxoplasma gondii* in ovine maternal and foetal tissues from experimentally infected pregnant ewes using real-time PCR. Veterinary Parasitology. 172:8–15.

[64] Jalal, S., Nord, C.E., Lappalainen, M. & Evengard, B. (2004). Rapid and sensitive diagnosis of *Toxoplasma gondii* infections by PCR. Research note, Clinical Microbiology and Infection. 10:937–939.

[65] Sousa, S., Ajzenberg, D., Canada, N., Freire, L., Corriera, da Costa, J.M., Daré, M.L., Thulliez, P. & Dubey, J.P. (2006). Biologic and molecular characterization of *Toxoplasma gondii* isolates from pigs from Portugal. Veterinary Parasitology. 135:133–136.

[66] Kasper, D.C., Sadeghi, K., Prusa, A.R., Reischer, G.H., Kratochwill, K., Förster-Waldl, E., Gerstl, N., Hayde, M., Pollak, A. & Herkner, K.R. (2009). Quantitative real-time polymerase chain reaction for the accurate detection of *Toxoplasma gondii* in amniotic fluid. Diagnostic Microbiology and Infectious Disease. 63:10–15.

[67] Richomme, C., Aubert, D., Gliot-Fromont, E., Ajzenberg, D., Mercier, A., Ducrot, C., Ferté, H., Delorme, D. & Villena, I. (2009). Genetic characterization of *Toxoplasma gondii* from wild boar (Sus scrofa) in France. Short communication, Veterinary Parasitology. 164:296–300.

[68] Luptakova, L., Valencakova, A., Balent, P., Malcekova, B. & Petrovova, E. (2012). Evaluation of detection of *Toxoplasma gondii* DNA in animal blood samples by quantitative PCR. Research article, Central European Journal of Biology. 7(3):431–435.

[69] Aigner, C.P., Silva, A.V., Sandrini, F., Osório, P.S., Poiares, L. & Largura, A. (2010). Real-time PCR- based quantification of *Toxoplasma gondii* in tissue samples of serologically positive outdoor chickens. Memorias Instituto Oswaldo Cruz, Rio de Janeiro, 105(7):935–937.

[70] Warnekulasuriya, M.R., Jphnson, J.D. & Holliman, R.E. (1998). Detection of *Toxoplasma gondii* in cured meats. International Journal of Microbiology. 45:211–215.

[71] Silva, A.V. & Langoni, H. (2001). The detection of *Toxoplasma gondii* by comparing cytology, histopatology, bioassay in mice, and the polymerase chain reaction (PCR). Veterinary Parasitology. 97:191–198.

[72] Jauregui, L.H., Higgins, J., Zarlenga, D., Dubey, J.P. & Lunney, J.K. (2001). Development of a real time PCR assay detection of *Toxoplasma gondii* in pig and mouse tissues. Journal of Microbiology. 39(6):2065–2071.

[73] Aspinall, T.V., Marlee, D., Hyde, J.E. & Sims, P.F.G. (2002). Prevalence of *Toxoplasma gondii* in commercial meat products as monitored by polymerase chain reaction- food for thought? International Journal for Parasitology. 32:1193–1199.

[74] García, J.L., Gennari, S.M., Machado, R.Z. & Navarro, I.T. (2006). *Toxoplasma gondii*: detection by mouse bioassay, histopathology, and polymerase chain reaction in tissues from experimentally infected pigs. Experimental Parasitology. 113:267–271.

[75] Tsutsui, V.S., Freire, R.L., García, J.L., Gennari, S.M. Vieira, D.P., Marana, E.R.M., Prudencio, L.B. & Navarro, I.T. (2007). Detection of *Toxoplasma gondii* by PCR and mouse bioassay in commercial cuts of pork from experimentally infected pigs. Arquivo Brasileiro de Medicina Veterinária e Zootecnia. 59:30–34.

[76] Asgari, Q., Sarnevesht, J., Kalantari, M., Adnani-Sadat, S.J., Hossein-Motazedian, M. & Sarkari, B. (2010). Molecular survey of *Toxoplasma* infection in sheep and goat from Fars province, Southern Iran. Tropical Animal Health and Production. DOI: 10.1007/s11250-010-9704-1.

[77] Juránková, J., Hurková-Hofmannová, L., Volf, J., Baláz, V. & piálek, J. (2014). Efficacy of magnetic capture in comparison with conventional DNA isolation in a survey of *Toxoplasma gondii* in wild house mice. European Journal of Parasitology. 50:11–15.

[78] Faucher, B., Miermont, F., Ranque, S., Franck, J. & Piarroux, R. (2011). Optimization of *Toxoplasma gondii* DNA extraction from amniotic fluid using NucliSENS easyMAG and comparison with QIAamp DNA minikit. European Journal of Clinical Microbiology &and Infectious Diseases. 31:1035–1039.

[79] Kompalic-Cristo, A., Frotta, C., Suárez-Mutis, M., Fernandes, O. & Britto, C. (2007). Evaluation of a real-time PCR assay based on the repetitive B1 gene for the detection of *Toxoplasma gondii* in human peripheral blood. Parasitology Research. 101:619–625.

[80] Hill, D.E., Chirukandoth, S., Dubey, J.P., Lunney, J.K. & Gamble, H.R. (2006). Comparison of detection methods for *Toxoplasma gondii* in naturally and experimentally infected swine. Veterinary Parasitology. 141:9–17.

[81] Lehmann, T., Blackston, C. R., Parmley, S. F., Remington, J. S. & Dubey, J. P. (2000). Strain typing of *Toxoplasma gondii*: comparison of antigen-coding and housekeeping genes. Journal of Parasitology. 86:960–971.

[82] Santos, C.B.A., Carvalho, A.C.F.B., Ragozo, A.M.A., Soares, M.R., Amaku, M., Yai, L.E.O., Dubey, J.P. & Gennari, S.M. (2005). First isolation and molecular characterization of *Toxoplasma gondii* from finishing pigs from São Paulo State, Brazil. Veterinary Parasitology. 131:207–211.

[83] Shaapan, R.M., Abo-Elmaaty, A.M., Razik, K.A.A. & Hafez, S.M.A. (2006). PCR and serological assays for detection of *Toxoplasma gondii* infection in sport horses in Cairo, Egypt. Asian Journal of Animal and Veterinary Advances. 7:158–165.

[84] Krijger, I.M., Cornelissen, J.B., Wisselink, H. & Meerburg, B.G. (2014). Prevalence of *Toxoplasma gondii* in common moles (Talpa europea). Acta Veterinaria Scandinavica. 56:48.

[85] Switaj, K., Master, A., Skrzypczak, M. & Zaborowski, P. (2005). Recent trends in molecular diagnostics for *Toxoplasma gondii* infections. European Society of Clinical Microbiology and Infectious Diseases. 11:170–176.

[86] Garibyan, L. & Avashia, N. (2013). Polymerase chain reaction. Journal of Investigative Dermatology. 133(6):1–4. DOI: 10.1038/jid.2013.1.

[87] Lewin, B. (2008). Genes, 9th edition. McGrawHill. 428–453.

[88] Welch, H.M. (2012). The polymerase chain reaction. Metastasis Research Protocols, Methods in Molecular Biology. 878:71–88. DOI: 10.1007/978-1-61779-854-2_5.

[89] Grunenwald, H. (2003). Optimization of Polymerase Chain Reactions. In: PCR Protocols. Bartlett, J., Stirling, D. 2nd Edition.Humana press. 21–23.

[90] Bonin, S. & Dotti, I. (2011). Nested-PCR. En G. Stanta (ed.). Guidelines for molecular análisis in archive tissues. Springer-Verlag Berlin Heidelberg. DOI: 10.1007/978-3-642-17890-0_22.

[91] Berger-Schoch, A.E., Herrmann, D.C., Schares, G., Müller, N., Bernet, D., Gottstein, B. & Frey, C.F. (2011). Prevalence and genotypes of *Toxoplasma gondii* in feline faeces (oocysts) and meat from sheep, cattle and pigs in Switzerland. Veterinary Parasitology. 177:290-297.

[92] Barkway, C.P., Pocock, R.L., Vrba, V. & Blake, D.P. (2011). Loop-mediated isothermal amplification (LAMP) assays for the species-specific detection of Eimeria that infect chickens. BMC Veterinary Research. 7:67.

[93] Kong, Q.M., Lu, S.H., Tong, Q.B., Lou, D., Chen, R., Zheng, B., Kumagai, T., Wen, L.Y., Ohta, N. & Zhou, X.N. (2012) Loop-mediated isothermal amplification (LAMP): early detection of *Toxoplasma gondii* infection in mice. Parasites & Vectors. 5:2.

[94] Robert-Gangneux F, Dardé ML. Epidemiology of and Diagnostic Strategies for Toxoplasmosis. (2012). Clinical Microbiology Reviews. 25(2):264–296.

[95] Sivaganesan, M., Haugland, R.A., Chern, E.C., Shanks, O.C. (2010). Improved strategies and optimization of calibration models for real-time PCR absolute quantification. Water Research. 44(16):4726–4735.

[96] Fallahi, S., Seyyed Tabaei, S.J., Pournia, Y., Zebardast, N. & Kazemi, B. (2014). Comparison if loop-mediated isothermal amplification (LAMP) and nested-PCR assay targeting the RE and B1 gene for detection of *Toxoplasma gondii* in blood samples of children with leukemia. Diagnostic Microbiology and Infectious Disease. 79(3):347–354.

[97] Zhang, H., Thekisoe, O.M., Aboge, G.O, Kyan, H., Yamagishi, J., Inoue, N., Nishikawa, Y., Zakimi, S. & Xuan, X. (2009). *Toxoplasma gondii:* sensitive and rapid detection of infection by loop-mediated isothermal amplification (LAMP) method. Experimental Parasitology. 122(1):47–50.

# 10

# Experimental Models of Ocular Toxoplasmosis

Aléx Martins Nasaré and Roberto Carlos Tedesco

**Abstract**

First described in *Ctenodactylus gundi* and simultaneously in rabbit, *Toxoplasma gondii*, an etiological agent of toxoplasmosis, affects different species of vertebrates and invertebrates, presenting different manifestations depending on the host. Ocular toxoplasmosis is one of the mean manifestations of toxoplasmosis in humans, affecting 2% of infected individuals in Europe and North America. Otherwise many aspects of ocular toxoplasmosis still await answer. One of the major factors limiting this process is the difficulty to obtain human samples, doing necessary the use of experimental models. By the way, animal models do not express reality of human disease. The present study defines a compilation of report cases and results that supports the choice of an ideal experimental animal model of ocular toxoplasmosis. Actual literature bears new researches contributing in the choice of a specific experimental animal model. Moreover, the choice must consider behavior, period of life, and maintenance in captivity and ocular toxoplasmosis manifestation. Previous studies contribute for a best-chosen experimental animal model, by the way fragmented information makes difficult to compare mostly animal models picked that do not present efficiency enough. In conclusion, experimental animal models are able to bring relevant information about the course of ocular toxoplasmosis.

**Keywords:** experimental model, ocular toxoplasmosis, animal model

## 1. Introduction

*Toxoplasma gondii* was first described in 1908 by Nicolle and Manceaux, presented into tissues of a north-African rodent, known as *Ctenodactylus gundi*, which after was mentioned to describe the specific epithet that compose specie. Simultaneously in Brazil, Splendore identified same parasite in rabbit tissues. *T. gondii*, etiological agent of toxoplasmosis and an obligatory intra-cellular parasite, affects different species of vertebrates and invertebrates. In addition, *T. gondii* presents three different infective forms that can infect hosts by ingestion of raw meat containing cysts or, food and water containing oocysts [1]. Infection can also affect the embryo, during pregnancy; with different levels of severity, depending on the specie and the period that infection occurs. Toxoplasmosis can present different manifestations, as fever, increase of lymph nodes, intraocular inflammation [2], encephalitis, and other systemic infections [3].

Ocular toxoplasmosis, a vision-threatening ocular disease, is the most common cause of infectious uveitis [4]. It is one of the mean manifestations of toxoplasmosis in humans, affecting up to 30% of the humans worldwide. In Europe and North America, development of ocular toxoplasmosis is around 2% of infected individual. In Brazil, uveitis is estimated to be caused by toxoplasmosis in 60–85% of lesions cases [5]. Highlighting Erechim, Southern Brazil with a high frequency of humans infected usually transmitted by ingestion of uncooked meat containing cysts [6]. Ocular toxoplasmosis was first described in 1923 by Jankû, and subsequently by Levaditi in 1928. Whereas it was just in 1952 that *T. gondii* had its relation to the retinochorioiditis Foerster in Weiss and Kim [7]. Accordingly, some authors, retinochorioiditis is a major cause of visual impairment in the USA, where it accounts around 30–50% of all cases of uveitis [8]. Otherwise many aspects of ocular toxoplasmosis still await answer.

One of the major factors limits is the difficult to obtain human infected material. Once *T. gondii* had a predilection by nervous tissues, locating itself in immune competent individuals in brain and eyes. So, it does necessary experimental animal models. But, animal models do not express reality of human disease. Therefore, the establishment of an ideal experimental model, that mimic the course of ocular toxoplasmosis, is fundamental as a springboard for finding answers of the disease. Considering particularities of each experimental animal model for each specific conduced study.

## 2. Ocular toxoplasmosis

Accordingly literature, the *T. gondii* reaches the bulb of the eye using the blood, normally causing a focal lesion and asymptomatic, but not well comprehended [9]. The eye is an immunologic privileged environment, as the brain. But, brain barrier is more studied than ocular barrier [10]. In previous studies, ocular toxoplasmosis infection has been formed principally by lymphocytes B. This increase in migration of lymphocytes is associated to high levels of IFN-$\gamma$ and IL-6 and low levels of IL-10, suggesting that cytokines alterations provide inflammation and retinochorioiditis. Other studies indicate that the severity of ocular toxoplasmosis is close related to intensity of inflammation and presence of IL-17. Thus toxoplasmosis infection relates pathogenesis to Th1 and Th17 cell. While IL-10, TGF-$\beta$, and IL-27 are cytokines with an important role into immune regulation of maintenance and inflammation of important sites, as eye environment [5, 7].

The most affected structure in ocular toxoplasmosis is the retina. Retina is the nervous tissue of the bulb of the eye, responsible for transduce photon stimulus into electric impulse. And for that transduction occurs, it is necessary that the integrity and well function of the 10 layers of retina tissue, identified in **Figure 1**, from the inner tissues to outer in the following order: inner limiting membrane, nerve fibers layer, ganglion cells, inner plexiform, inner nuclear layer, outer plexiform and nuclear layers, outer limiting membrane, segments of photoreceptors, and retinal pigmented epithelium. In evidence, toxoplasmic retinochorioiditis affects straight the retina as a structure, but most damaged layers are nuclear plexiform and ganglion layers, as well as the segments of photoreceptor, once RPE presents a migration, causing a discontinuity forming great interstitial lacunae. Also is observed inflammatory cells in the inner plexiform layers, also responsible for none well function of retina tissue [11].

The retina is the first area involved, furthermore choroids, vitreous humor, and anterior chamber might be also involved, but never will it happen before retina. The most common sign of acute ocular toxoplasmosis is a focal and in major times, unilateral retinal lesion [12].

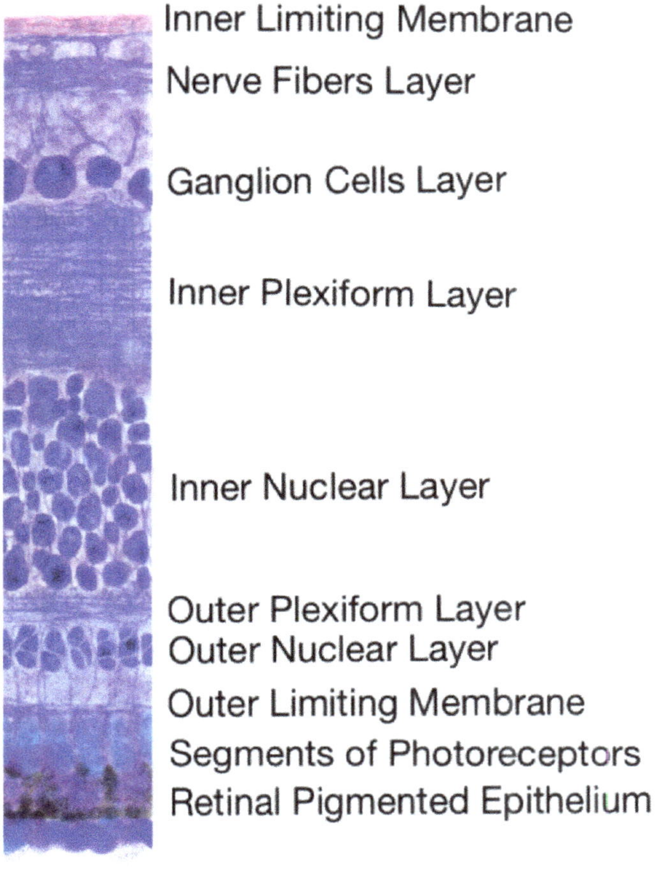


**Figure 1.** Retinal scheme containing 10 layers that compose this tissue.

But, in some individuals it was observed too, bilateral lesion, occlusive vasculitis, diffuse necrotizing retinitis and scleritis. Retinochorioiditis is commonly observed in congenital and acquired toxoplasmosis [13] resulting in acute disease and infection reactivation. It is possible to affect one or both eyes, presenting it in three different forms. Forms can be didactically differentiated (**Figure 2**) as punctual, multiple, and satellite lesions. In other worlds, punctual lesion might indicate primary infection, while multiple and satellite lesions, might indicate reactivation of disease. In addition, satellite lesions it is characterized by a combination of an active lesion with a healed retinal scar [10]. By the way, it is not dependent if it is acquired or congenital toxoplasmosis [4].

Clinical finds may be influenced by clonal type of *T. gondii*. There are three predominant clonal types, based on virulence studies [14]. But virulent strains appear to have their origin in one genetically homogeneous lineage. Studies based one murine model infers that type II would be responsible for the majority of ocular lesions. Furthermore, recent studies shows that type I, is atypical and with an important role in ocular lesions [14–16]. In Europe, type II strains are responsible for majority of human infections. In South America, a recombinant strain is associated to ocular toxoplasmosis [4]. Studies of Howe and Sibley, in 1995 and Belfort-Neto and collaborators in 2007 correlate type II with an important role in acquired infection, while type I clonal lineage may be responsible for the congenital toxoplasmosis, even so type I and atypical strains may play a role in acquired infection [14]. For instance, type III has been reported only 9% of toxoplasmosis patients in France and United States [17]. However, even with few information relating clonal type with virulence and frequency, just an insufficient part is known, needing more studies in this area.

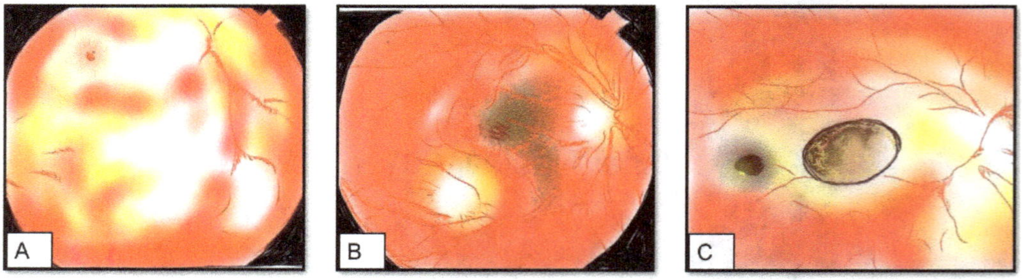


**Figure 2.** Ophthalmoscopy scheme differentiation of retinal lesions; (A) punctual lesion; (B) multiple lesions; and (C) satellite lesion.

## 3. Acquired toxoplasmosis

Acquired toxoplasmosis occurs principally for ingesting of raw meat, vegetables, and water contemned with oocysts of *T. gondii*. Acquired toxoplasmosis normally can affect the eye in acute form, beyond 10% of the cases, but the majority is naïve, transitory, and frequently asymptomatic [18]. Loss vision in acquired toxoplasmosis is normally due from destruction of retina tissue, specially the macula. Furthermore, might be worse by reactivation, months or years after [19].

## 4. Congenital toxoplasmosis

Congenital toxoplasmosis is a result of an infection in prenatal presenting clinic morphologies before birth, or just along the first quarter of gestational period, been present in the forms of anencephaly, hematological abnormalities, loss vision, and blindness or even death [4, 20]. But the majority of manifestations are rare, been subclinical at birth. It can be possible to present lesions along the life. Congenital ocular toxoplasmosis can present itself neonatal, or lately, but it is more common in the last quarter of gestational period. Retinal destruction is a very frequent sequel of congenital disease [8] presenting a predilection for macular involvement [4]. A congenital ocular lesion appears to be the highest risk of systemic infection when compared to acquire ocular toxoplasmosis. Congenital ocular toxoplasmosis has been estimated to affect 3000 kids born in the USA each year. It affects 70–90% of patients, been the most common manifestation of disease. By the way, great majority of kids appears asymptomatic. Report cases indicate that some of them develop chorioretinal lesions, from scars until vision loss [7].

## 5. Experimental models of ocular toxoplasmosis

First animal model of toxoplasmosis was guinea pig, established by Markham in 1937. But just in 1951, the first animal model for ocular toxoplasmosis was established by Hogan, using intracarotid injection in rabbits. Following same lineage, in 1953, Frenkel managed an intraperitoneal injection in hamster. Lately nonhuman primates, cats, pigs, and dogs started been used as model [4]. Accordingly history of experimental animal models for toxoplasmosis, author and method used exposed in following time line (**Figure 3**).

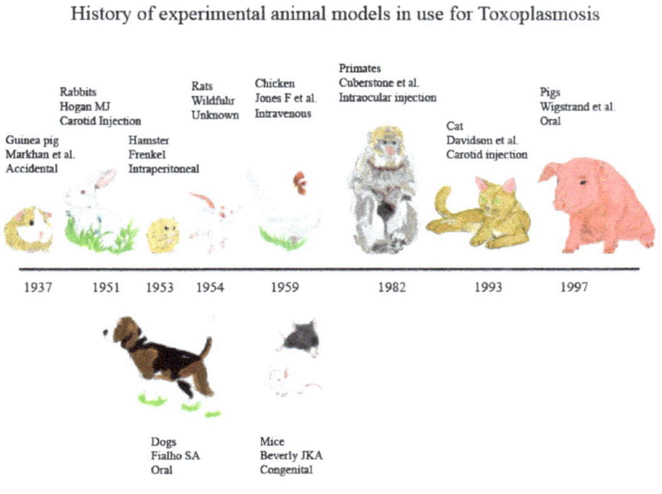


**Figure 3.** Schematic time line with historic of experimental animal models for toxoplasmosis, independent on development of ocular toxoplasmosis.

In impossibility to obtain sample from human with acute ocular infection, animal models has been developed to supply and find answers [4]. In spite of, any animal model of ocular toxoplasmosis must consider some criteria: parasite entry, onset of disease and manifestation, self-limitation of ocular inflammation, and model of recurrence, parasite strain used, and experimental manipulation of disease processing and treatment [10]. Ocular toxoplasmosis animal models should answer how disease happens in humans, as close as possible, from entry of parasite to development of disease. Furthermore, strains of parasite is so important as route of infection, once some strains show certain defect achieving system of host. The most used strains are: RH, ME-49, Beverly, PLK, and Fukaya. Strains from type I was isolated from patients and animals. Type II lesser extent type I strains are used in animal models of ocular infection.

*T. gondii* parasitizes the host, without producing clinical disease. After penetrating intestinal epithelial cells. *T. gondii* may spread to other organs by lymphatics and blood system, multiplying in any cell of the organism. As long *T. gondii* may cause an infection and severe disease in animals, causing great losses in some species, like sheep and goats, generating embryonic death, abnormalities, and others.

It is important to highlight that toxoplasmosis affects individuals in different forms, and in some cases do not express the disease how it is described in literature, otherwise it is of major importance to express how parasite is able to hand on the intermediate and definitive host. In immunosuppressed host, toxoplasmosis may lead them to death, unless accomplished of correct treatment. Actually known as corticosteroid, sulfadiazine, and pyrimethamine. Those medics relapse disease, doing necessary in some experimental models. Besides, pathogenicity of *T. gondii* is determined by virulence of the strain and resistance of the host, in some cases even hosts habits.

Nowadays, it is known that some variation of mice is more susceptible than other, seeing the severity of infection course. Adult rats do not become ill, differently from the youngers from the same species, which can dies of toxoplasmosis. Ungulates are the most resistant hosts to toxoplasmosis, whereas some marsupials, and nonhuman primates are highly susceptible to *T. gondii* infection [21]. In literature animals like pig, ordinarily there are not many descriptions as experimental models, moreover as case report. Like young pigs, which have high mortality, while adult pigs are resistant. Notwithstanding, infected pigs are described with pneumonia, myocarditis, encephalitis, and placental necrosis. Other species as mink, rabbits, birds, and other domesticated and wild animals, show sporadic and widespread outbreaks of toxoplasmosis [22]. Many authors have described toxoplasmosis in different species along the years, and this allows conclude how spread is toxoplasmosis.

Retinochorioiditis in laboratory animals may vary, because interferences with parasite proliferation and viability, and the inoculation route (perioral, intraocular, intraperitoneal, conjunctival, or parenteral administration [23].

## 6. Methods of infection

Any experimental animal model of ocular toxoplasmosis has a set of specific features: specie, parasite strain, stage and concentration of parasites per milliliter of the inoculum, and infection route. Also important, parasite entry must be rigorously chosen. Parasite entry groups: intracarotid injection; intraperitoneal and oral infection, and presents different recurrences of the disease. Intracarotid injection is performed in bigger experimental models like nonhuman primates, cats, and rabbits. Animals must be anesthetized, accordingly Institutional Animal Care and Use Committee, and the right common carotid artery has to be isolated surgically. Using a 27-gauge hypodermic needle, the inoculum must be performed [24].

Intraocular injection allows purport an ocular toxoplasmosis, and has been used in nonhuman primates, guinea pigs, rabbits, and mice. It is possible to perform intracamerally, periretinally, or intraretinally. The disadvantage of this method is that it can cause mechanical damage to retina, which may interfere in results of the course of the disease. First experiments, using this method consisted on retinal injections through the pars plana, crossing the vitreous cavity. Before introducing needle it was necessary a sclerotomy in the pars plana. Place where the needle was introduced [25]. Notwithstanding, administration by instillation, consist of an application over the surface of the eye, and it has shown close results to intraocular injection and in addition maintains integrity of ocular tissue [2]. Instillation is conduced using one drop of solution containing a determined concentration of parasites directly on eye surface.

The most used method, intraperitoneal injection consists of an inoculum inside the peritoneal cavity. This method is easy to perform and successfully leads to ocular toxoplasmosis and, it has many reports in hamsters and mice. Perioral via is described in literature, by introducing a solution containing oocytes in determined concentration inside the mouth of the animal. Equally important gavage is executed with an instrument that certified that experimental animal model received the right dosage, introducing a solution containing oocytes direct into the stomach of experimental model. But it does not reproduce the ocular toxoplasmosis in majority of cases, further results, or depending on the strain no result. Nevertheless performing perioral demonstrated promising results. For congenital ocular toxoplasmosis experimental models, still been an inoculum in pregnant mice, or embryonated eggs. Normally, pregnant mice are infected via intraperitoneal or perioral. Alternatively, an injection of Tachyzoite free forms in embryonated eggs, allow simulating directly embryo infection.

## 7. Diagnose in experimental model

In experimental model, identification of toxoplasmosis can be made finding *T. gondii* cysts into the biopsies, with a specific color reaction and immunohistochemical, or polymerase chain reaction (PCR) technique [13]. Nowadays, PCR is used even when is not found the cysts on biopsies. Diagnose of toxoplasmic retinochorioiditis in experimental animal model, is already described in literature, as a combination of three techniques: ELISA, PCR, and immune-staining. By the way, PCR has been replaced by real-time PCR (qPCR), that increases the sensibility of diagnose in 97% and considers that results are further than PCR [14]. Eventually, enzyme-linked immunosorbent assay (ELISA) is one of the most used tests, identifying immunodominant antigens during *T. gondii* infection. However, it can be used only as a complementary diagnose, once identify antigens and not the parasite. Actually, ELISA has been replaced by flow cytometry. Flow cytometry allows to measure the concentration of substances further and in a less sample dilution. Besides, nowadays there are some specific commercial kits that provide good results, multianalyses in a short period.

## 8. Guinea pig model

Guinea pigs were one of the first experimental animal models used for this purpose, in an accidental experiment [26]. While working with the submaxillary gland virus of guinea pigs, Markham had noted that some of animals were dying after experiments. Asymptomatic and temperature abruptly fell. However, they have rarely been used for further investigation of the disease after first experiments, with little information about. In a study of acquired transmission, a conjunctiva penetration of tachyzoites in this model was preceded, and authors found invasion of conjunctiva epithelia and goblet cells within 15 minutes post infection [27]. Replicating study within 4 hours was possible to identify a high concentration of antibodies. In conclusion, *T. gondii* evokes a mild to moderate inflammatory response. In spite of, the instillation and infection perioral have associated lymphoid tissue, been considered part of the mucosal immune system, and invasions mimic the three forms of parasite forms (tachyzoites, bradyzoites, and sporozoites). In accordance with previous studies, guinea pig might be a good experimental animal model of ocular toxoplasmosis, once it is susceptible to *T. gondii* infection and also it is resistant to great number of parasites [28].

## 9. Rabbit model

Rabbits are known to have a genetically determined low resistance against infection. With exacerbated inflammation accordingly to virulence and antigenicity of the parasite strain. Toxoplasmosis in this animal model was described first by Hogan in 1951 [29]. Infection with RH strains is able to produce chorioretinal lesions similar those described in cats and humans, however, concomitantly meningoencephalitis and rapid death. This describe how susceptible is this model. The most common route of infection in this experimental animal model is intravitreal inoculum, developing retinochorioiditis, equally in nonhuman primates. In rabbits as the same in nonhuman primates model is possible to observe pigmented scars after disease remission.

Intraocular infection combined with ophthalmoscopy in rabbits is easy to perform. The infection is described as a dissemination of retinochorioiditis, vitreal infiltration, and retinal detachment [30]. First affecting retina before choroid, differing from *Felidae* model. By the way, this route of infection might cause some trauma in the ocular tissue interfering on results. Instillation on the ocular surface must supplant best this method. In studies, which were described perioral infection, animal model presented low seroprevalence, and did not presented parasites, when histologically analyzed. Tissues like brain, diaphragm, and heart are considered the most damaged. But with no ocular signal described.

## 10. Hamster model

As experimental model, hamsters had experimental ocular toxoplasmosis, described by Frenkel in 1953 [31], using RH strains showed necessity of therapy while CJ did not generate ocular lesions. In fact the use of ME-49 strains do, intraperitoneal or perioral may influence on ocular toxoplasmosis [7].

Golden Hamster, when infected with RH or CJ strains of *T. gondii*, normally presents sporadic ocular disease, and without treatment with sulfadiazine and pyrimethamine, animals succumb to encephalitis. In contrast, when using ME-49 strain, Golden hamster became an excellent model for ocular toxoplasmosis [32]. Disease may vary among hamsters, but all develop ocular disease, usually limited to retina with loss of layers. All the animals can develop in both eyes the disease among 2 or 3 weeks post inoculum, resolving spontaneously over time, as in humans. As an advantage, eye of this model are large enough to allow fundus photography, in spite of lesions are different from humans, becoming bilateral and multifocal. Hamsters infected orally show development of ocular toxoplasmosis within 4–8 weeks after infection even when intraperitoneal infection is performed, causing retinochorioiditis. Therefore, hamster's disease does not result in pigmentation, showing itself atrophic and bilateral [7].

## 11. Dog model

There are few studies in experimental dog model, but Fialho's study is one of the first studies using dogs as experimental models, with mean alterations: ocular lesions [33]. In dogs are present retinitis, choroiditis and pseudocyst in ciliary epithelium [34]. During days post inoculation, there was only as a clinical sign a submandibular lymph node enlargement. Considering that gavage, intraperitoneal and intravenous demonstrated similar finds. With nonrelevant difference. Indicating that the immune response was observed in all animals. Similar to humans, dogs present ocular toxoplasmosis evolution from simple papillary edema to blindness and ocular necrosis. Morphological alterations in this experimental model are highly considered, once in humans are described in literature as late manifestation of toxoplasmosis, acquired or congenital. It is also demonstrated in experimental dog model [34]. Accordingly author's results can be reproduced in only 30 days. Turning dogs excellent experimental models. By the way, its maintenance and costs turn this experimental animal model expensive and labored. Once it is seem as a pet animal. Not been easily accepted as an experimental model, for the society and committee for the use of laboratory animals.

## 12. Murine model

In majority toxoplasmosis in murine model, shows itself as asymptomatic, and widely prevalent, but clinically is relatively rare [21]. They are easily accessible, with complete genome sequenced, exist many knock-outs and a large number of immunological reagents available.

Beverly JKA introduced mice as animal model in 1959, for congenital experiments [35]. Furthermore, it presents certain resistance to toxoplasmic encephalitis that is controlled by gene action. On the other hand, some vary lineage, like C57BL/6 do not have this haplotype generating spontaneously eye lesions [8]. C57BL/6 shows a high parasite load after 7 days of reinfection associated with deterioration of retinal architecture. When mice are infected by instillation or intraocular injection, both methods unleash ocular toxoplasmosis. Highlighting that instillation must replace with excellence infection of bulb of the eye, obtaining in a short period of time an infection, approaching in 7 days [2]. Considering period of obtaining results, NMRI mice infected, with same strain of *T. gondii* demonstrate bilateral ocular toxoplasmosis in 14–21 days, while Swiss-Webster mice, parasite loads did not peak upon reinfection. BALB/c is considered resistant to the infection, showing itself as asymptomatic. In the same way, it must be noticed that diagnosis of migrant of retinal pigmented epithelium is more difficult in albino mice. Otherwise murine congenital toxoplasmosis there is significant opaque cataract formation [7].

Rats as an experimental model described by Wildfuhr, in 1954 [36], but with little information about this author's studies, present high resistance to toxoplasmic infection, because of this, that experimental animal model is used only when compared to human adults disease.

Murine model mimics likely time of exposure, establishment of cysts in humans and is easy of manipulation. Instead, it has the disadvantages of producing different degrees of severity and ocular lesions and hard monitoring, because of size of the eye [24]. Hence with many advantages, murine model may offer a great spread of methods and variable results, but it is necessary such a great number of animals to perform statistically relevant analyses.

## 13. Bird model

As a natural host of T. gondii, chicken was first described as an experimental model for toxoplasmosis in 1959 by Jones et al. [37]. Level of infection in chicken may be under detectable levels, and low parasitemia makes diagnosis in this model by microscopy difficult, needing ELISA or more sensible methods [38]. In some studies, already has been demonstrated that dose of parasites influence on studies, finding parasites in liver and heart, but none was found in brain cells. Doses higher than $10^3$ parasites per milliliter, showed high mortality, indicating in these case lower dosages. Many species of birds can act as a reservoir for *T. gondii*, apparently with or without symptoms [39]. But some studies relating to gender prove that female chicken present more seroprevalence than male, probably associated to behavior manner [38].

On the other hand, embryonated eggs have actually shown itself as good model to test pathogenicity of strains of *T. gondii*, but not all animals in study have demonstrated alteration in ocular structure. Embryos of chicken are able to reproduce projections of retinal layers, detachment of retinal pigmented epithelium, alterations in disposition of photoreceptor, inflammatory infiltrate and alteration in gene expression, important for the development of retina [40].

It is also possible to see migration of RPE, suggesting a potential role of RPE phagocytosis. Evolution of retinochorioiditis in embryo models is related to the period of infection and strain of parasite, and it has a major tachyzoites proliferation in last periods [23].

Chicken embryo has shown itself, as an excellent performance when compared to other congenital ocular toxoplasmosis animal model, although does not exclude them. Its maintenance, usability, stereo environment, and easy to obtain, qualify this model as a great experimental model [40] and can present great studies when correlated to the control of environmental contamination, by controlling prevalence of infected chickens [38].

## 14. Nonhuman primate model

This experimental animal model of ocular toxoplasmosis, was first described in a bid of replace rabbit model proposed by Nozik and O'Connor in 1968 [25]. First experiment in this model was described using intraocular inoculum containing RH strains of *T. gondii*, even so it was possible to mimic a retinochoroidal inflammation, there was not retinal necrosis, with no evidence of systemic illness, not even detachments of retinal layer. In nonhuman primates, it is possible to see a remission of the disease [10]. Furthermore, intraretinal infection is easy to perform in monkeys, and ophthalmoscopy can easily be done due to the size of eye of this experimental model. In spite of, it is already known that New world monkeys, *Carabide* are highly susceptible to clinical toxoplasmosis when compared to Old world monkeys, as *Cercopithecide*, that present itself resistant. Monkeys from the Old world seem resistant to infection comprehending that it might not been a good experimental model for ocular toxoplasmosis, whereas monkeys from New world look like useful. In contrast, as a disadvantage, these experimental animal models are costly and require proper housing conditions, which sometimes cannot be granted in most laboratories.

## 15. *Felidae* model

Clinical toxoplasmosis has been diagnosed in wild *felidaes* but, in great majority of cases, the parasite was identified only in feces. First report of cats as experimental model was made in 1993 by Davidson et al. Cats were infected via carotid injection containing ME-49 strains of *T. gondii*. This experiment induced an increase in rectal temperature, and focal areas of choroidal and retinal inflammation, highlighting bilateral lesions. Equally important within 4 weeks, blood-retinal barrier has been established in most posterior segments lesion. Unlike humans, choroiditis is more pronounced in this model than retinitis during the course of the disease. Another relevant information about this model is that oocysts are detectable in feces from 24 days post inoculation but with a low reproducibility [24].

In addition, an advantage of this method of infection for this experimental model is the low concentration of tachyzoites inoculated via carotid, showing retinal inflammation, different from human. In humans, this characteristic is about a reactivation of congenital infection, multifocal, and self-limiting.

Routes of inoculation as subcutaneous and intraperitoneal, performed with a large number of tachyzoites of RH strains, leads cat too fast to death. Oral administration produces only sporadic ocular lesions, but has shown as not a good via. After exposure, there is dissemination of *T. gondii* to various extraintestinal tissues, like in humans, but most cats present immunity development and express disease only when immune-suppressed or immune-competent. It can present itself as a good model for understanding biology of parasite, but do not understand disease in humans [24].

## 16. Pig model

Pigs present a potential infection for humans, from eating under-cooked meat [22]. This experimental animal model infected orally [41] or by intramuscular injection presented apathetic and lethargic among 2 and 9 days post infection. Besides, it is possible to see some aggressiveness attitude during chronic phase. By the way, nonlesion was allowed to identify. Using RH strains of *T. gondii*, animals can present eye discharge and temperature embracing form of *T. gondii*. When using ME-49 strains, this experimental animal model demonstrated increase in band neutrophils. Even those neutrophils are not crucial for toxoplasmosis control; but seem to exert some important role during ocular toxoplasmosis infection, when compared to RH strains immune response. RH strains trigger a lower immune response than ME-49. On the other hand, ME-49 strains reach blood system faster by perioral method than RH via intramuscular inoculum, and can mimic the biological activity of parasite as in immunocompromised humans chronically infected, indicating that the pig experimental model may be a good model to understand chronic toxoplasmosis in immune competent humans [42].

## 17. Sea mammals model

Many sea mammals are described with toxoplasmosis. In Philadelphia, at a zoo, a case of a sea lion that has died was discovered during necropsy, with cysts of *T. gondii* in heart and stomach. In 1985, a fur seal died of toxoplasmic encephalitis. More after serological studies reported a prevalence of 7.6% of toxoplasmosis in harbor seals and dolphins in Canada. Thereafter, congenital toxoplasmosis was reported in sea mammals in Australia and in Beluga whales from an estuary at St. Lawrence. In general, there are many case reports in this model. Furthermore, there are no relevant study using sea mammals as experimental models for ocular toxoplasmosis, but they might be, an important fount of information for controlling marine infection of environment. Previous studies suggest that coastal pollution from human activities is a source of *T. gondii*. Actually, concentration of oocysts by shellfish can occur, and once sporulated, oocysts can survive in marine water for a long period of time, turning shellfish a source of infection to marine environment [22].

## 18. Ungulates model

Since 1992, ungulates and nondomestic ruminants have been reported clinically; at the same time, nonexperimental study describes clinically infection by toxoplasmosis. Actually, reports of a *Saiga antelope*, deer, and other animals showed fatal in these cases. Otherwise, there is no report of ungulates as pronghorn, once it is highly susceptible to *T. gondii* infection [22]. Expressing that ungulates are not good experimental models for toxoplasmosis, once it is extremely sensible to this protozoan infection.

## 19. Marsupials model

Toxoplasmosis is a serious disease of Australian marsupials, local zoo report countless death, as suddenly die, without clinical or neurological signs, loss of vision, diarrhea, or respiratory distress. Virtually any organ can be affected [43]. Even so, some species of wallabies were identified with high levels of antibodies, like adult black-faced kangaroos, this allows to comprehend that not all exposed wallabies die of toxoplasmosis. But, some tests of vaccine (S-48) with live, or modified and nonpersistent strain of *T. gondii* showed itself lethal in Tammar wallabies, describing how susceptible is this specie. Marsupials as New World Monkeys look to be unusually susceptible to toxoplasmosis [7]. Actually the approach is preventing contamination of food and water, needing more studies that are able to immunize those models, with no founds until now [22].

## 20. Conclusion

Experimental animal models do not express disease how it happens in humans. However, they are able to bring relevant information about the course of ocular toxoplasmosis. Mice in general are the most usual models nowadays. Adult birds do not express the disease, being a reservoir with no clinical manifestation, but avian embryos allow studies about congenital ocular toxoplasmosis, while hamsters provide information about infection. Nonhuman primates, instead the route of infection, may present important facts of the disease, while cat as the definitive host also presents ocular alteration. Other models do not have experimental description, by the way, case report help to fill the blanks for new contributions of methods, experimental model, and strain of parasite. The choice of an ideal experimental animal model is extremely important to understand and contribute for improvements on prospective treatments.

## Author details

Aléx Martins Nasaré* and Roberto Carlos Tedesco

*Address all correspondence to: alex.nasare@hotmail.com

Federal University of São Paulo, São Paulo, Brazil

## References

[1] Jones LA, Alexander J, Roberts CW. Ocular toxoplasmosis: in the storm of the eye. Parasite Immunology. 2006;28:635–642.

[2] Tedesco RC, Smith RL, Corte-Real S, Calabrese KS. Ocular toxoplasmosis in mice: comparison of two routes of infection. Parasitology. 2005;131:303–307. DOI: 101017/S003118200500781X

[3] Dubey JP. Advances in the life cycle of *Toxoplasma gondii*. International Journal of Parasitology. 1998;28:713–717.

[4] Dukaczewska A, Tedesco R, Liesenfeld O. Experimental models of ocular infection with *Toxoplasma gondii*. European Journal of Microbiology and Immunology. 2015;4:293–305. DOI: 10.1556/1886.2015.00045

[5] de Souza W, Belfort Jr. R. Toxoplasmose e *Toxoplasma gondii*. 1st ed. Rio de Janeiro. Editora: Fiocruz. 2014. pp. 181–196. ISBN: 978-85-7541-437-8

[6] Belfort-Neto R, Nussenblatt V, Rizzo L, Muccioli C, Silveira C, Nussenblatt R, Khan A, Sibley LD, Belfort Jr. R. High prevalence of unusual genotypes of *Toxoplasma gondii* infection pork meat samples from Erechim, Southern Brazil. Annals of the Brazilian Academy of Sciences. 2007;79:111–114.

[7] Weiss LM, Kim K. *Toxoplasma gondii:* the model apicomplexan – perspective and methods. 2nd ed. Massachusetts. Academic press. 2013. pp. 161-192. ISBN: 978-9-12-39648 1-6

[8] Roberts F, McLeod R. Pathogenesis of toxoplasmic retinochoroiditis. Parasitology Today. 1999;15:51–57. DOI: 10.1016/S0169-4758(98)01377-5

[9] Bossi P, Caumes E, Paris L, Dardé M, Bricaire F. *Toxoplasma gondii*-associated Guillain Barré syndrome in an immunocompetent patient. Journal of Clinical Microbiology. 1998;36(12):3724–3725.

[10] Maenz M, Schlüter D, Liesenfeld O, Schares G, Gross U, Pleyer U. Ocular toxoplasmosis past, present and new aspects of an old disease. Progress in Retinal and Eye Research. 2014;39:77–106. DOI: 10.1016/j.preteyeres.2013.12.005

[11] Tedesco RC, Smith RL, Corte-Real S, Calabrese KS. Ocular toxoplasmosis: the role of retinal pigment epithelium migration in infection. Parasitology Research. 2004;92:467–472. DOI: 10.1007/S00436-003-1031-2

[12] Holland GN, O'Connor GR, Belfort Jr. R, Remington JS. Toxoplasmosis. In: Pepose JS, Holland GN, Wilhelmus KR. Ocular infection and immunity. St. Louis: Mosby. 1996. pp. 1183–1223.

[13] Arcelus MP, Salinas A, Layana AG. Manifestaciones retinianas de las enfermedades infecciosas. Anales del Sistema Sanitario de Navarra. 2008;31:57–68.

[14] Commodaro A, Belfort RN, Rizzo LV, Muccioli C, Silveira C, Claudio JR, Burnier MN Jr., Belfort R. Ocular toxoplasmosis – an update and review of the literature. The Memórias do Instituto Oswaldo Cruz. 2009;104:345–350.

[15] Dubey JP, Graham DH, Blackston CR, Lehmann T, Gennari SM, Ragozo AMA, Nishi SM, Shen SK, Kwok OCH, Hill DE, Thulliez P. Biological and genetic characterization of *Toxoplasma gondii* isolates from chicken (*Gallus domesticus*) from São Paulo, Brazil: unexpected findings. International Journal of Parasitology. 2002;32:99–105.

[16] Dubey JP, Jones JL. *Toxoplasma gondii* infection in humans and animals in the United States. International Journal of Parasitology. 2008;38:1257–1278.

[17] Nowakowska D, Colón I, Remington JS, Grigg M, Golab E, Wilc-zynski J, Sibley LD. Genotyping of *Toxoplasma gondii* by multiplex PCR and peptide-based serological testing of samples from infants in Poland diagnosed with congenital toxoplasmosis. Journal of Clinical Microbiology. 2006;44:1382–1389.

[18] Nussenblatt RB, Whitcup SM. Uveitis: fundamentals and clinical practice. 4th ed. San Louis: Mosby. 1996. p. 480.

[19] Petrilli AMN. Uveítes na infância [thesis]. São Paulo: Escola Paulista de Medicina. 1987.

[20] Holand GN. Ocular toxoplasmosis: a global reassessment. Part I: epidemiology and course of disease. American Journal of Ophthalmology. 2003;136:973–988.

[21] Dubey JP, Beatie CP. Toxoplasmosis of animals and man. Boca Raton: CRC press. 1988. p. 220. ISBN: 0849346185

[22] Hill DE, Chirukandoth S, Dubey JP. Biology and epidemiology of *Toxoplasma gondii* in man and animals. Animal Health Research Reviews. 2005;6(1):41–61. DOI: 10.1079/AHR2005100

[23] Moraes AMM, Pessôa CN, Vommaro RC, de Souza W, de Mello FG, Hokoç JN. Cultured embryonic retina systems as a model for the study of underlying mechanisms of *Toxoplasma gondii* infection. Investigative Ophthamology and Visual Science. 2004;45:2813–2821.

[24] Davidson MG, Lappin MR, English RV, Tompkins MB. A feline model of ocular toxoplasmosis. Investigative Ophthalmology and Visual Science. 1993;34:3653–3660.

[25] Culbertson WW, Tabbara KF, O'Connor GR. Experimental ocular toxoplasmosis in primates. Archives of Ophthalmology. 1982;100:321–323.

[26] Markham FS. Spontaneous Toxoplasma encephalitis in the guinea pig. American Journal of Hygiene. 1937;26:193–196.

[27] Pavesio CE, Lightman S. *Toxoplasma gondii* and ocular toxoplasmosis: pathogenesis. British Journal of Ophthalmology. 1996;80:1099–1107.

[28] Skorich DN, Chiappino ML, Nichols BA. Invasion of the guinea pig conjunctiva by *Toxoplasma gondii*. Investigative Ophthalmology and Visual Science. 1988;29(12):1871–1880.

[29] Hogan MJ. Ocular Toxoplasmosis. New York: Columbia University Press. 1951.

[30] Garweg JG, Kuenzli H, Boehnke M. Experimental ocular toxoplasmosis in navie and primed rabbits. Ophthalmology. 1998;212:136–141.

[31] Frenkel JK. Ocular lesions in hamsters with chronic Toxoplasma and Besnoitia infection. American Journal of Ophthalmology. 1955;39:203–225.

[32] Pavesio CE, Chiappino ML, Gormley P, Setzer PY, Nichols BA. Acquired retinochoroiditis in hamsters inoculated with ME 49 strain Toxoplasma. Investigative Ophthalmology Visual Science. 1995;36:2166–2175.

[33] Fialho, S.A. Toxoplasmoseocular: contribuiçãoaoestudo clínico e experimental [thesis]. Rio de Janeiro. Tese (Doutorado em Medicina)—Faculdade Nacional de Medicina da Universidade do Brasil, 1953; p. 139.

[34] de Abreu CB, Navarro IT, dos Reis ACFM, de Souza MSB, Machado R, Marana ERM, Prudêncio LB, Mattos MR, Tsutsui. Ocular toxoplasmosis in young Dogs inoculated with *Toxoplasma gondii.* Ciência Rural. 2002;32(5):807–812. ISSN: 0103-8478

[35] Beverly JKA. Congenital transmission of toxoplasmosis through successive generations of mice. Nature. 1959;4671:1348–1349.

[36] Wildfuhr G. Toxoplasmose. Nature. Jena: Gustav Fischer, Villengang 2. 1954. pp. 176.

[37] Jones FE, Melton ML, Lunde MN, Eyles DE, Jacobs L. Experimental toxoplasmosis in chickens. The Journal of Parasitology. 1959;45:31–37.

[38] Ibrahim HM, Abdel-Gha ar F, Osman GY, El-Shourbagy SH, Nishikawa Y, Kha ab RA. Prevalence of Toxoplasma gondii in chicken samples from delta of Egypt using ELISA, histopathology and immunohistochemistry. Journal of Parasitic Diseases. 2016;40(2): 485-90 DOI: 10.1007/s12639-014-0530-7

[39] Dubey JP. Tachyzoite-induced life cycle of *Toxoplasma gondii* in cats. Journal of Parasitology. 2002;88:713–717.

[40] Nasare AM, Tedesco RC, Cristovam PC, Cenedese MA, Galisteo Jr. AJ, Andrade Jr HF, Gomes JAP, Guimarães EV, Barbosa HS, Alonso LG. *Toxoplasma gondii* infection of chicken embryos causes retinal changes and modulates *HSP90B1* gene expression: a promising ocular toxoplasmosis model. European Journal of Microbiology and Immunology. 2015;5(4):316–320. DOI: 10.1556/1886.2015.00024

[41] Wingstrand A, Lind P, Haugegaard J, Henriksen SA, Bille-Hansen V, Sørensen V. Clinical observations, pathology, bioassay in mice and serological response at slaughter in pigs experimentally infected with *Toxoplasma gondii.* Veterinary Parasitology. 1997;72:129–140.

[42] Miranda FJB, de Souza DB, Frazão-Teixeira E, de Oliveira FC, de Melo JC, Mariano CMA, Albernaz AP, de Carvakho ECQ, de Oliveira FCR, de Souza W, DaMatta RA.

Experimental infection with the *Toxoplasma gondii* ME-49 strain in the Brazilian BR-1 mini pig is a suitable animal model for human toxoplasmosis. The Memórias do Instituto Oswaldo Cruz. 2015;110(1):95–100. DOI: 10.1590/0074-02760140318

[43] Canfield PJ, Hartley WJ, Dubey JP. Lesions of toxoplasmosis in Australian marsupials. Journal of Comparative Pathology. 1990;103:159–167.

# 11

# IgY-Technology Applied to Studies of *Toxoplasma gondii* Infection

Alvaro Ferreira Júnior, Jandra P. Santos,

Paula B. Bassi, Joely F.F. Bittar and

Eustáquio R. Bittar

**Abstract**

In this chapter, we describe relevant aspects of immunoglobulin Y (IgY) technology for *Toxoplasma gondii* applications, including comparison of avian IgY antibody with mammalian IgG antibody, egg yolk IgY production and isolation procedures, important applications for IgY antibody, and state of the art and perspectives for IgY-technology in *T. gondii* studies. *T. gondii* is a worldwide public health problem. IgY-technology provides an alternative antibody (IgY) to mammalian Immunoglobulin G (IgG) antibody. IgY-technology involves the chicken immunization, yolk IgY isolation, antibody characterization, and purified IgY application to several kinds of methods. Immunized chicken transfers a specific IgY from blood to egg yolk. Phylogenetic distance between chickens and mammals influences the generation of antibody repertoires recognizing an antigen profile. IgY is not bound to rheumatoid factor or mammalian complement protein and thus avoids the false-positive results. Yolk IgY isolation is carried out by simple procedures that are accessible for any laboratory and, also, for IgY isolation at large-scale production. IgY-technology provides antibodies for proteomic studies, diagnostic assays, and immunotherapy. Although IgY-technology is promising, there is a reduced number of investigations with IgY and *T. gondii*. Future perspectives involve the use of IgY-technology for the screening of new *T. gondii* antigens for diagnostics, therapy, or vaccine, development of innovative techniques for toxoplasmosis diagnostics and may be an immunotherapy for toxoplasmosis.

**Keywords:** antibodies, chicken, toxoplasmosis, immunoassay, immunotherapy

## 1. Introduction

*Toxoplasma gondii* is the toxoplasmosis agent in human and animals and is a worldwide public health problem. Alternative approach that offers possibility to improve diagnostics, treatment, or control of toxoplasmosis should be accepted as a protective approach to hosts at risk of infection by *T. gondii*. Immunoglobulin Y (IgY)-technology was designed in 1980s with the aim to reduce the suffering procedures to obtain a high-quality antibody, replace animal model for antibody production and refine the kind of applications for purified antibodies. IgY-based antibody production derived from chicken egg yolk antibody is named immunoglobulin Y (IgY). Hens transfer IgY from blood to egg yolk protecting their offspring. Isolation of yolk IgY avoids bleeding the chicken and reduces the number of painful procedures. Hens can lay approximately one egg each day during a period of 2 years. IgY antibody is functional and is equivalent to mammal IgG antibody. Both avian and mammalian antibodies have structure similarity. They have two identical light chains and two identical heavy chains bounded to each other by disulfide bonds. In the amino terminal extremity, they have the fragment antigen-binding (Fab). In the carboxy terminal region, they have the fragment crystallizable (Fc) that is associated to biological antibody functions as interaction with cells or molecules from immune system. Virtually, any substance can be the target of an antibody response and the response to even a single epitope comprises many different antibody molecules, each with a subtly different specificity for the epitope and a unique affinity, or binding strength. The total number of antibody specificities available for an individual is known as the antibody repertoire. The number of antibody specificities present at a particular time is limited by the total number of B cells in an individual, as well as by each individual's previous encounters with antigens. Albeit, they are equivalent in function and structure, the phylogenetic distance and the way to generate antibody specificities produce difference in epitope recognition repertoire between avian and mammalian host. Additionally, modifications in amino acid sequence of IgY antibody result in advantages, comparing to IgG, as follows: IgY does not bound to rheumatoid factor, Fc receptor or mammalian complement proteins that can avoid false-positive results, and many others. Isolation of yolk antibodies begins by removing lipid fraction from yolk and obtaining a water-soluble fraction, and further procedures including salt-based precipitation, gel filtration, or affinity chromatography provide a high-purity IgY-enriched fraction. Purified IgY antibody can be applied to several kinds of techniques including screening new antigens by phage display, enzymatic or florescence immunoassays, diagnostics, and, also, passive immunization for therapy against gastrointestinal pathogens in humans and animal hosts. Future perspective using IgY-technology as a tool for *T. gondii* investigation should include development of new antigen libraries as an innovative source of possible targets for diagnostics, therapy, or vaccination. In addition, create new diagnostic platforms for diagnosing *T. gondii* infection. Finally, the potential protective effect of IgY to be used in prevention or toxoplasmosis therapy by passive immunization should be explored. In this chapter, we describe relevant aspects of IgY-technology to *T. gondii* investigations, including comparing avian IgY antibody with mammalian IgG antibody, egg yolk IgY production and isolation procedures, important applications for IgY antibody, and state of the art and perspectives for IgY technology in *T. gondii* studies.

## 2. Overview in IgY technology

### 2.1. Comparing avian IgY antibody with mammalian IgG antibody

#### *2.1.1. General history*

In the early 1893, Klemperer published his observation that there must be neutralizing proteins (i.e., antibodies) in the yolk of eggs laid by immunized chickens. In 1980s, when animal welfare came to be regarded as a serious ethical claim for the scientific community, the extraction of specific antibodies from the egg yolk was considered as an alternative to the blood-taking methods. In this context, phylogenetic distance between chickens and mammals, mechanisms of antibody repertoire diversification, and the way in which chickens deposit IgY immunoglobulin in the egg yolk provide a number of advantages compared to mammals as animal model for antibody production. In an additional manner, the one-step purification of antibodies from egg yolk in large amounts provides a virtually continuous supply; the epitope repertoire recognition of IgY antibodies potentially grants access to new specificities; the absence of cross-reactivity with mammalian epitopes avoids false-positive interference and improves the performance of immunological assays. The generation and application of avian antibodies has caused a surge of interest in a wide variety of applications within the life sciences [1].

#### *2.1.2. Structure characterization of IgY and IgG antibodies*

Structurally, avian IgY antibody is similar to mammalian IgG antibody (**Figure 1**). Two identical light chains and two identical heavy chains that are bounded by disulfide bonds compose the antibody's molecular structure [2]. Both chains are formed by the sequences of amino acids (approximately 110 amino acids) named domains which are numerically ordered from the amino terminal region ($NH_3^+$) to the carboxy terminal region ($COO^-$). The amino terminal domain, named variable domains, presents a variable amino acid composition sequence by the occurrence of mutational events during the B lymphocyte-produced immune response. For both light chain and heavy chain, variable domains (VL and VH) have three regions with higher variation rate in amino acid sequence named complementarity determining region (CDR). Complementarity determining regions (CDRs) are completely bounded to epitopes (antigenic determinant) during a specific humoral response. In the direction to carboxy terminal extremity, after the variable domain, there are the constant domains. The light chain has one constant domain (CL); however, the number of constant domains for the heavy chain varies with antibody isotypes. IgY heavy chain, named upsilon (Greek letter $\upsilon$), has four constant domains (CH), and IgG heavy chain, named gamma (Greek letter $\gamma$), has three domains (CH) [2, 3].

The fragment antigen-binding (Fab) is positioned in amino terminal extremity and is composed by the entire light chain (VL and CL) and both VH and CH1 domains. The IgY fragment crystallizable (Fc) is formed by CH2, CH3, and CH4 domains and IgG Fc by the hinge region is formed by CH2 and CH3 domains. There was proposed that IgY CH2 domain must be

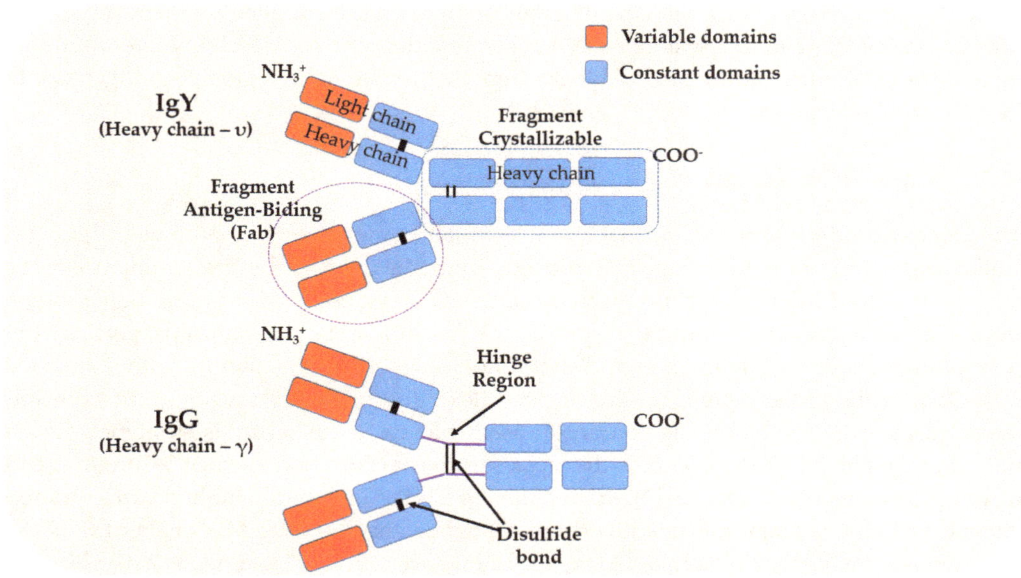


**Figure 1.** Schematic general structure of the egg yolk antibody (IgY) and the mammalian IgG antibody.

converted to IgG hinge region, which provides a higher mobility to the mammalian Fab than to its avian equivalent. Regarding heavy chain, the chicken has two other classes of antibodies (Immunoglobulin M [IgM], heavy chain μ, and IgA, heavy chain α) and mammals have other four classes of antibodies (IgM, heavy chain μ; Immunoglobulin A [IgA], heavy chain α; Immunoglobulin E [IgE], heavy chain ε; and Immunoglobulin D [IgD], heavy chain σ) [2, 3].

### *2.1.3. Generation of antigen recognizing repertoire in chicken and mammals*

In the genome of a germ-line cell, the genetic information for an immunoglobulin (Ig) polypeptide chain is contained in multiple gene segments scattered along a chromosome. During the development of bone marrow-derived lymphocytes, these gene segments are assembled by recombination that leads to the formation of a complete gene [4]. The vertebrate B-cell repertoire is capable of generating up to 10(9) different antibody molecules. To generate diversity, mammals depend on combinatorial and functional variations that occur during the gene rearrangement events to produce complete heavy and light chain Ig genes. This gene rearrangement process goes continuously in the bone marrow, where each developing B cell assembles a unique heavy and light chain Ig gene from families of functional V (variable), D (diversity), and J (joining) gene segments. In contrast, chickens have only single functional V and J segments for the heavy and light chain loci, and chicken Ig gene rearrangement occurs only during a brief period of embryonic development. A specialized organ involved in avian B-cell development, the bursa of Fabricius, provides the microenvironment necessary for the amplification of B cells that have undergone productive Ig gene rearrangements. Within the bursa, B cells also acquire somatic diversity among the rearranged V gene segments of the heavy and light chain Ig loci. Somatic diversification of chicken V gene segments occurs by intrachromosomal gene conversion, a DNA recombination process which involves unidirectional transfer of nucleotide sequence blocks from the families of V region pseudogenes into the functional rearranged VH and VL genes [5].

#### *2.1.4. Molecular characterization of IgY and IgG antibodies*

Phylogenetic studies have shown that the IgY antibody, homolog of mammalian IgG, has similarities with both mammalian IgG and IgE antibodies. IgY is the predominant isotype in sera, produced after IgM in the primary antibody response, and it is the main isotype produced in the secondary immune response. IgY has different biochemical properties from those of mammalian IgG antibodies and shares homology while functioning with them. Due to the lack of the hinge region, IgY has limited flexibility to its Fab resulting in to precipitate antigens at physiological salt concentrations. Chicken IgY in serum is monomeric, with molecular weight (MW) 165–206 kDa, the mean serum concentration average 5–7 mg/mL and in yolk approximately 25 mg/mL [2]. Mammalian IgG is the Ig found in highest concentration in blood and plays a major role in antibody-mediated defenses. It has a MW of about 180 kDa. Its serum level is approximately 8–16 mg/mL in human and 17–27 mg/mL in cattle [3]. The amount of antibodies obtainable from rabbit is approximately 200 mg, IgG/bleeding (40 mL blood) with 5% of specific antibody, and from chicken is approximately 100 mg/egg (5–7 eggs/week) with 2–10% of specific antibody. IgY sampling is not invasive, which confers advantage on IgG; also, yolk antibody does not interfere with rheumatoid factor or activate mammalian complement [1].

### 2.2. IgY production

The IgY technology–based layout to produce polyclonal antibodies is displayed in **Figure 2**. First step is the chicken immunization followed by the yolk IgY extraction, the antibody characterization, and finally IgY applications in various kinds of assays. Chickens are a suitable model to produce IgY by immunization with nucleic acid [6], protein [7], lipid, and carbohydrates [8]. In addition, an immune humoral response must be elicited by immunization with recombinant proteins [9] or peptides [10]. To improve the specific IgY response it is demanded the use of adjuvants like Freund's adjuvants for immunization procedures, which is the most frequently used adjuvant. Intramuscularly way is a common way for chicken immunization to produce specific IgY. Alternatively, subcutaneous way provides satisfactory amounts of specific antibody [1].

### 2.3. IgY purification

Regarding its constitution, yolk can be viewed as an oil-water emulsion with a watery portion containing proteins and a dispersal portion of so-called yolk-granules and lipid-drops [11]. The concentration and distribution of immunoglobulins Y (IgY) in the serum and egg are 6 and 25 mg/ml, respectively. The concentrations of specific antibodies in the yolk are similar to the antibody profile of the serum. To isolate yolk IgY, distinct procedures may be used alone

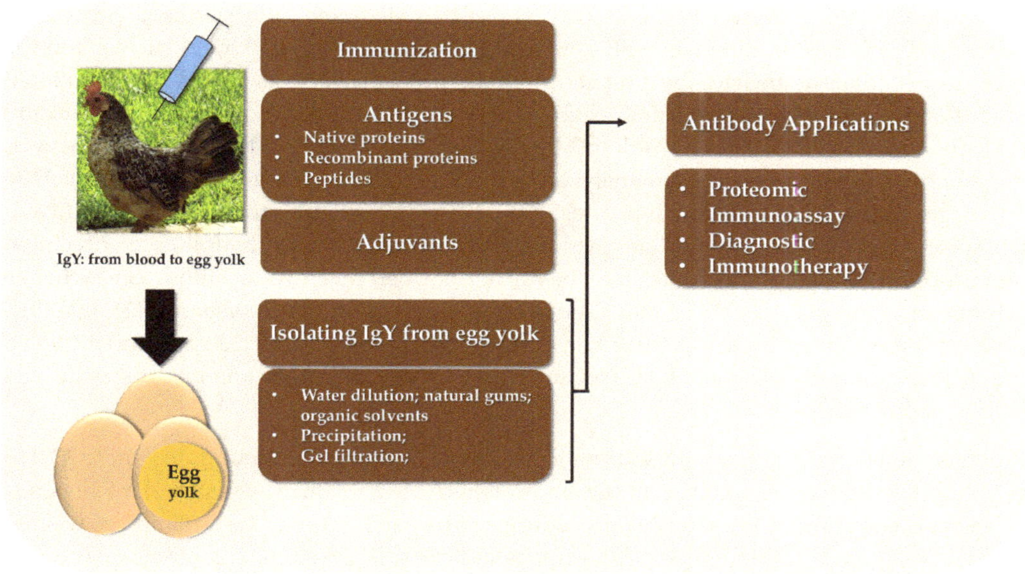


**Figure 2.** General layout to produce specific IgY antibodies. From immunization with different antigens added to adjuvants, isolating egg yolk antibody to IgY applications.

or in combination according to the following criteria: amount, purity, and biological activity. The yolk antibody extraction begins by separating yolk and egg white. After removal of the vitellin membrane, the yolk is put into a measuring cylinder. The next steps in IgY extraction are devoted to removing the lipid content and obtaining a water soluble phase (WSP) antibodies enriched [12]. The consequent purification procedures vary widely in type and combination and from laboratory to laboratory. The degree of IgY purity depends on desired application; for example, for oral administration, the whole yolk can be used, and on the other hand, for a reagent, isolated IgY from the mixture of yolk molecules is necessary [1].

### 2.3.1. *Removing lipid from yolk*

A high quality removing lipid method is the first step to efficiently isolate IgY antibodies from egg yolk. Several natural gums, as carrageenan and xanthan gum, were found to be effective for removal of yolk lipoprotein as a precipitate, resulting in a water-soluble fraction with very low lipid concentration [13, 14]. Optionally, organic solvents (chloroform) have been used as a mean to remove yolk lipid content at the initial step of IgY isolation [1, 14]. The water-dilution method is a widespread procedure for the yolk lipid removal, which provides IgY-enriched water-soluble fraction [14–16].

### 2.3.2. *Isolating IgY by precipitation methods*

The extraction of yolk antibodies by the use of polyethylene glycol precipitation (PEG, MW 6000) was, firstly, developed by Polson et al. [17]. The IgY-extraction by means of PEG-precipitation is very cost-effective and results in highly specific antibody with stable titers up to 1:1,000,000 [18]. Afterwards, PEG 6000 was widely accepted as a standard procedure. Pulverized PEG 6000 is added to WSP until the final concentration of 3.5% is stirred, and the protein precipitate is pelleted by first centrifugation. Finally, PEG is added to supernatant until it brings the final concentration to 12%. The mixture is stirred thoroughly and a second centrifugation PEG method can result in a high IgY antibody concentration per egg; however, it may not be homogeneous when analyzed by SDS-polyacrylamide gel electrophoresis [19]. To improve the quality of extraction, after PEG 12% precipitation, saturated ammonium sulfate solution can be added to IgY enriched fraction [20]. Additionally, by following precipitation procedures, the IgY antibodies may be further purified by DEAE cellulose ion-exchange column chromatography [21] or ionic-liquid based aqueous biphasic systems [22]. IgY-PEG 6000 can be extracted by using three consecutive precipitation steps: 3.5, 8.5, and 12% is a recent adaptation to Polson et al. [17] technique and produces a high amount of specific egg yolk antibodies [23].

Proteins can be precipitated with sodium sulfate ($Na_2SO_4$, NaS) or ammonium sulfate [$(NH_4)SO_4$, AmS]. Since the precipitation of certain proteins from a mixture by NaS or AmS depends on the concentration of the salt, this procedure can be used not only for isolation of desired proteins but also for elimination of the undesired ones. A precipitate is obtained through centrifuging, taken up in a certain amount of desired buffer or distilled water, and finally dialyzed [1]. NaS and AmS precipitations are economical and environmentally correct procedures for yolk antibody extraction [24]. The major problem in separating IgY is to remove the high concentrations of lipids in egg yolk, which can be obtained by water dilution method [15], followed by IgY salt-based precipitation in the antibody-enriched fraction [25]. NaS or AmS precipitation provides fractions with low protein content compared to original yolk, but with a high specific activity [26]. Salt-based yolk antibody precipitation is promising to be a more efficient and useful purification method for the large-scale IgY from egg yolk preparation [16, 27].

The isolation of IgY from yolk using of combination of different methods results in a high amount of specific antibodies with elevated purity. Sequential precipitation with 31% ammonium sulfate and 12% polyethylene glycol (PEG) produces IgY antibodies with above 95% purity and there is no loss in immunoreactivity [28]. The salt-based egg antibody precipitation combined with thiophilic acid chromatography provides a simple and efficient mean of IgY from egg yolk [29, 30]. Association between AmS and ethanol to IgY precipitation results in a high quantity of antibodies with great purity [31]. Specific antisnake venom IgY with neutralizing effect for therapeutic proposes can be isolated by AmS precipitation followed to ion exchange chromatography [32, 33]. The inhibiting growth activity of IgY anti-*Streptococcus mitis* was preserved by extracting yolk antibodies by precipitation with PEG 6000 and AmS and further isolation by DEAE cellulose ion exchange column chromatography [34]. Similarly, growth inhibition of *Staphylococcus aureus* and *Escherichia coli* was obtained with yolk antibodies isolated by NaS and AmS precipitations [35].

#### *2.3.3. Isolating IgY by gel filtration*

The separation of IgY antibodies according to their molecular weight through gel filtration is a further stage of purification of yolk antibodies but rarely reported except in the desalting of preparation through columns instead through a dialysis [1]. Gel filtration by Sephacryl S300 and Sephadex G50 or G75 provides a high-purity IgY separation but further protein concentration procedures for separated antibody samples are desired [16, 36, 37]. On the other hand, the ion-exchange chromatography is a widespread method to separate proteins from mixtures and it is also used for immunoglobulins isolation. IgY antibodies are bound electrostatically to an ion-exchange matrix with a reverse charge. According to the strength of binding, the antibodies are detached by increasing concentrations of ions of the buffers [1, 32, 33, 34].

#### 2.3.4. *Isolating IgY by affinity chromatography*

The isolation of yolk IgY antibodies by affinity chromatography consist in attach an antibody ligand on a matrix. The extraction of mammalian IgG-isotypes by affinity chromatography can be obtained by immobilized *S. aureus* A protein or B protein from the *Streptococci* of the C- or G-group. IgY antibodies bind neither with protein A nor with protein G [1]. Recently, protein M (a transmembrane protein from human mycoplasma) has been demonstrated as a promising ligand for purifying polyclonal, monoclonal, or engineered IgY antibodies [38]. Synthetic IgY-ligands were developed to improve yolk antibody isolating mainly by reducing the purification steps and increasing the amount and purity of recovered IgY [39, 40]. Attaching the IgY-induced antigen to matrix provides another way to extract a high-purity IgY by affinity chromatography [41, 42]. The chromatographic thiophilic interaction provides a simple one-step method capable of recovering IgY at concentration close to 100% of initial yolk antibody amount [29, 43].

### 2.4. IgY applications

#### 2.4.1. *Proteomic*

IgY antibodies are suitable for a wide application protocols like proteomic, diagnostics, and therapy. The immunodepletion for humans or animal fluids by using specific IgY-attached columns enables the detection of new protein spots, increases resolution, and highly improves the intensity of low-abundance proteins by two-dimensional polyacrylamide gel electrophoresis (2D-PAGE) [44, 45]. Other possibility for the use of IgY to proteomic studies is screening random peptide phage display library to detect new epitope candidates to be applied for diagnostic methods to widespread parasitic human diseases [46]. Additionally, using phage-displayed chicken single-chain antibody fragment libraries provides useful diagnostic and research reagents. Libraries constructed, using mRNA from an immune source, are enriched in affinity-matured sequences. Repertoires focused on a number of defined targets can be constructed using lymphocyte mRNA from chickens immunized with a mixture of several different antigens from *Plasmodium falciparum*, *Trypanosoma* sp., or human viruses [47, 48].

#### 2.4.2. *Immunoassay*

Development of IgY-based immunoassay is a widespread field to apply yolk antibodies. Enzyme-linked immunosorbent assay (ELISA), western blotting (WB), immunofluorescence

(IF), and immunohistochemistry (IHC) methods are the most common applications for IgY [1]. Relevant to consider that antigenic targets recognition by the use of antibodies can show some differences according to the method used. Regarding the conformational epitope structure, the performance of antibodies recognizing a given epitope by WB can represent nothing about the same antibody performance in ELISA with the same antigen [49]. IgY antibody shows advantages comparing to the mammal IgG use in immunoassay. In this context, the rheumatoid factor (RF) is a major source of interference in many immunoassays using mammalian polyclonal or monoclonal antibodies by interacting with IgG and causing false-positive results. IgY antibodies do not react with RF avoiding false-positive results in ELISA [50].

#### *2.4.2.1. Enzyme-linked immunosorbent assay*

IgY-based ELISA does not demand expressive modifications from the most common procedures and reagents used to carry out this protocol [16, 51]. Egg yolk IgY can be labeled with horseradish peroxidase for use in immunoenzymatic assays [52]. Some possibilities for application of yolk antibodies-based ELISA are: screening molecules related to drug-drug interactions [53]; sandwich ELISA to capture bacterial toxins [54]; screening animal diseases by using recombinant antigens [55]; characterization of maternal IgY transferred to egg yolk [56]; coproantigen to capture ELISA for intestine human parasite [57]; screening antibiotic residues in food samples [58]; detection of blood circulating helminth antigens by immunomagnetic bead ELISA [59]; potential for clinical application diagnosing cancer antigen [60].

#### *2.4.2.2. Immunofluorescence assay*

IgY antibodies can be applied to immunofluorescence and flow cytometry assays. IgY-based immunofluorescence experiment allows the detection of antigenic targets on cells and tissues samples [61]. Considering that IgY antibodies do not induce Fc-dependent activation of complement, they must be used to clarify the pathogeny of mammalian autoimmune diseases by immunofluorescence assay [62]. Chicken IgY and rabbit IgG conjugations with fluorescein isothiocyanate (FITC) comparatively used to examine strains of *Campylobacter fetus* revealed that both conjugates have a high percentage rate of detection; IgY has less background due to unspecific fluorescence than IgG. Additionally, IgY is a cheap, bloodless, and very productive method [63]. FITC-labeled anti-*Mycobacterium avium* subspecies *paratuberculosis* can target the pathogen inside the cytoplasm of infected macrophages [64]. Frozen liver fragments were diagnosed with cytomegalovirus antigens by using IgY-based confocal microscopy confirming the yolk antibody as suitable reagent for immunofluorescence assay [65].

#### *2.4.2.3. Flow cytometry assay*

IgY antibodies are suitable reagents for flow cytometry and as well as certain monoclonal antibodies, for example, to study human and rabbit platelet physiology [66]. When using phage display-based single chain variable fragments (scFvs), polyclonal IgY production and further the flow cytometry assays it is possible to develop immunoreagents for the isolation and characterization of stem cells, molecular diagnostics and therapeutics of lung cancers [67, 68].

#### *2.4.2.4. Immunochromatographic assay*

The immunochromatographic assay (ICA) requires no instruments and has a detection time of less than 10 minutes and it is portable and easy to perform in the field. The development of IgY-based strip could be a promising on-site tool for screening infection or disease outbreaks. IgY-gold complexes depositing onto the conjugate pad as detector reagents showed high specificity [69, 70].

#### *2.4.2.5. Using IgY for passive immunization*

The passive immunization is a protective method, which has been tested for many years and shown to be effective [71]. Passive immunization with pathogen-specific egg yolk antibodies (IgY) is emerging as a potential alternative to antibiotics for the treatment and prevention of several human and animal diseases. Laying hens are an excellent source of high-quality polyclonal antibodies, which can be collected noninvasively from egg yolks. The use of IgY offers several advantages such as it is environmentally friendly, nontoxic, reduces the numbers of animals required for antibody production, stability in the orogastrointestinal tract, and its safety profile [71–74]. A major obstacle to its implementation is its relatively high cost, which is dependent, among other things, mainly on two factors: the efficacy of antibody production, and the use of specific pathogen-free (SPF) birds for antibody production to avoid the possible of pathogens transference from commercial layers. Alternatively, treatment of the extracted IgY with formalin can negate the need for SPF birds and shows no interference with the Fab specific antigen-binding or Fc-complement activation of the antibody [75].

Regarding the IgY concentration in egg yolk and blood of laying hens, a recent study provides evidence that there is a significant circaseptan rhythm in yolk IgY and circaquattran rhythm in serum IgY. Additionally, the serum IgY concentration reached to maximum in the morning, decreased to minimum during the daytime, and increased again at night revealing a significant circadian rhythm, which may reflect in yolk antibody concentration [76].

The microencapsulation with a methacrylic acid copolymer may be an effective method of protecting purified yolk IgY from gastrointestinal inactivation, enabling its use for oral passive immunotherapy [77]. The use of chitosan-alginate microcapsules to protect IgY from gastrointestinal environment conditions provides significant resistance to pepsin hydrolysis and may enable intact IgY to reach target microorganisms within the lower digestive tract [78]. Another approach protecting IgY from degradation in gastric pH can be the incorporation of antibodies to hydrogel containing acrylamide and acrylic acid with promising results for IgY oral delivery [79].

Oral administration of IgY antibodies has been tested for many years with promising results [80] to different pathogens as human rotavirus [81]; dental plaque formation by *Streptococcus mutans* [82, 83]; enteropathogenic *E. coli* [84]; *Helicobacter pylori* [85, 86]; *Cryptosporidium parvum* [87, 88]; canine parvovirus [89]; *Porphyromonas gingivalis* [90]; *Pseudomonas aeruginosa* [91]; shrimp's white spot syndrome virus [92]; *Eimeria acervulina* [93]; *E. tenella* and *E. maxima* [94, 95]; H5N1 e H1N1 in mice [96]; *Vibrio cholerae* [97]; rotavirus and norovirus [98]; *Campylobacter jejuni* [99–101]; and botulinum neurotoxins [102]. Immunotherapy as a passive immunization method to neutralize venom using purified IgY proved to be efficient for therapy protocol [103–107].

### 2.5. State of art the use of IgY for Toxoplasma gondii studies

Currently, there are a limited number of studies about IgY antibody production against *T. gondii*, either native or recombinant antigens. *T. gondii* is a worldwide public health and veterinary problem.

Hassl et al. [108] first described the production of anti-*T. gondii* IgY. They used total soluble antigens that are immunogenic to comparatively produce rabbit IgG and chicken IgY. The results indicated differences between the specificities of egg yolk IgY antibodies and rabbit IgG serum antibodies, although both animal species had been immunized with identical antigen preparations. Ferreira Junior et al. [16] have produced comparative mice IgG and chicken IgY against soluble antigens from tachyzoites of *T. gondii*. They purified yolk antibodies by water dilution method, sodium sulfate precipitation, and molecular weight exclusion chromatography. Specific antibody characterization was due to both indirect ELISA and Western blotting methods and applied to immunofluorescence assays by immunohistochemistry and immunocytochemistry assays. Using the Western blotting method, the antigenic bands recognition profile were different between mice and chicken antibodies. IgY antibodies detected parasites in cytoplasm of infected cells and in brain samples of infected mice.

Hoto et al. [109] experimentally infected turkeys with tachyzoites and oocyst, and chickens with oocyst from *T. gondii* and investigated the humoral response against recombinant *T. gondii* antigens (rGRA1, rGRA6, rGRA9, rSAG1, and r SUB1) in a line blot assay. They found that infection with oocyst induced a stronger, permanent long-lasting antibody response compared to tachyzoite-infected animals.

Studying the heat shock protein of *T. gondii* (TgHSP70), a parasite virulence factor that is expressed during parasite stage conversion, Barenco et al [110] produced a polyclonal IgY against the recombinant TgHSP70 and tested it to detect native heat shock protein in brain samples from *T. gondii*-infection resistant (BALB/c) and susceptible (C57BL/6) mice after dexamethasone (DXM)-induced infection reactivation. In parallel, they investigated the TgHSP70-specific humoral response. They found higher specific antibody titers in serum samples of BALB/c compared with C57BL/6 mice. C57BL/6 mice presented high expression of TgHSP70 in the brain with the progression of infection and under DXM treatment. They conclude that these data suggest that the TgHSP70 release into the bloodstream depends on the death of the parasites mediated by the host immune response, whereas the increased TgHSP70 expression in the brain depends on the multiplication rate of the parasite.

More recent study with IgY and *T. gondii* was published by Cakir-Koc [111]. In this investigation, specific IgY antibodies were produced against the surface antigen 1 (SAG1) protein of *T. gondii* and the antibody activity was carried out by ELISA. Specific and higher amounts of IgY antibody against SAG1 were obtained. Regarding the advantages of IgY antibody and the importance of SAG1 for the diagnosis of toxoplasmosis, anti-SAG1 IgY would be a promising reagent in research, diagnostics, and immunotherapy against toxoplasmosis.

### 2.6. Future perspectives for the use of IgY for *Toxoplasma gondii* investigations

Although there are a reduced number of papers with IgY and *T. gondii*, the yolk IgY antibody has been demonstrated as an efficient tool for application for various kinds of different methods. Regarding phylogeny distance between chicken and mammals, which reflects differences in antigens profile recognition, IgY technology may be applied for the screening of new antigen libraries by random phage display method and the selection of candidate targets for therapy, diagnostics, or vaccine. In this context, polyclonal IgY and scFvs may be a promising alternative for proteomic studies. In the field of diagnostic methods, yolk IgY might be used as an alternative to mammalian IgG for rapid test to detect phase disease-associated circulating antigens, ELISA, flow cytometry test, and fluorescence techniques. Enzyme-labeled or fluorophore-labeled IgY as a primary antibody is employed to detect *T. gondii* antigens in fixed tissue samples or parasite-cultured cells. Speculating about a possible therapy for oral infection by *T. gondii*, IgY protecting the definitive and the intermediary hosts against infection may be an efficient tool for public health to control human and animal toxoplasmosis.

## Author details

Alvaro Ferreira Júnior*, Jandra P. Santos, Paula B. Bassi, Joely F.F. Bittar and Eustáquio R. Bittar

*Address all correspondence to: alvaro.junior@uniube.br

Veterinary Medicine School, University of Uberaba, Minas Gerais, Brazil

## References

[1] Behn I, Erhard M, Hlinak A, Staak C, editors. Chicken Egg Yolk Antibodies, Production and Application – IgY-Technology. Berlin Heidelberg: Springer-Verlag: 2001. p. 255. ISBN: 3540666796

[2] Schat KA, Kaspers B, Kaiser P, editors. Avian Immunology. 2nd ed. San Diego: Elsevier; 2013. p. 456. eBOOK ISBN: 9780123972729

[3] Tizard I. Veterinary Immunology. 9th ed. China: Elsevier; 2013. p. 551. ISBN: 9781455703623

[4] Tonegawa S. Somatic generation of antibody diversity. Nature. 1983;**302**:575-581

[5] McCormack WT, Tjoelker LW, Thompson CB. Avian B-cell development: Generation of an immunoglobulin repertoire by gene conversion. Annual Review Immunology. 1991;**9**:219-241

[6] Bachtiar EW, Bachtiar BM, Soejoedono RD, Wibawan IW, Afdhal A. Biological and immunogenicity of IgY anti *S. mutans* ComD. The Open Dentistry Journal. 2016;**10**:308-314. DOI: 10.2174/1874210601610010308

[7] Lee CH, Lee YC, Leu SJ, Lin LT, Chiang JR, Hsu WJ, Yang YY. Production and characterization of neutralizing antibodies against Bungarus multicinctus snake venom. Applied and Environmental Microbiology. 2016. Sep 23. pii: AEM.01876–16 (Epud ahead of print) DOI: 10.1128/AEM.01876-16.

[8] Zhen YH, Fang R, Ding C, Jin LJ, Li XY, Diao YP, Shu XH, Ma XC, Xu YP. Efficacy of specific IgY for treatment of lipopolysaccharide-induced endotoxemia using a mouse model. Journal of Applied Microbiology. 2011;**6**:1524-1532. DOI: 10.1111/j.1365-2672.2011.05155.x

[9] Nasiri K, Zibaee S, Nassiri M, Tahmoorespur M, Haghparast A. Production of specific IgY antibody to the recombinant FanC protein produced in *Escherichia coli*. Iranian Journal of Basic Sciences. 2016;**19**:883-889

[10] Hodek P, Hrdinova J, Macova I, Soucek P, Mrizova I, Burdova K, Kizek R, Hudecek J, Stiborova M. Preparation and application of anti-peptide antibodies for detection of orphan cytochromes P450. Neuro Endocrinology Letters. 2015;**36**(Suppl 1):38-45

[11] Anton M. Egg yolk: Structures, functionalities and processes. Journal of the Science of Food and Agriculture. 2013;**93**:2871-2880. DOI: 10.1002/jsfa.6247

[12] Lee HY, Abeyrathne ED, Choi I, Suh JW, Ahn DU. Sequential separation of immunoglobulin Y and phosvitin from chicken egg yolk without using organic solvents. Poultry Science. 2014;**93**:2668-2677. DOI: 10.3382/ps.2014-04093

[13] Hatta H, Kim M, Yamamoto T. A novel isolation method for hen egg yolk antibody, "IgY". Agricultural and Biological Chemistry. 1990;**54**:2531-2535

[14] Ren H, Yang W, Thirumalai D, Zhang X, Schade R. A comparative evaluation of six principal IgY antibody extraction methods. Alternatives to Laboratory Animals: ATLA. 2016;**44**:11-20

[15] Akita EM, Nakai S. Production and purification of Fab' fragments from chicken egg yolk immunoglobulin Y (IgY). Journal of Immunological Methods. 1993;**162**:155-164

[16] Ferreira Júnior a, Santiago FM, Silva MV, Ferreira FB, Macedo Júnior AG, Mota CM, Faria MS, Silva Filho HH, Silva DA, Cunha-Júnior JP, Mineo JR, Mineo TW. Production, characterization and applications for *Toxoplasma gondii*-specific polyclonal chicken egg yolk immunoglobulins. Plos One. 2012;**7**:e40391. DOI 10.1371/journal.pone.0040391

[17] Polson A, von Wechmanr MB, van Regenmortel MH. Isolation of viral IgY antibodies from yolks of immunized hens. Immunological Communications. 1980;**9**:475-493

[18] Pauly D, Chacana PA, Calzado EG, Brembs B, Schae R. IgY Technology: Extraction of chicken antibodies from egg yolk by polyethylene glycol (PEG) precipitation. Journal of Visualized Experiments: JoVE. 2011;**51**:3084. DOI: 10.3791/3084

[19] Carroll SB, Stollar BD. Antibodies to calf thymus RNA polymerase II from egg yolks of immunized hens. The Journal of Biological Chemistry. 1983;**258**:24-26

[20] Lemamy GJ, Roger P, Mani JC, Robert M, Rochefort H, Brouillet JP. High-affinity antibodies from hen's-egg yolks against human mannose-6-phosphate/insulin-like growth-factor-II receptor (M6P/IGFII-R): Characterization and potential use in clinical cancer studies. International Journal of Cancer. 1999;**80**:896-902

[21] Selvan K, Sentila R, Michael A. Generation and characterization of chicken egg yolk antibodies against Propionibacterium acnes for the prevention of acne vulgaris. Indian Journal of Dermatology. 2012;**57**:15-19. DOI: 10.4103/0019-5154.92669

[22] Taha M, Almeida MR, Silva FA, Domingues P, Ventura SP, Coutinho JA, Freire MG. Novel biocompatible and self-buffering ionic liquids for biopharmaceutical applications. Chemistry (Weinheim an der Bergstrasse, Germany). 2015;**21**:4781-4788. DOI: 10.1002/chem.201405693

[23] Borhani K, Mobarez AM, Khabiri AR, Behmanesh M, Khoramabadi N. Production of specific IgY *Helicobacter pylori* recombinant OipA protein and assessment of its inhibitory effects towards attachment of *H. pylori* to AGS cell line. Clinical and Experimental Vaccines Research. 2015;**4**:177-183. DOI: 10.7774/cevr.2015.4.2.177

[24] Schwarzkopf C, Thiele B. Effectivity of different methods for the extraction and purification of IgY. ALTEX. 1996;**13**:35-39

[25] Ruan GP, Ma L, He XW, Meng MJ, Zhu Y, Zhou MQ, Hu ZM, Wang XN. Efficient production, purification, and application of egg yolk antibodies against human HLA-A*0201 heavy chain and light chain (beta2m). Protein Expression and Purification. 2005;**44**:45-51. DOI: 10.1016/j.pep.2005.03.013

[26] Cook CL, Pao W, Firca JR, Anderson BE, Fryer JO. Simple purification methods for an alphagalactose-specific antibody from chicken eggs. Journal of Bioscience and Bioengineering. 2001;**91**:305-310

[27] Ko KY, Ahn DU. Preparation of immunoglobulin Y from egg yolk using ammonium sulfate precipitation and inoexchange chromatography. Poultry Science. 2007;**86**:400-407

[28] Rajic A, Stehmann C, Autelitano DJ, Vrkic AK, Hosking CG, Rice GE, Ilag LL. Protein depletion using IgY from chickens immunized with human protein cocktails. Preparative Biochemistry and Biotechnology. 2009;**39**:221-247. Doi: 10.1080/10826060902952915

[29] Hansen P, Scoble JA, Hanson B, Hoogenraad NJ. Isolation and purification of immunoglobulins from chicken eggs using thiophilic interaction chromatography. Journal of Immunological Methods. 1998;**215**:1-7

[30] Ortiz-Bueno AM, León-Chávez BA, Ruiz-Tagle A, Lozano-Zarain O, Castro-Caballero L, Achanzar WE, Bramblia E. Production of metallothionein polyclonal antibodies using chickens as model. Applied Biochemistry and Biotechnology. 2009;**158**:502-511. DOI: 10.1007/s12010-008-8349-2

[31] Kim WK, Patterson PH. Production of an egg yolk antibody specific to microbial uricase and its inhibitory effects on uricase activity. Poultry Science. 2003;**82**:1554-1558

[32] Meenatchisundaram S, Parameswari G, Michael A, Ramalingam S. Neutralization of the pharmacological effects of Cobra and Krait venoms by chicken egg yolk antibodies. Toxicon: Official Journal of the International Society on Toxicology. 2008;**52**:221-227. DOI: 10.1016/j.toxicon.2008.04.179

[33] Araújo AS, Lobato ZI, Chávez-Olórtegui C, Velarde DT. Brazilian IgY-Bothrops antivenom: Studies on the development of a process in chicken egg yolk. Toxicon: Official Journal of the International Society on Toxicology. 2010;**55**:739-744. DOI: 10.1015/j.toxicon.2009.11.004

[34] Meenatchisundaram S, Shanmugam V, Anjali VM. Development of chicken egg yolk antibodies against *Streptococcus mitis* – purification and neutralizing efficacy. Journal of Basic and Clinical Pharmacy. 2011;**2**:109-114

[35] Tobias FL, Garcia LN, Kanashiro MM, Medina-Acosta E, Brom-de-Luma JG, de Almeida CM, Azevedo Junior RR, Lemos M, Vieira-da-Motta O. Growth inhibition of *Staphylococcus aureus* and *Escherichia coli* strains by neutralizing IgY antibodies from ostrich egg yolk. Brazilian Journal of Microbiology. 2012;**43**:544-551. DOI: 10.1590/S1517-83822012000200015

[36] Fu CY, Huang H, Wang XM, Liu YG, Wang ZG, Cui SJ, Gao HL, Li Z, Li JP, Kpng XG. Preparation and evaluation of anti-SARS coronavirus IgY from yolks of immunized SPF chickens. Journal of Virological Methods. 2006;**133**:112-115

[37] Zolfagarian H, Dounighi NM. Study on development of Vipera lebetina snake anti-venom in chicken egg yolk for passive immunization. Human Vaccines and Immunotherapeutics. 2015;**11**:2734-2739. DOI: 10.4161/21645515.2014.985492

[38] Jiang X, Diraviyam T, Zhang X. Affinity purification of egg yolk immunoglobulins (IgY) using a human mycoplasma protein. Journal of Chromatography. B, Analytical Technologies in the Biomedical and Life Sciences. 2016;**1012-1013**:37-41. DOI: 10.1016/j.jchromb.2016.01.012

[39] Verdoliva A, Baslie G, Fassina G. Affinity purification of immunoglobulins from chicken egg yolk using a new synthetic ligand. Journal of Chromatography. B, Biomedical Sciences and Applications. 2000;**749**:233-242

[40] Dong D, Liu H, Xiao Q, Li R. Affinity purification of egg yolk immunoglobulins (IgY) with a stable synthetic ligand. Journal of Chromatography. B, Analytical Technologies in the Biomedical and Life Sciences. 2008;**870**:51-54. DOI: 10.1016/j.jchromb.2008.05.036

[41] Chen CC, Tu YY, Chen TL, Chang HM. Isolation and characterization of immunoglobulin in yolk (IgY) specific against hen egg white lysozyme by immunoaffinity chromatography. Journal of Agricultural and Food Chemistry. 2002;**50**:5424-5428

[42] Sui J, Lin H, Cao L. Affinity purification of specific anti-Listeria monocytogenes egg yolk antibodies (IgY) using amino-activated cells as receptor. Journal of Immunoassay and Immunochemistry. 2011;**32**:131-144. DOI: 10.1080/15321819.2010.545160

[43] Constantinoiu CC, Molly JB, Jorgensen WK, Coleman GT. Purification of immunoglobulins from chicken sera by thiophilic gel chromatography. Poultry Science. 2007;**86**:1910-1914

[44] Fahiminyia S, Roche S, Gérard N. Improvement of 2D-PAGE resolution of human, porcine and canine follicular fluid: Comparison of two immunodepletion columns. Reproduction in Domestic Animlas = Zuchthygiene. 2012;**47**:e67-e70. DOI: 10.1111/j.1439-0531.2011.01939

[45] Tan Sh, Mohamedali A, Kapur A, Baker MS. Ultradepletion of human plasma using chicken antibodies: A proof of concept study. Journal of Proteome Research. 2013;**12**:2399-2413. DOI: 10.1021/pr3007182

[46] Manhani MN, Ribeiro VS, Cardoso R, Ueira-Vieria C, Goulart LR, Costa-Cruz JM. Specific phage-display peptides discriminate diferente forms of neurocysticercosis by antibody detection in the serum samples. Parasite Immunology. 2011;**33**:322-329. DOI: 10,1111/j.1365-3024.2011.01283.x

[47] Chiliza TE, Van Wyngaardt W, Du Plessis DH. Single-chain antibody fragments from a display library derived from chickens immunized with a mixture of parasite and viral antigens. Hybridoma. 2008;**27**:413-421. DOI: 10.1089/hyb.2008.0051

[48] Lee YC, Leu SJ, Hung HC, Wu HH, Huang IJ, Hsieh WS, Chiu WT, Hsieh MS, Cheng TF, Yang YY. A dominant antigenic epitope an SARS-CoV spike protein identified by an avian single-chain variable fragment (scFv)-expressing phage. Veterinary Immunology and Immunopathology. 2007;**117**:75-85. DOI: 10.1016/j.vetimm.2007.02.001

[49] Uhlen M, Bandrowski A, Carr S, Edwards A, Ellenberg J, Lundberg E, Rimm DL, Rodriguez H, Hiltke T, Snyder M, Yamamoto T. A proposal for validation of antibodies. Nature Methods. 2016;**13**:823-827. DOI: 10.1030/nmeth.3995

[50] Larsson A, Karlsson-Parra A, Sjoquist J. Use of chicken antibodies in enzyme immunoassays to avoid interference by rheumatoid factors. Clinical Chemistry. 1991;**37**:411-414.

[51] da Silva Raposo R, Santarém VA, Merigueti YF, Rubinsky-Elefant G, de Lima Cerazo LM, Pereira L, Zampieri BP, da Silva AV, Laposy CB. Kinetic and avidity of IgY anti-Toxocara antibodies in experimentally infected chickens. Experimental Parasitology. 2016;**171**:33-41. DOI: 10.1016/j.exppara.2016.09.009

[52] Ruan GP, Ma L, Meng XL, Wang XN, Lin Y, Wu ZQ, He XW, Wang JF, Zhu y. Quantification of antibody (IgY) titers in hen eggs following immunization and their use in detecting cell surface molecules on nitrocellulose membranes. Journal of Immunoassay and Immunochemistry. 2007;**28**:35-45. DOI: 10.1080/15321810601026083

[53] Jiang Z, Jiang X, Li C, Xue H, Zhang X. Development of an IgY antibody-based immunoassay for the screening of the CYP2E1 inhibitor/enhancer from herbal medicines. Frontiers in Pharmacology. 2016;**7**:502. DOI: 10.3389/fphar.2016.00502

[54] Nagaraj S, Ramlal S, Kingston J, Batra HV. Development of IgY based sandwich ELISA for the detection of staphylococcal enterotoxin G (SEG), an egc toxin. International Journal of Food Microbiology. 2016;**237**:136-141. DOI: 10.1016/j.ijfoodmicro.2016.08.009

[55] Zhang X, Diraviyam T, Li X, Yao G, Michael A. Preparation of chicken IgY against recombinant E2 protein of bovine viral diarrhea virus (BVDV) and development of ELISA and ICA for BVDV detection. Bioscience, Biotechnology and Biochemistry. 2016;**80**:2467-2472. DOI: 10.1080?09168451.2016.1217144

[56] Murai A, Kakiuci M, Hamano T, Kobayashi M, Tsudzuki M, Nakano M, Matsuda Y, Horio F. An ELISA for quantifying quail IgY and characterizing maternal IgY transfer to egg yolk in several quails strains. Veterinary Immunology and Immunopathology. 2016;**175**:16-23. DOI: 10.1016/j.vetimm.2016.04.013

[57] Teimoori S, Arimatsu Y, Laha T, Kaewkes S, Sereerak P, Sripa M, Tangkawattana S, Brindley PJ, Sripa B. Chicken IgY-based coproantigen capture ELISA for diagnosis of human pisthorchiasis. Parasitology International. 2016;pii:S1383-5769(16)30093-9. DOI: 10.1016/I.PARINT.2015.10.011

[58] He J, Hu J, Thirumalai D, Schade R, Du E, Zhang X. Development of indirect competitive ELISA using egg yolk-derived immunoglobulin (IgY) for the detection of gentamicin residues. Journal of Environmental Science and Health. Part. B, Pesticides, Food Contaminants, and Agricultural Wastes. 2016;**51**:8-13. DOI: 10.1080/03601234.2015.1080479

[59] Nie G, Wang T, Lu S, Liu W, Li Y, Lei J. Detection of Clonorchis sinensis circulating antigen in sera from Chinese patients by immunomagnetic bead ELISA based on IgY. PloS One. 2014;**9**:e113508. DOI: 10.1371/journal.pone.0113208

[60] Grzywa R, Lupicka-Slowik A, Walczak M, Idzi M, Bobrek K, Boivin S, Gawel A, Stefaniak T, Oleksyszyn J, Sienczyk M. Highly sensitive detection of cancer antigen 15-3 using novel avian IgY antibodies. ALTEX. 2014;**31**:43-52. DOI: 10.14573/altex.1309181

[61] Camenisch G, Tini M, Chilov D, Kvietikova I, Srinivas V, Caro J, Spielmann P, Wenger RH, Gassmann M. General applicability of chicken egg yolk antibodies: The performance of IgY immunoglobulins raised against the hypoxia-inducible factor 1 alpha. FASEB Journal. 1999;**13**:81-88

[62] Sesarman A, Mihai S, Chiriac MT, Olaru F, Sitaru AG, Thurman JM, Zillikens D, Sitaru C. Binding of avian IgY to type VII collagen does not activate complement and leucocytes and fails to induce subepidermal blistering in mice. The British Journal of Dermatology. 2008;**158**:463-471. DOI: 10.1111/j.1365-2133.2007.08388.x

[63] Cipolla A, Cordeviola J, Terzolo H, Combessies G, Bardón J, Ramón N, Martínez A, Medina D, Morsella C, Malena R. *Campylobacter fetus* diagnosis: Direct immunofluorescence comparing chicken IgY and rabbit IgG conjugates. ALTEX. 2001;**18**:165-170

[64] Shin SJ, Lee SS, Manning EJ, Collins MT. Production of and applications foa a polyclonal IgY diagnostic reagent specific for *Mycobacterium avium* subsp. *paratuberculosis*. Journal of Microbiology. 2009;**47**:600-609. DOI: 10.1007/s12275-009-0052-7

[65] Bentes GA, LAnzarini NM, Lima LR, Manso PP, da Silva Ados S, Mouta Junior Sda S, Guimarães JR, de Moraes MT, Pelajo-Machado M, Pinto MA. Using immunoglobulin Y as an alternative antibody for the detection of hepatitis A virus in frozen

liver sections. Memórias do Instituto Oswaldo Cruz. 2015;**110**:577-579. DOI: 10.1590/0074-02760140457

[66] Santoro ML, Barbaro KC, Flores da Rocha TR, Soares Torquato RJ, Hirata IY, Sano-Martins IS. Simultaneous isolation of platelet factor 4 and glycoprotein IIb-IIIa complex from rabbit platelets, and characterization of specific chicken antibodies to assay them. Journal of Immunological Methods. 2004;**284**:55-72

[67] Leu SJ, Lee YC, Shih NY, Huang IJ, Liu KJ, Lu HF, Huang SY, Yang YY. Generation and characterization of anti-alpha-enolase single-chain antibodies in chicken. Veterinary Immunology and Immunopathology. 2010;**137**:251-260. Doi: 10.1016/j.vetimm.2010.06.001

[68] Bowes T, Hanley SA, Liew A, Eglon M, Mashayekhi K, O'Kennedy R, Barry F, Taylor WR, O'Brien T, Griffin MD Finlay WJ, Greiser U. Developing cell-specific antibodies to endothelial progenitor cells using avian immune phage display technology. Journal of Biomolecular Screening. 2011;**16**:744-754. DOI: 10.1177/1087057111407067

[69] Zhang L, Li D, Liu L, Zhang G. Rapid immunochromatographic test strip to detect swimming crab Portunus trituberculatus reovirus. Diseases of Aquatic Organisms. 2015;**117**:21-29. DOI: 10.3354/dao02921

[70] He J, Wang Y, Sun S, Zhang X. Evaluation of chicken IgY generated against canine parvovirus viral-like particles and development of enzyme-linked immunosorbent assay and immunochromatographic assay for canine parvovirus detection. Viral Immunology. 2015;**28**:489-494. DOI: 10.1089/vim.2015.0030

[71] Dias da Silva W, Tambourgi DV. IgY: A promising antibody for use in immunodiagnostic and in immunotherapy. Veterinary Immunology and Immunopathology. 2010;**135**:173-180. DOI: 10.1016/j.vetimm.2009.12.011

[72] Lee J, Kang HE, Woo HJ. Stability of orally administered immunoglobulin in the gastrointestinal tract. Journal of Immunological Methods. 2012;**384**:143-147. DOI: 10.1016/j.jim.2012.06.001

[73] Rahman S, Van Nguyen S, Icatlo FC Jr, Umeda K, Kodama Y. Oral passive IgY-based immunotherapeutics: A novel solution for prevention and treatment of alimentary tract diseases. Human Vaccines and Immunotherapeutics. 2013;**9**(5):1039–1048. DOI: 10.4161/hv.23383

[74] Gadde U, Rathinam T, Lillehoj HS. Passive immunization with hyperimmune egg-yolk IgY as prophylaxis and therapy for poultry diseases – A review. Animal Health Research Reviews. 2015;**16**:163-176. DOI: 10.1017/S1466252315000195

[75] Aizenshtein E, Yosipovich R, Kvint M, Shadmon R, Krispel S, Shuster E, Eliyahu D, Finger A, Banet-Noach C, Shahar E, Pitcovski J. Practical aspects in the use of passive immunization as an alternative to attenuated viral vaccines. Vaccine. 2016;**34**:2513-2518. DOI: 10.1016/j.vaccine.2016.03.051

[76] He JX, Thirumalai D, Schade R, Zhang XY. Chronobiological studies of chicken IgY: Monitoring of infradian, circadian and ultradian rhythms of IgY in blood and yolk of chickens. Veterinary Immunology and Immunopathology. 2014;**160**:266-272. DOI: 10.1016/j.vetimm.2014.05.016

[77] Kovacs-Nolan J, Mine Y. Microencapsulation for the gastric passage and controlled intestinal release of immunoglobulin Y. Journal of Immunological Methods. 2005;**296**:199-209. DOI: 10.1016/j.jim.2004.11.017

[78] Li XY, Jin LJ, McAllister TA, Stanford K, Xu JY, Lu YN, Zhen YH, Sun YX, Xu YP. Chitosan-alginate microcapsules for oral delivery of egg yolk immunoglobulin (IgY). Journal of Agricultural and Food Chemistry. 2007;**55**:2911-2917. DOI: 10.1021/jf062900q

[79] Bellingeri RV, Picco NY, Alustiza FE, Canova JV, Molina MA, Acevedo DF, Barbero C, Vivas AB. pH-responsive hydrogels to protect IgY from gastric conditions: In vitro evaluation. Journal of Food Science and Technology. 2015;**52**:3117:3122. DOI: 10.1007/s13197-014-1337-3

[80] Muller S, Schubert A, Zajac J, Dyck T, Oelkrug C. IgY antibodies in human nutrition for disease prevention. Nutrition Journal. 2015;**14**:109. Doi: 10.1186/s12937-015-0067-3

[81] Hatta H, Tsuda K, Akachi S, Kim M, Yamamoto, Ebina T. Oral passive immunization effect of anti-human rotavirus IgY and its behavior against proteolytic enzymes. Bioscience, Biotechnology and Biochemistry. 1993;**57**:1077-1081

[82] Hatta H, Tsuda K, Ozeki M, Kim NM, Yamamoto T, Otake S, Hirasawa M, Katz J, Childers NK Michalek SM. Passive immunization against dental plaque formation in humans: Effect of a mouth rinse containing egg yolk antibodies (IgY) specific to *Streptococcus mutans*. Caries Research. 1997;**31**:268-274

[83] Smith DJ, King WF, Godiska R. Passive transfer of immunoglobulin Y antibody to *Streptococcus mutans* glucan binding protein B can confer protection against experimental dental caries. Infection and Immunity. 2001;**69**:3135-3142. DOI: 10.1128/IAI.69.5.3135-3124.2001

[84] Amaral JA, Tino de Franco M, Carneiro-Sampaio MM, Carbonare SB. Anti-enteropathogenic *Escherichia coli* immunoglobulin Y isolated from eggs laid by immunised Leghorn chickens. Resaerch in Veterinary Science. 2002;**72**:229-234. DOI: 10.1053/rvsc.2002.0551

[85] Suzuki H, Nomura S, Masaoka T, Goshima H, Kamata N, Kodama Y, Ishii H, Kitajima M, Nomoto K, Hibi T. Effect of dietary anti-*Helicobacter pylori*-urease immunoglobulin Y on *Helicobacter pylori* infection. Alimentary Pharmacology and Therapeutics. 2004; v.20 (Suppl 1):185–192. DOI: 10.1111/J.1365.2036.2004.02027.x

[86] Borhani K, Mohabati Mobarez A, Khabiri AR, Behmanesh M, Khoramabadi N. Inhibitory effects of rHP-NAP IgY against *Helicobacter pylori* attachment to AGS cell line. Microbial Pathogenesis. 2016;**97**:231-235. DOI: 10.1016/j.micpath.2016.06.004

[87] Kobayashi C, Yokoyama H, Nguyen SV, Kodama Y, Kimata T, Izeki M. Effect of egg yolk antibody on experimental *Cryptosporidium parvum* infection in scid mice. Vaccine. 2004;**23**:232-235. DOI: 10.1016/j.vaccine.2004.05.034

[88] Omidian Z, Ebrahimzadeh E, Shahbazi P, Asghari Z, Shayan P. Application of recombinant *Cryptosporidium parvum* P23 for isolation and prevention. Parasitology Research. 2014;**113**:229-237. DOI: 10.1007/s00436-013-3648-0

[89] Van Nguyen S, Umeda K, Yokoyama H, Tohya Y, Kodama Y. Passive protection of dogs against clinical disease due to canine parvovirus-2 by specific antibody from chicken egg yolk. Canadian Journal of Veterinary Research. 2006;**70**:62-64

[90] Hamajima S, Maruyama M, Hijika T, Hatta H, Abiko Y. Egg yolk-derived immunoglobulin (IgY) against *Prophyromonas gingivalis* 40-kDa outer membrane protein inhibits coaggregation activity. Archives of Oral Biology. 2007;**52**:697-704. DOI: 10.1016/J.archoralbio.2006.12.013

[91] Nilsson E, Kollberg H, Johannesson M, Wejaker PE, Carlander D, Larsson A. More than 10 years' continuous oral treatment with specific immunoglobulin Y for the prevention of *Pseudomonas aeruginosa* infections: A case report. Journal of Medicinal Food. 2007;**10**:375-378. DOI: 10.1089/jmf.2006.214

[92] Lu Y, Liu J, Jin L, Li X, Zhen Y, Xue H, You J, Xu Y. Passive protection of shrimp against white spot syndrome virus (WSSV) using specific antibody from egg yolk of chickens immunizaed with inactivated virus or a WSSV-DNA vaccine. Fish and Shellfish Immunology. 2008;**25**:604-610. DOI: 10.1016/j.fsi.2008.08.010

[93] Lee SH, Lillehoj HS, Park DW, Jang SI, Morales A, Garcia D, Lucio E, Larios R, Victoria G, Marrufo D, Lillehoj EP. Induction of passive immunity in broiler chickens against Eimeria acevulina by hyperimmune egg yolk immunoglobulin Y. Poultry Science. 2009;**88**:562-566. DOI: 10.3382/ps.2008-00340

[94] Lee SH, Lillehoj HS, Park DW, Jang SI, Morales A, Garcia D, Lucio E, Larios R, Victoria G, Marrufo D, Lillehoj EP. Protective effect of hyperimmune egg yolk IgY antibodies against *Eimeria tenella* and *Eimeria maxima* infections. Veterinary Parasitology. 2009;**163**:123-126. DOI: 10.1016/j.vetpar.2009.04.020

[95] Xu J, Ren C, Wang S, Liu D, Cao L, Tao J. Protection efficacy of multivalent egg yolk immunoglobulin against *Eimeria tenella* infection in chickens. Iranian Journal of Parasitology. 2013;**8**:449-458

[96] Nguyen HH, Tumpey TM, Park HJ, Byun YH, Tran LD, Nguyen VD, Kilgore PE, Czerkinsky C, Katz JM, Seong BL, Song JM, Kim YB, Do HT, Nguyen T, Nguyen CV. Prophylatic and therapeutic efficacy of avian antibodies against influenza virus H5N1 and H1N1 in mice. PLoS One. 2010;5:e10152. DOI: 10.1371/journal.pone.0010152

[97] Hirai K, Arimitsu H, Umeda K, Yokota K, Shen L, Ayada K, Kodama Y, Tsuji T, Hirai Y, Oguma K. Passive oral immunization by egg yolk immunoglobulin (IgY) to *Vibrio cholerae* effectively prevents clolera. Acta Medica Okayama. 2010;**64**:163-170

[98] Dai YC, Zhang XF, Tan M, Huang P, Lei W, Fang H, Zhing W, Jiang X. A dual chicken IgY against rotavirus and norovirus. Antiviral Research. 2013;**97**:293-300. DOI: 10.1016/j.antiviral.2012.12.011

[99] Al-Adwani SR, Crespo R, Shah DH. Production and evaluation of chicken egg-yolk-derived antibodies against *Campylobacter jejuni* colonization-associated proteins. Foodborne Pathogens and Disease. 2013;**10**:624-631. DOI: 10.1089/fpd.2012.1313

[100] Hermans D, Van Steendam K, Verbrugghe E, Verlinden M, Martel A, Seliwiorstow T, Heyndrickx M, Haesebrouck F, De Zutter L, Deforce D, Pasmans F. Passive immunization to reduce *Campylobacter jejuni* colonization and transmission in broiler chickens. Veterinary Research. 2014;**45**:27. DOI: 10.1186/1297-9716-45-27

[101] Paul NC, Al-Awani S, Crespo R, Shah DH. Evaluation of passive immunotherapeutic efficacy of hyperimmunized egg yolk powder against intestinal colonization of *Campylobacter jejuni* in chickens. Poultry Science. 2014;**93**:2779-2787. DOI: 10.3382/ps.2014-04234

[102] You Z, Yang H, Xin W, Kang L, Gao S, Wang J, Zhang T, Wang J. Preparation of egg yolk antibodies aginst BoNT/B ant their passive protection in mouse models. Human Vaccines and Immunotherapeutics. 2014;**10**:2321-2327. DOI: 10.4161/hv.29433

[103] Almeida CM, Kanashiro MM Rangel Filho FB, Mata MF, Kipnis TL, da Silva WD. Development of sanke antivenom antibodies in chickens and their purification from yolk. The Veterinary Record. 1998;**143**:579-584

[104] Meenatchisundaram S, Parameswari G, Michael A, Ramalingam S. Studies on pharmacological effects of Russell's viper and Saw-scaled viper venom and its neutralization by chicken egg yolk antibodies. International Immunopharmacology. 2008;**8**:1067-1073. DOI: 10.1016/j.intimp.2008.03.017

[105] de Andrade FG, Eto SF, Navarro dos Santos Ferraro Ac, Gonzales Marioto DT, Vieira NJ, Cheirubim AP, de Paula Ramos S, Venâncio EJ. The production and characterization of anti-bothropic and anti-crotalic IgY antibodies in laying hens: A long term experiment. Toxicon. 2013;**66**:18-24. DOI: 10.1016./j.toxicon.2013.01.018

[106] Alvarez A, Montero Y, Jimenez E, Zerpa N, Parrilla P, Malavé C. IgY antibodies anti-Tityus caripitensis venom: Purification and neutralization efficacy. Toxicon. 2013;**74**:208-214. DOI: 10.1016/j.toxicon.2013.08.058

[107] Navarro D, Vargas M, Herrera M, Segura Á, Gómez A, Villata M, Ramírez N, Williams D, Gutiérrez JM, León G. Development of a chicken-derived antivenom against the taipan snake (*Oxyuranus scutellatus*) venom and comparison with an equine antivenom. Toxicon. 2016;**120**:1-8. DOI: 10.1016/j.toxicon.2016.06.018

[108] Hassl A, Aspock H, Flamm H. Comparative studies on the purity and specificity of yolk immunoglobulin Y isolated from eggs laid by hens immunized with *Toxoplasma gondii* antigen. Zentralblatt fur Bakteriologie. Mikrobiologie, und Hygiene. Series A, Medical Microbiology, Infectious Disease, Virology, Parasitology. 1987;**267**:247–253

[109] Hoto A, Buschtons S, Bangoura B, Zoller B, Koethe M, Spekker-Bosker K, Hotop SK, TEnter Am, Daubener W, Straubinger RK, Groβ U. Humoral immune responses in chickens and turkeys after infection with *Toxoplasma gondii* by using recombinant antigens. Parasitology Research. 2014;**113**:1473-1480. DOI: 10.1007/s00436-014-3788-x

[110] Barenco PV, Lourenço EV, Cunha-Júnior JO, Almeida KC, Roque-Barreira MC, Silva DA, Araújo EC, Coutinho LB, Oliveira MC, Mineo TW, Mineo JR, Silva NM. *Toxoplasma gondii* 70 kDa heat shock protein: Systemic detection is associated with the death of the parasites by the immune response and its increased expression in the brain is associated with parasite replication. PLoS One. 2014;**9**:e96527. DOI: 10.1371/journal.pone.0096527

[111] Cakir-Koc R. Production of anti-SAG1 IgY antibody aginst *Toxoplasma gondii* parasites and evaluation of antibody activity by ELISA method. Parasitology Research. 2016;**115**:2947-2952. DOI: 10.1007/s00436-016-5047-9

# 12

# Effective Diagnostic Marker for Serodiagnosis of *Toxoplasma gondii* Infection: New Developments and Perspectives

Zeehaida Mohamed and Khalid Hajissa

**Abstract**

Toxoplasmosis is a prevalent parasitic infection caused by an obligate intracellular parasite *Toxoplasma gondii*. Various methods have been established in the laboratory diagnosis of toxoplasmosis. Among these methods, serological tests are common and provide satisfactory results. However, producing reliable reagents and standard antigen remains difficult and expensive. Replacing native antigens in all current diagnostic kits with standard and reliable reagents are speculated to achieve more sensitive and specific detection that can significantly improve the assay performance. This review provides updated data on toxoplasmosis serodiagnosis. It focuses on the recent trends of producing reliable and standard antigens that have been used in the serological tests of toxoplasmosis, as well as the future direction in this field.

**Keywords:** ELISA, serodiagnosis, multiepitope peptide, recombinant antigen, sensitivity, specificity, toxoplasmosis

## 1. Introduction

Toxoplasmosis is one of the most prevalent parasitic infections caused by an obligate intracellular parasite *Toxoplasma gondii*. This parasite can infect almost all warm-blooded animals including humans. The effect of *T. gondii* on public health and animal production is significantly evident worldwide. Therefore, it became one of the well-studied parasites because of its medical and veterinary importance. Although the prevalence rate of toxoplasmosis is approximately one-third of the world's human population, *T. gondii* infection in immunocompetent individuals is usually asymptomatic, even though some patients may experience fever and other non-specific clinical signs [1]. In immunocompromised patients, this disease may be serious or even fatal; furthermore, primary invasion during pregnancy may endanger the life of the fetus as well as the infected mothers [1, 2]. Accurate diagnosis of the acquired infection by highly sensitive and specific methods is crucial for proper management of animal and human toxoplasmosis and represents the key step in the prevention and treatment of the disease [3].

Various methods have been established in the laboratory diagnosis of toxoplasmosis. Among these methods, serological tests are common and provide satisfactory results. However, producing reliable reagents remains laborious and expensive. Acquiring a specific and effective reagent that can be used in the serodiagnosis is necessary. In the present review, we provide updated data on toxoplasmosis serodiagnosis. The review focuses on the recent trends of producing reliable and standard antigens that have been used in the serological tests of toxoplasmosis, as well as the future direction in this field.

## 2. Serodiagnosis

Various direct and indirect detection methods have been established to detect *T. gondii* infectious agent or anti-*Toxoplasma* antibodies [4]. In particular, different sets of detection methods have also been developed and evaluated to achieve accurate diagnosis [5]. There are several diagnostic approaches which are applicable to detect the parasitic agents include: histological identification, isolation of the organism in tissue culture [4], and recovery of the parasite DNA by the polymerase chain reaction (PCR) [6, 7] or by a combination of these techniques, whereas the serodiagnostic tests are mainly designated to detect the different classes of antibodies or antigens [8].

Despite the various methods of toxoplasmosis investigation, the routine laboratory diagnosis in both humans and animals depends mainly on conducting various serological investigations to detect specific anti-*Toxoplasma* antibodies in serum samples [5, 9]. It remains the primary approach to achieve satisfactory results [10]. The production and appearance of each antibody isotype are correlated with the immune response after the infection, thus, the determination whether the host has got *Toxoplasma* infection or not can be achieved simply by monitoring the immune response especially humoral immunity. The disease symptoms are non-specific and not enough to characterize accurate diagnosis because of clinical signs mimicry between toxoplasmosis and several other infections [5, 11]. Many serological tests have been designed to measure different types of antibody, which show unique increases and decreases during or after infection [12]. All immunoglobulin isotypes have been used successfully in *T. gondii* serodiagnosis, including IgG, IgM IgA, and IgE [10]. Specific *T. gondii* IgM is considered as early and sensitive diagnostic marker that correlates with the occurrences of acute toxoplasmosis. Particularly, IgM can be detected in serum only 1 week following the infection.

However, it may remain in the serum for several months or years [8]. Thus, the interpretation of the serology results sometimes becomes more difficult. Furthermore, the presence of IgM antibodies in the maternal circulation even 18 months after invasion influence the accuracy of this diagnostic approach because determining whether an antibody is from active or previous infection is crucial during gestation [13]. If an antibody is from a previous infection, no consequences for the fetus normally occur. If the infection occurs during pregnancy, the clinician should decide on administering anti-parasitic treatment to avoid disease complication in the unborn child [5, 11]. Recent studies have shown that the use of IgM alone for the establishment of acute toxoplasmosis is insufficient [8].

Detection of IgG antibodies in patients may aid diagnosis. IgG antibodies can be detected within 1–2 weeks following infectionacquisition, and normally peak within 1–2 months, and decline at various rates, but usually persist lifelong at residual titers [5, 11]. High levels of this antibody indicate previous infection. Therefore, measuring of IgG antibody is a common diagnostic marker that helps clinicians to decide whether a patient has chronic infection or not. However, this antibody still has difficulty in distinguishing previous infection from a recent infection. Consequently, an auxiliary test based on the IgG avidity has been established to differentiate acute from chronic infection in an asymptomatic patient [5, 11]. In recent years, precise dating and infection have been proven to be obtained by using IgE and IgA. However, they produced during the first weeks of infection, and disappear early [9]. There are various serological procedures have been established for the detection of anti *T. gondii* antibodies; these include Sabin-Feldman dye test (SFDT), indirect fluorescent assay (IFA), agglutination tests, and enzyme-linked immunosorbent assays (ELISAs), or a combination of these methods are also required for determining recent and previous infections [9, 10, 12].

## 3. Sabin-Feldman dye test (SFDT)

It was a greatest advancement in the field of toxoplasmosis diagnosis when Sabin and Feldman described the dye test as a novel diagnostic test 60 years ago [14]. Though SFDT is the first assay developed for the laboratory investigation of *T. gondii* infection [10], but still considered as "gold standard" with high sensitivity and specificity [15]. The principle of the assay is based on incubating live tachyzoites with patient serum and complement. Subsequently, if the serum contains specific antibodies against *T. gondii*, it will immediately coat the parasite and the tachyzoite will be lysed by the complement system and fail to stain with dye methylene blue. The number of unstained (dead) and stained (live) tachyzoites will be counted and used to establish the end-point titer [10, 15, 16]. In comparison with other diagnostic tests, SFDT has the potential to detect both IgM and IgG. On the other hands, the assay has certain limitations. For example, application of live parasite is considered a biohazard; thus, it can be only applied in a few laboratories. The antibody titers also do not give strong clues to determine whether the infection is acute or chronic [15, 16].

## 4. Indirect fluorescent assay (IFA)

IFA is one of the most simple, sensitive, safe, and widely used assays in the usual detection of anti-*Toxoplasma* antibodies [17]. It has been established as an alternative diagnostic method in response to overcome the biohazard of using live tachyzoites in SFDT [10]. Diluted serum specimens are incubated with killed *Toxoplasma* tachyzoites fixed on a glass slide to allow specific antigen-antibody interaction [8]. The interaction will then detected by addition of fluorescent-labeled anti-human IgG or IgM antibodies, and the result is viewed under a fluorescence microscope [18]. Although IFA is relatively inexpensive, fluorescence microscope is required, and the individual differences in result reading are considered as one of the test limitation. Furthermore, false-positive results may occur in case the sera contain rheumatoid factors or antinuclear antibodies [10]. Nevertheless, high levels of *T. gondii*-specific IgG in some acute acquired toxoplasmosis patients may interfere with the IgM and cause false negative results [19].

## 5. Agglutination tests

Different agglutination tests, including direct agglutination test (DAT), indirect hemagglutination test (IHAT), and latex agglutination test (LAT), are applied in toxoplasmosis serology [9, 12, 20]. Development of DAT assists tremendously in identifying of anti-*T. gondii* antibody in humans and animal sera [12]. Fulton achieved this test in 1965; the important features of this test are the absence of secondary antibody and no special equipment needed. The principle of DAT starting with coating of microtiter plates with formalinized *Toxoplasma* tachyzoites. Diluted patient sera will then added. Accordingly, the agglutination will occur if anti-*Toxoplasma* antibodies are present in the tested sera. However, precipitated tachyzoites will be noticed at the bottom of the wells if the sample is negative [21]. The test is very simple and has proved to be very sensitive and inexpensive, although a large quantity of antigen is required. Despite that DAT is only used for detection of IgG antibodies, non-specific agglutination can be induced by occurrences of IgM antibodies [12, 20].

In the IHAT test, red blood cells (RBCs) are sensitized with *T. gondii* soluble antigen. Subsequently, sensitized cells will then incubated with patient sera. Accordingly, the RBCs will agglutinate if the sera contain anti-*T. gondii* antibodies. Furthermore, IHAT is also simple to perform and inexpensive and can be used for both humans and animals [8]. In the LAT, tachyzoite particle is fixed to latex beads. When the beads are incubated with patient sera containing specific IgG antibody, visible agglutination reaction will occur [22]. The disadvantage of this assay is the low sensitivity and specificity, particularly in immunocompromised patients; moreover, non-specific IgM can generate false-positive result [9, 20].

### 5.1. Enzyme-linked immunosorbent assay (ELISA)

ELISA is highly sensitive and specific analytical assay for quantitative detection of antibodies or virtually all types of antigenically active molecule. Application of ELISA in the diagnosis of toxoplasmosis has been established since 1976 [23]. Since developed up to now, it has been one of the most common biochemical techniques used in research and clinical laboratories, including detection of anti *T. gondii* antibodies [8, 24]. In this assay, a microtiter plate is coated with antigens, and then diluted patients sera are applied. If the serum contains anti-*Toxoplasma* antibodies, it will bind directly to coated antigen, and the presence of *Toxoplasma*-specific antibody will detect by using anti-human enzyme-conjugate (secondary antibody). Any unbound reagents are removed in the washing steps. Finally, the substrate is added, and subsequently, color reaction develops (which is relatively correlated with the quantity of the antibody). Interpretation of the ELISA results normally depends on the assessment of color change spectrophotometrically [25].

ELISA can easily determine a positive or negative sample by correlating the optical density of the serum with the control after a threshold value is established [25]. In general, the advantages of ELISA test are as follows: it shows high sensitivity which allows quantitative and semi-quantitative antibody measurements, automatically adopted and is inexpensive [26]. Furthermore, the assay is simple and easy to carry out and can be used to investigate a large number of serum samples in a short period of time [4]. Moreover, it can be used to detect both IgG and IgM antibodies [25]. The disadvantage of the ELISA includes standardization of used antigens [26]. A photometer is also necessary to assess the results, otherwise, it is difficult to distinguish between negative reaction and weak positive reaction by visual examination, and this may increase the cost of the test [25]. Generally, detection of anti-*T. gondii* IgM antibody possesses a high degree of accuracy according to the reports; however, it might sometimes give false-positive result [27]. It is most probably due to the presence of rheumatoid factor in serum, and on the other hands, it is common to get false-negative results due to specific IgG competitive inhibition [28].

### 5.2. Production of reliable and standard antigen for serological diagnosis

Establishing of *T. gondii* serology is an essential diagnostic tool, which gives satisfactory results. However, producing specific and standard antigens is a real challenge. Currently, most commercial serological kits use crude *Toxoplasma* antigens prepared through mouse passages or cell culture systems [29, 30]. The soluble native antigen of *T. gondii* parasite has been applied as a diagnostic marker in various seroepidemiological studies [4], a researcher used crude native antigen of type I and II, for example [1]. Crude *T. gondii* tachyzoite antigen applied in an indirect ELISA yielded sensitivity and specificity of 95.75 and 85.11%, respectively [31]. A significant variation between laboratories exists in the process of producing native antigen. Furthermore, antigen contamination with non-parasitic materials is also possible because of the lack of standard method for antigen purification [32]. Moreover, the use of ve pathogens in antigen preparation process needs extra care because of biological hazards generated by the parasite [33]. Therefore, serological tests that use tachyzoite crude antigens seem difficult to standardize [32]. To overcome this limitation and improve the serodiagnostic tests, recombinant antigen may be used as an alternative diagnostic marker, and it could replace the native antigens [34].

## 6. Recombinant antigens

Application of the recombinant antigens in serodiagnostic kits reduces the native antigen production time and significantly reduces the antigen production cost. Furthermore, better test standardization is achieved when recombinant antigen is used [35]. Moreover, the particular antigenicity of specific antigen can be easily investigated, and with the ability to combine more than one antigen to evaluate their diagnostic value, definitely this will facilitate the standardization of diagnostic assays [29]. If the synthesis of any selected antigens during the parasite life cycle is related to acute or chronic phase of infection, application of this particular antigen as discriminating tool leads to significant improvement in *Toxoplasma* diagnosis [35]. The use of recombinant DNA technology to obtain identical antigenic protein helps in overcoming the biohazard problem related to native antigens production and is greatly beneficial to reduce time, cost and labor consumption. Interestingly, one of the most advantageous of using recombinant antigen in the development of diagnostic tests is that the potential to determine precise protein composition, with reduced non-parasitic material. In addition, more than one antigen can be combined in a single test [32].

Recently, several *T. gondii* antigenic genes have been successfully cloned and expressed using various expression systems. Many reports indicate the successful use of recombinant antigen in toxoplasmosis serodiagnostic tests [33]. The antigens that have been extensively involved in the progress of *T. godii* diagnosis improvement include the surface antigens (SAGs) [36], dense granule antigens (GRAs) [36], microneme antigens (MICs) [37], and rhoptry antigens (ROPS) [33]. More details about the application of *T. gondii* recombinant antigens in the diagnostic studies are illustrated in **Table 1**. Most previous and current studies approved that recombinant protein technology significantly improves the serodiagnosis of *T. gondii* infection. Moreover, the uses of recombinant antigen allow not only the detection of anti-*T. gondii* antibodies but also differentiation between recently acquired and previous infections, resulting in reduced medical complication risk of the disease in immunocompromised patients, especially pregnant women [32]. The potential ability of specific *T. gondii* recombinant antigen to identify the clinical phases of the disease was extensively studied, in the attempts to discriminate acute from chronic infection. The performance of recombinant antigen seems to be sensitive enough and promising in differentiating acute versus chronic infection [35, 38]. Although there is no clear definition of either chronic or acute infection, identification of recently acquired infection normally relies on the detection of specific IgM in patients serum; however, IgM might persist for a long time after infection. Thus, the results may not be precise to indicate recent infection, unless the serum is subjected to additional method such as the IgG avidity, definitely this will improve the accuracy of identification of the infection occurrence. Performance of IgG avidity assay by using *T. gondii* recombinant antigens may be useful for identification of toxoplasmosis phases.

| Antigen | Diagnostic test | Sensitivity % | Specificity % | Reference |
|---|---|---|---|---|
| SAG1 | ELISA (IgG) | 100 | 100 | [39] |
| | Rapid diagnostic test (RDT) | 100 | 99.4 | [40] |
| SAG2 | ELISA (IgG) | 100 | 89.4 | [41] |
| SAG3 | ELISA (IgG) | 95.4 | 91.2 | [41] |
| GRA1 | ELISA (IgG) | 100 | 100 | [42] |
| GRA2 | Western blot | 100 | 90 | [43] |
| GRA5 | Western blot | 100 | 46.8 | [38] |
| GRA7 | ELISA (IgG) | 93.2 | 94.0 | |
| ROP1 | ELISA (IgG) | 100 | 100 | [44] |
| ROP8 | Western blot | 90 | 94 | [33] |

**Table 1.** Recombinant antigens of *T. gondii* as serodiagnostic markers.

## 7 Epitope-based antigen

The epitope or antigenic determinant is an antigenic part of a protein that possesses the potential ability to be recognized by T and B cells receptors or the antibodies binding sites [45]. The epitope is classified into two categories based on their primary structure: linear (continuous) epitope if the amino acids sequences in the epitope are continuous or conformational (discontinuous) epitope which composed from discontinuous sections of amino acid [46]. Attempts to achieve high sensitive and specific diagnostic assay usually assume that replacing the native antigen in all current diagnostic kits by standard and reliable reagents can significantly increase the assay performance [30]. In recent years, it has been demonstrated that the use of peptide-based antigen can meet the demand to standardize the serodiagostic test of toxoplasmosis and increase the sensitivity and specificity of these assays. Furthermore, the ability to distinguish between previous and recently acquired infection can be also achieved [47].

Theoretically, epitope or multiepitopes show numerous advantages compared with crude native antigen because they apply only the antibody-binding sites of the antigen, which definitely increase the accuracy of the test. The applied antigen composition in the serodiagnostic test will be known precisely, the ability to apply more than one identified epitope, easily standardization of the assays, application of only antigen epitope will reduce the biohazard problems in using live pathogens [30]. Nowadays, the use of a diagnostic marker that contains a high density of antibody binding site increases the chances of antibody detection in serum samples and provides the potential to acquire inexpensive diagnostic methods with a high degree of specificity and sensitivity. Therefore, a great possibility to improve diagnostic tests performance exists if multiepitope peptide is applied [48]. Application of multiepitopes antigen in diagnostic tests has been conducted successfully in several studies, employing multiepitope peptide in hepatitis C [49], influenza virus [50], leishmaniasis [51], leprosy

[52], *Trypanosoma cruzi* [53], leptospirosis, and *Mycobacterium tuberculosis* [54, 55] as well as *T. gondii* infection [30]. In all these studies, multiepitope proteins were proposed to enhance the test sensitivity. Identification of specific peptide epitope targeted by the host immunoglobulin allows better understanding of the immune response toward the parasite, as well as the development of accurate diagnostic tool, for development of diagnostic kit multiepitope antigen, appears as most promising antigens that can be used in routine toxoplasmosis screening [56].

Recently, bioinformatics tools are widely applied for epitope identification in protein analysis. Consequently, various epitope peptides are used to develop diagnostic antigen and epitope-based vaccines [47]. By using software-based prediction techniques, the SAG1 B cell epitope of *T. gondii* has been analyzed. Consequently, 11 selected peptides were successfully synthesized. The potential antigenicity of these peptides was evaluated by ELISA using pig sera collected from different periods of post infection. Four of 11 peptides showed high reactivity and were identified by all sera, whereas the rest of the peptides interacted with selected sera only [57]. When the same procedure was applied to *T. gondii* GRA1, 3 of 11 peptides were successfully recognized by all sera. The study suggested that these epitopes can activate the host immune system and generate constant immune response because its immunoreactivity was not affected when evaluated using sera collected from different time periods following the infection [47].

The involvement of GRA1 immunodominant B cell epitope in inducing antibody production by the human immune system was previously identified [58], whereas the immunodominant epitope on GRA1 was also located and accessed using pig sera. The result indicates high immunoreactivity as well as the capability of the peptide to improve the toxoplasmosis serodiagnostic tests [56]. The newly synthesized immunodominant epitopes of *T. gondii* antigens (SAG1, SAG2, SAG3, GRA5, GRA6, and P35) appear to be the most promising diagnostic reagents can be applied in routine toxoplasmosis screening The demonstrated multiepitope peptides can successfully replace the recombinant antigens for differentiating the recently acquired infection from the previous infection; thus, it can serve as an effective tool for human serodiagnosis [30].

The advantage of using epitope peptide in serodiagnostic tests can easily increase the assay sensitivity by applying different peptides. Alternatively, the use of multiepitope peptide that expresses a high density of conserved antigenic determinant can contribute in achieving a high degree of sensitivity and specificity [48, 53]. Multiepitope peptide has been evaluated to obtain specific and standard antigens for serodiagnosis of *T. gondii* infection. Findings showed promising results for developing more accurate assays with high degree of sensitivity and specificity and can differentiate between chronic and acute phases of infection [30, 46]. Multiepitope antigen expressed in *Escherichia coli* system provides the potential to replace the currently used crude antigen. This antigen can also contribute in developing accurate and inexpensive diagnostic assay with high degree of sensitivity and specificity. Therefore, recombinant multiepitope peptide appears as an attractive starting point for future development of *T. gondii* serodiagnosis and immunization [30, 48].

## 8. Concluding remarks

The diagnosis of *T. gondii* infection is still a huge challenge to the medical knowledge and clinical acumen of physicians. Currently, the serological diagnosis plays a vital role in the identification of both human and animal toxoplasmosis. However, the insufficient accuracy of current diagnostic tests due to the lack of standardization in the production of the *T. gondii* whole-cell lysate necessitates the exploration of standard diagnostic reagents. Nowadays, it is speculated that application of recombinant multiepitope antigens in toxoplasmosis serodiagnostic methods would significantly improve the sensitivity and specificity of these methods. Accordingly, the increased usage of the bioinformatics and recombinant DNA technology will dramatically assist in designing and producing of novel epitope-based antigen, which will be crucial to acquire effective serodiagnostic methods for toxoplamosis.

## Author details

Zeehaida Mohamed[1]* and Khalid Hajissa[2]

*Address all correspondence to: zeehaida@usm.my

1 Department of Medical Microbiology & Parasitology, School of Medical Sciences, Universiti Sains Malaysia, Kubang Kerian, Kelantan, Malaysia

2 Department of Zoology, Faculty of Science and Technology, Omdurman Islamic University, Omdurman, Sudan

## References

[1] Sun X, Lu H, Jia B, Chang Z, Peng S, Yin J, et al. A comparative study of *Toxoplasma gondii* seroprevalence in three healthy Chinese populations detected using native and recombinant antigens. Parasit. Vectors. 2013;6:241.

[2] Gatkowska J, Hiszczynska-Sawicka E, Kur J, Holec L, Dlugonska H. *Toxoplasma gondii*: an evaluation of diagnostic value of recombinant antigens in a murine model. Exp. Parasitol. 2006;114(3):220–7.

[3] Terkawi MA, Kameyama K, Rasul NH, Xuan X, Nishikawa Y. Development of an immunochromatographic assay based on dense granule protein 7 for serological detection of *Toxoplasma gondii* infection. Clin. Vaccine Immunol. 2013;20(4):596–601.

[4] Sudan V, Jaiswal AK, Shanker D. Recent trends in the diagnosis of toxoplasmosis. Clin. Rev. Opin. 2013;5(2):11–7.

[5] Montoya JG. Laboratory diagnosis of *Toxoplasma gondii* infection and toxoplasmosis. J. Infect. Dis. 2002;185(Suppl1):S73–S82.

[6] Sarkari B, Asgari Q, Bagherian N, Esfahani SA, Kalantari M, Mohammadpour I, et al. Molecular and serological evaluation of Toxoplasma gondii infection in reared Turkeys in Fars Province, Iran. Jundishapur J. Microbiol. 2014;7(7): e11598. doi: 10.5812/jjm.11598

[7] Burg JL, Grover CM, Pouletty P, Boothroyd J. Direct and sensitive detection of a pathogenic protozoan, *Toxoplasma gondii*, by polymerase chain reaction. J. Clin. Microbiol. 1989;27(8):1787–92.

[8] Liu Q, Wang Z-D, Huang S-Y, Zhu X-Q. Diagnosis of toxoplasmosis and typing of *Toxoplasma gondii*. Parasit. Vectors. 2015;8(1):292.

[9] Robert-Gangneux F, Darde ML. Epidemiology of and diagnostic strategies for toxoplasmosis. Clin. Microbiol. Rev. 2012;25(2):264–96.

[10] Rorman E, Zamir CS, Rilkis I, Ben-David H. Congenital toxoplasmosis—prenatal aspects of *Toxoplasma gondii* infection. Reprod. Toxicol. 2006;21(4):458–72.

[11] Lopes FMR, Gonçalves DD, Mitsuka-Breganó R, Freire RL, Navarro IT. *Toxoplasma gondii* infection in pregnancy. Braz. J. Infect. Dis. 2007;11(5):496–506.

[12] Dubey JP. The history of *Toxoplasma gondii*—the first 100 years. J. Eukaryot. Microbiol. 2008;55(6):467–75.

[13] Bortoletti Filho J, Araujo Júnior E, Carvalho NdS, Helfer TM, Nogueira Serni Pdo, Nardozza LMM, et al. The Importance of IgG avidity and the polymerase chain reaction in treating toxoplasmosis during pregnancy: current knowledge. Interdiscip. Perspect. Infect. Dis. 2013;2013. Volume 2013 (2013), Article ID 370769, 5 pages. http://dx.doi.org/10.1155/2013/370769

[14] Sabin AB, Feldman HA. Dyes as microchemical indicators of a new immunity phenomenon affecting a protozoon parasite (*Toxoplasma*). Science. 1948;108(2815):660–3.

[15] Grillo R, Gross U, Hayde M, Holliman R, Ho-Yen D, Janitschke K, et al. The past and present role of the Sabin±Feldman dye test in the serodiagnosis of toxoplasmosis. Bull. World Health Organ. 1999;77(11); 929-935.

[16] Udonsom R, Buddhirongawatr R, Sukthana Y. Is Sabin-Feldman dye test using *T. gondii* tachyzoites from animal inoculation still the best method for detecting *Toxoplasma gondii* antibodies?. Southeast Asian J. Trop. Med. Public Health. 2010;41(5):1059.

[17] Saraei M, Shojaee S, Esmaeli A, Jahani-Hashemi H, Keshavarz H. Evaluation of confounders in toxoplasmosis indirect fluorescent antibody assay. Iran J. Parasitol. 2010;5(4):55.

[18] Bouer A, Werther K, Machado RZ, Nakaghi ACH, Epiphanio S, Catão-Dias JL. Detection of anti-*Toxoplasma gondii* antibodies in experimentally and naturally infected non-human primates by Indirect Fluorescence Assay (IFA) and indirect ELISA. Rev. Bras. Parasitol. Vet. 2010;19(1):26–31.

[19] Remington JS, Araujo FG, Desmonts G. Recognition of different Toxoplasma antigens by IgM and IgG antibodies in mothers and their congenitally infected newborns. J. Infect. Dis. 1985;152(5):1020–4.

[20] Daniel G. Development of a MODoclonal-Antibody Based Antigen Detection Enzyme Linked Immunosorbent Assay (ELISA) for the Diagnosis of Ruman Toxoplasmosis. In: Department of Microbiology & Immunology McGill University M, editor. 2001.

[21] Desmonts G, Remington JS. Direct agglutination test for diagnosis of Toxoplasma infection: method for increasing sensitivity and specificity. J. Clin. Microbiol. 1980;11(6):562–8.

[22] Mazumder P, Chuang H, Wentz MW, Wiedbrauk DL. Latex agglutination test for detection of antibodies to *Toxoplasma gondii*. J. Clin. Microbiol. 1988;26(11):2444–6.

[23] Voller A, Bidwell D, Bartlett A, Fleck D, Perkins M, Oladehin B. A microplate enzyme-immunoassay for toxoplasma antibody. J. Clin. Pathol. 1976;29(2):150–3.

[24] Döskaya M, Caner A, Can H, İz SG, Gedik Y, Döskaya AD, et al. Diagnostic value of a Rec-ELISA using *Toxoplasma gondii* recombinant SporoSAG, BAG1, and GRA1 proteins in murine models infected orally with tissue cysts and oocysts. PLoS One. 2014.9

[25] Seefeldt SL, Kirkbride CA, Dubey JP. Comparison of enzyme-linked immunosorbent assay, indirect fluorescent antibody test, and direct agglutination test for detecting *Toxoplasma gondii* antibodies in naturally aborted ovine fetuses. J. Vet. Diagn. Invest. 1989;1(2):124–7.

[26] Shaapan R, El-Nawawi F, Tawfik M. Sensitivity and specificity of various serological tests for the detection of *Toxoplasma gondii* infection in naturally infected sheep. Vet. Parasitol. 2008;153(3):359–62.

[27] Liesenfeld O, Press C, Montoya JG, Gill R, Isaac-Renton JL, Hedman K, et al. False-positive results in immunoglobulin M (IgM) toxoplasma antibody tests and importance of confirmatory testing: the Platelia Toxo IgM test. J. Clin. Microbiol. 1997;35(1):174–8.

[28] Fuccillo D, Madden D, Tzan N, Sever J. Difficulties associated with serological diagnosis of *Toxoplasma gondii* infections. Diagn. Clin. Immunol. 1986;5(1):8–13.

[29] Cóceres VM, Becher ML, De Napoli MG, Corvi MM, Clemente M, Angel SO. Evaluation of the antigenic value of recombinant *Toxoplasma gondii* HSP20 to detect specific immunoglobulin G antibodies in *Toxoplasma* infected humans. Exp. Parasitol. 2010;126(2):263–6.

[30] Dai J, Jiang M, Wang Y, Qu L, Gong R, Si J. Evaluation of a recombinant multiepitope peptide for serodiagnosis of *Toxoplasma gondii* infection. Clin. Vaccine Immunol. 2012;19(3):338–42.

[31] Titilincu A, Mircean V, Anamaria I, Cozma V. Development of an Indirect ELISA Test Using Tachyzoite Crude Antigen for Sero-Diagnosis of Sheep Toxoplasma gondii Infection. Bull. Univ. Agric. Sci. Vet. Med. Cluj-Napoca Vet. Med. 2009;66(2). http://dx.doi.org/10.15835/buasvmcn-vm:66:2:4164

[32] Holec-Gąsior L. *Toxoplasma gondii* recombinant antigens as tools for serodiagnosis of human toxoplasmosis–the current status of studies. Clin. Vaccine Immunol. 2013:CVI. 00117–13.

[33] Sonaimuthu P, Fong MY, Kalyanasundaram R, Mahmud R, Lau YL. Sero-diagnostic evaluation of *Toxoplasma gondii* recombinant Rhoptry antigen 8 expressed in *E. coli*. Parasit. Vectors. 2014;7(1):297.

[34] Cai Y, Wang Z, Li J, Li N, Wei F, Liu Q. Evaluation of an indirect ELISA using recombinant granule antigen Gra7 for serodiagnosis of *Toxoplasma gondii* infection in cats. J. Parasitol. 2015;101(1):37–40.

[35] Ferrandiz J, Mercier C, Wallon M, Picot S, Cesbron-Delauw M-F, Peyron F. Limited value of assays using detection of immunoglobulin G antibodies to the two recombinant dense granule antigens, GRA1 and GRA6 Nt of *Toxoplasma gondii*, for distinguishing between acute and chronic infections in pregnant women. Clin. Diagn. Lab. Immunol. 2004;11(6):1016–21.

[36] Sun X, Wang Z, Li J, Wei F, Liu Q. Evaluation of an indirect ELISA using recombinant granule antigen GRA1, GRA7 and soluble antigens for serodiagnosis of Toxoplasma gondii infection in chickens. Res. Vet. Sci. 2015;100;161-164.

[37] Yang D, Liu J, Hao P, Wang J, Lei T, Shan D, et al. MIC3, a novel cross-protective antigen expressed in *Toxoplasma gondii* and *Neospora caninum*. Parasitol. Res. 2015;114(10):3791–9.

[38] Ching XT, Lau YL, Fong MY, Nissapatorn V, Andiappan H. Recombinant dense granular protein (GRA5) for detection of human toxoplasmosis by Western Blot. Biomed. Res. Int. Volume 2014 (2014), Article ID 690529, 8 pages. http://dx.doi.org/10.1155/2014/690529

[39] Bel-Ochi NC, Bouratbine A, Mousli M. Enzyme-linked immunosorbent assay using recombinant SAG1 antigen to detect *Toxoplasma gondii*-specific immunoglobulin G antibodies in human sera and saliva. Clin. Vaccine Immunol. 2013;20(4):468–73.

[40] Chong C-K, Jeong W, Kim H-Y, An D-J, Jeoung H-Y, Ryu J-E, et al. Development and clinical evaluation of a rapid serodiagnostic test for toxoplasmosis of cats using recombinant SAG1 antigen. Korean J. Parasitol. 2011;49(3):207–12.

[41] Khanaliha K, Motazedian MH, Kazemi B, Shahriari B, Bandehpour M, Sharifniya Z. Evaluation of recombinant SAG1, SAG2, and SAG3 antigens for serodiagnosis of toxoplasmosis. Korean J. Parasitol. 2014;52(2):137–42.

[42] Holec-Gąsior L, Ferra B, Hiszczyńska-Sawicka E, Kur J. The optimal mixture of *Toxoplasma gondii* recombinant antigens (GRA1, P22, ROP1) for diagnosis of ovine toxoplasmosis. Vet. Parasitol. 2014;206(3):146–52.

[43] Ching XT, Lau YL, Fong MY, Nissapatorn V. Evaluation of *Toxoplasma gondii*-recombinant dense granular protein (GRA2) for serodiagnosis by western blot. Parasitol. Res. 2013;112(3):1229–36.

[44] Wang Z, Ge W, Huang S-Y, Li J, Zhu X-Q, Liu Q. Evaluation of recombinant granule antigens GRA1 and GRA7 for serodiagnosis of *Toxoplasma gondii* infection in dogs. BMC Vet Res. 2014;10(1):158.

[45] Saha S, Raghava G. Prediction of continuous B-cell epitopes in an antigen using recurrent neural network. Proteins. 2006;65(1):40–8.

[46] Van Regenmortel M. Synthetic peptide vaccines and the search for neutralization B cell epitopes. Open Vaccine J. 2009;2:33–44.

[47] Wang Y, Wang G, Ou J, Yin H, Zhang D. Analyzing and identifying novel B cell epitopes within *Toxoplasma gondii* GRA4. Parasit. Vectors. 2014;7(1):474.

[48] De Souza MQ, Galdino AS, dos Santos JC, Soares MV, Nóbrega YCd, Álvares AdCM, et al. A recombinant multiepitope protein for hepatitis B diagnosis. Biomed. Res. Int. Volume 2013 (2013), Article ID 148317, 7 pages. http://dx.doi.org/10.1155/2013/148317

[49] Dipti CA, Jain S, Navin K. A novel recombinant multiepitope protein as a hepatitis C diagnostic intermediate of high sensitivity and specificity. Protein. Expr. Purif. 2006; 47(1):319–28.

[50] Stoloff GA, Caparros-Wanderley W. Synthetic multi-epitope peptides identified in silico induce protective immunity against multiple influenza serotypes. Eur. J. Immunol. 2007; 37(9):2441–9.

[51] Menezes-Souza D, de Oliveira Mendes TA, Nagem RAP, de Oliveira Santos TT, Silva ALT, Santoro MM, et al. Mapping B-Cell Epitopes for the peroxidoxin of Leishmania (Viannia) braziliensis and its potential for the clinical diagnosis of tegumentary and visceral leishmaniasis. PLoS One. 2014;9(6):e99216.

[52] Duthie MS, Hay MN, Morales CZ, Carter L, Mohamath R, Ito L, et al. Rational design and evaluation of a multiepitope chimeric fusion protein with the potential for leprosy diagnosis. Clin. Vaccine Immunol. 2010;17(2):298–303.

[53] Camussone C, Gonzalez V, Belluzo MS, Pujato N, Ribone ME, Lagier CM, et al. Comparison of recombinant *Trypanosoma cruzi* peptide mixtures versus multiepitope chimeric proteins as sensitizing antigens for immunodiagnosis. Clin. Vaccine Immunol. 2009; 16(6):899–905.

[54] Lin Xa, Chen Y, Yan J. Recombinant multiepitope protein for diagnosis of leptospirosis. Clin. Vaccine Immunol. 2008;15(11):1711–4.

[55] Cheng Z, Zhao JW, Sun ZQ, Song YZ, Sun QW, Zhang XY, et al. Evaluation of a novel fusion protein antigen for rapid serodiagnosis of tuberculosis. J. Clin. Lab. Anal. 2011; 25(5):344–9.

[56] Wang Y, Wang G, Zhang D, Yin H, Wang M. Identification of novel B cell epitopes within *Toxoplasma gondii* GRA1. Exp. Parasitol. 2013;135(3):606–10.

[57] Wang Y, Wang G, Zhang D, Yin H, Wang M. Screening and identification of novel B cell epitopes of *Toxoplasma gondii* SAG1. Parasit. Vectors. 2013;6:125.

[58] Beghetto E, Pucci A, Minenkova O, Spadoni A, Bruno L, Buffolano W, et al. Identification of a human immunodominant B-cell epitope within the GRA1 antigen of *Toxoplasma gondii* by phage display of cDNA libraries. Int. J. Parasitol. 2001;31(14):1659–68.

# 13

# Prevalence, Genetic Diversity, Tissue Distribution, and Risk Factors Contributing to *T. gondii* Burden in Domestic Pigs

Małgorzata Jennes and Eric Cox

**Abstract**

*Toxoplasma gondii* is an obligatory intracellular parasite of mammals, including humans and domestic animals. The infection with this parasite has severe clinical consequences, as it causes abortion or fetal abnormalities, encephalitis in immunocompromised humans, ocular toxoplasmosis with chorioretinitis, and it may contribute to Alzheimer disease. Therefore, an efficient control of *T. gondii* by prevention of the transmission to humans is strongly recommended. Pork is considered as an important source of toxoplasmosis, due to the frequent consumption of the raw or undercooked porcine meat products, a high susceptibility of pigs to the infection, and because of the numerous risk factors, contributing to the prevalence of toxoplasmosis in the pig population. The cellular and humoral immune responses, such as IgM, IgG, IFN-gamma, and interleukin-10 or -12 production, associated with the acute and chronic infection in pigs, do not prevent development of the tissue cysts, which persist lifelong within the intermediate host. Therefore, the prevalence of *T. gondii* in the pig population might be an useful indication of the risk associated with the consumption of the porcine meat.

**Keywords:** *Toxoplasma gondii*, pigs, meat, risk factors, parasitic burden

## 1. Introduction

*Toxoplasma gondii* is an obligate and worldwide-distributed intracellular parasite, causing disease in all warm-blooded animals, which includes aquatic and terrestrial mammals and birds. The prevalence of toxoplasmosis in humans reaches, depending on the study, 33–50% of the worldwide population, regardless of the geographical location or the economic status of the inhabitants [1, 2]. The pig is, among other domestic and wild mammals, a common intermediate host for *T. gondii*. At the same time, it can trigger human infection via the consumption of raw, undercooked, or cured porcine meat products [3]. Therefore, pork is indicated as one of the major meat sources associated with human food borne *T. gondii* infection, together with *Salmonella* and *Campylobacter* [4].

Although the exact prevalence of this food pathogen, in consumption of meat, is difficult to establish, the subsequent infection rate of humans has been estimated as an average of 300 consumers per 1 infected animal [5]. In addition, nearly all tissues from a pig are used directly for the consumption or processed in other meat products without freezing or cooking, increasing in that way the chance of the transmission of the disease [1].

The naturally infected domestic pigs are considered one of the sources for toxoplasmosis in humans. The lack of an obligatory screening method for the detection of antibodies or the viable parasite in the edible tissues, respectively on farm level or in slaughterhouses, increases the risk that infected animals enter the food chain. The worldwide prevalence of 0.4–93% varies significantly between continents and countries, being determined by diverse serological techniques using different cutoff values. Overall, the results strongly depend on the detection method, the age, and the size of the sampled population. In the developed countries, a spectacular drop in the prevalence of toxoplasmosis was observed in pigs, raised indoor in a strict confinement. Interestingly, next to the management system, many other factors can contribute to the increased risk of infection in pigs in the modern farms. The rodent control is of pivotal importance, together with the proper carcass disposal. The increasing age of the animals, small size of the herd, free range or backyard pigs rather than the strict confinement housing, source of water, and feeding of goat whey to the pigs are frequently listed risk factors. Reversely, organic or biofarms increase the chance of the transmission to pigs, and indirectly, toward humans.

## 2. Prevalence of *T. gondii* in domestic pig

The global incidence of the porcine toxoplasmosis per continent and country is shown in **Table 1**, taking into account the origin and the age of the animals, the farm management, and the serologic assay applied [48, 49]. According to the report from European Food Safety Agency published in 2012 [50], describing the number of the foodborne zoonotic outbreaks between 2008 and 2010, the highest proportion of positive samples in PCR or serology for *T. gondii* across all countries was reported for sheep and goats. However, the clinical manifestation of toxoplasmosis is particularly obvious in these two species due to abortion, so it is also more likely to be confirmed, compared with other animal species, in which the more subtle signs of infection (particularly in the acute phase of the disease) may be missed. Referring to the same report, the prevalence of *T. gondii*-specific antibodies in the porcine serum samples collected in all the EU-states was 2.2% [50].

In general, the seroprevalence of *T. gondii* dropped significantly during the last decades in Europe and in the USA. Corresponding to that, a low (0.0–0.4%) to moderate (36%) prevalence was estimated on conventional pig farms in European countries [43, 48]. In the USA, a higher

| Country | Origin | Prevalence (%) | Assay | Reference [No.] |
|---|---|---|---|---|
| Argentina | Sows | 37.80 | MAT | Venturini et al. (2004) [6] |
| Brazil | Farm | 25.50 | In-house ELISA | de Sousa et al. (2014) [7] |
| | Slaughter | 19.50 | IFAT | Cademartori et al. (2014) [8] |
| | Indoor raised | 11.50 | In-house ELISA | Luciano et al. (2011) [9] |
| | Free range | 20.60 | | |
| | Farm | 13.40 | MAT | Piassa et al. (2010) [10] |
| Canada | Finisher | 0.74 | ELISA kit[4] | Poljak et al. (2008) [11] |
| Chile | Slaughter | 8.80 | ELISA kit[4] | Munoz-Zanzi et al. (2012) [12] |
| China | Finishers | 4.60 | IHAT | Chang et al. (2013) [13] |
| | Farm | 29.60 | In-house ELISA | Du et al. (2012) [14] |
| | Slaughter | 12.00 | IHAT | Wu et al. (2012) [15] |
| | Finishers | 24.50 | In-house ELISA | Tao et al. (2011) [16] |
| | Mixed farm | 53.40 | ELISA kit[5] | Yu et al. (2011) [17] |
| | Sows | 14.40 | IHAT | Huang et al. (2010) [18] |
| Czech Republic | Slaughter | 36.00 | ELISA kit[2] | Bartova and Sedlak (2011) [19] |
| France | Slaughter | 2.00 | ELISA kit[3] | Roqueplo et al. (2011) [20] |
| Germany | Finisher | 4.10 | In-house ELISA | de Buhr et al. (2008) [21] |
| | Sows | 16.50 | IFAT | Damriyasa et al. (2004) [22] |
| Ireland | Finishers | 4.70 | LAT | Halova et al. (2013) [23] |
| Italy | Indoor raised | 16.10 | IFAT, 1/16 | Veronesi et al. (2011) [24] |
| | Slaughter | 16.30 | ELISA kit[1] | Villari et al. (2009) [25] |
| Latvia | Finishers | 0.40 | In-house ELISA | Deksne and Kirjusina (2013) [26] |
| | Free ranged | 6.20 | | |
| Malaysia | Sows | 0.00 | IFAT | Chandrawathani et al. (2008) [27] |
| Mexico | Backyard | 17.20 | MAT | Alvarado-Esquivel et al. (2012) [28] |
| | Farm | 0.50 | | |
| Nepal | Slaughter | 11.70 | In-house ELISA | Devleesshouwer et al. (2013) [29] |
| Panama | Indoor raised | 32.10 | IFAT | Correa et al. (2008) [30] |
| Peru | Slaughter | 27.70 | Western blot | Saavedra et al. (2004) [31] |
| Poland | Slaughter | 26.40 | MAT | Sroka et al. (2008) [32] |
| Portugal | Farm | 9.80 | MAT | Lopes et al. (2013) [33] |
| Romania | Backyard | 30.50 | IFAT | Pastiu et al. (2013) [34] |
| | Sows | 12.40 | | |
| | Finishers | 0.00 | | |

| Country | Origin | Prevalence (%) | Assay | Reference [No.] |
|---|---|---|---|---|
| Serbia | Slaughter | 9.20 | MAT | Klun et al. (2011) [35] |
| Slovakia | Slaughter | 2.16 | ELISA kit[1] | Turcekowa et al. (2013) [36] |
| | Sows | 4.26 | | |
| Spain | Finisher | 9.70 | MAT | Garcia-Bocanegra et al. (2010) [37] |
| | Sows | 24.20 | | |
| Switzerland | Finishers | 14.00 | ELISA kit[3] | Berger-Schoch et al. (2011) [38] |
| | Adult | 3.60 | | |
| | Free range | 13.00 | | |
| Taiwan | Slaughter | 10.10 | LAT | Tsai et al. (2007) [39] |
| The Netherlands | Organic | 10.9 | In-house ELISA | Kijlstra et al. (2008) [40] |
| | Indoor raised | 0.40 | | van der Giessen et al. (2007) [41] |
| | Organic | 2.70 | | |
| | Free range | 5.60 | | |
| | Organic | 3.00 | ELISA-kit[3] | Meerburg et al. (2006) [42] |
| | Indoor raised | 0.00 | LAT | Kijlstra et al. (2004) [43] |
| | Free range | 4.70 | | |
| | Organic | 1.20 | | |
| USA | Indoor raised | 2.60 | ELISA kit[4] | Hill et al. (2010) [44] |
| | Outdoor raised | 6.80 | In-house ELISA | Gebreyes et al. (2008) [45] |
| | Indoor raised | 1.10 | | |
| | Free range | 25.00 | ELISA kit[4] | Dubey et al. (2008) [46] |
| | Slaughter | 16.40 | Western blot | Saavedra et al. (2004) [31] |
| Vietnam | Finisher | 23.00 | MAT | Huong et al. (2007) [47] |
| | Sows | 32.30 | | |
| | Free range | 35.70 | | |

Adapted from Guo et al. [48].

[1]Institut Pourquier, Montpellier, France; [2]ID Screen Toxoplasmosis Indirect, ID-Vet, Grabels, France; [3]p30-ELISA; [4] SafePath Laboratories, Carlsbad, CA; [5]Haitai Biological Pharmaceuticals Co., Ltd., Zhuhai, People's Republic of China.

**Table 1.** Global seroprevalence of *T. gondii* in domestic pigs.

(25%) prevalence was detected in the free range animals than in the outdoor- (6.8%) or indoor-ranged finishers (2.8%) [46, 51]. In the Netherlands, a spectacular drop was seen for the finishers (from 54 to 1.9%; Ref. [72]) and for the seropositive sows (30.9–5.6%; Ref. [41]). In the most industrialized countries, the prevalence is not higher than 5% [2]. Nevertheless, the low prevalence cannot however, prevent the high transmission rate to humans, as even as low as 1% is equal to 1 million *T. gondii* seropositive animals, infecting potentially 300 million humans [52]. To date, there is no obligatory screening or notification system for the detection of seropositive animals on farms or in slaughterhouses within the EU-states. These observations and the possible reasons of the decreased prevalence are discussed in detail under Section 5 (Risk factors associated with porcine toxoplasmosis).

## 3. Genetic diversity

Because of the high clinical relevance, the parasite has been isolated from many naturally infected animals and humans, and molecular analysis of the parasitic genome was performed using restriction fragment length polymorphism (RFLP), PCR, or random amplified polymorphism DNA [53]. The obtained data led to genetic identification of the isolated parasites; and therefore, allowed to distinguish three major multilocus genotypes of *T. gondii*. The genetic lines named I, II, and III correspond to the genetic analysis of the polymorphic surface antigen 2 locus (*SAG2*) [54] and are characterized by a different degree of virulence and pathogenicity in LD50 in mice. Type I is considered as the most virulent genotype, followed by type III and type II. The latter is the most prevalent type present in animal reservoir and human population throughout Europe. Additionally, next to the typical three lineages, some of the strains obtained from South America, Africa, and Asia show an atypical genome or a mixed genotype of the existing ones. These strains are often characterized by an increased virulence in mice [2, 55]. Concerning the genotypes of pigs' isolates, the majority of the strains circulating within the porcine population in North America belong to the genotypes II and III or has a mixed allele composition, while in Europe, genotype II seems to be the most predominant clonal type [56, 57]. In South America, on the contrary, genotype I or mixed types are prevalent in domestic pigs [58].

## 4. Immune responses and tissue distribution upon acute and chronic toxoplasmosis

Upon infection with the parasite, the humoral and cellular immune responses are initiated, while clinically toxoplasmosis in pigs proceeds mainly asymptomatic. Only occasionally, pigs develop clinical signs. Following experimental inoculation of pigs with any infectious stage of *T. gondii* (oocysts, tissue cysts, or tachyzoites), a range of antibodies develops against the parasitic antigens. The time interval between the inoculation and the first detection of the immunoglobulins or cytokines varies depending on the virulence of the used strain, the infectious stage, and the applied dose [37, 59–62].

Secondly, a significant Th1-immune response can be observed as an increase of IFN-$\gamma$ production after inoculation of pigs with a well-defined number of the infectious *T. gondii* strains [61, 63–65]. This increase is positively correlated with the duration of the experiment and can be detected in the serum collected from the infected animals in the supernatant from cultured PBMCs, and also as IFN-$\gamma$ mRNA expression in PBMCs and intestinal lymphoid tissues. The IFN-$\gamma$ production associated with the induced toxoplasmosis in pigs was in this case the result of the activation of the innate and acquired immune system. These immune responses were investigated *in vitro* by determining the cytokine profile until 14 [61], 40 [63], or 56 dpi [66].

Next to IFN-$\gamma$, other cytokines are involved in the immune response. The infection of pigs with the VEG-strain oocysts induced a Th-1 immune response shortly after the inoculation, with the production of IL-15 and TNF-$\alpha$ mRNA [61]. Subsequently, a Th-2 response profile with IL-10 as anti-inflammatory cytokine was detected after the acute phase of the infection, dominated by IFN-$\gamma$ production [63].

During the acute phase of the infection, the immune responses are directed against the disseminating tachyzoites, while throughout the chronic toxoplasmosis they also target the latent cysts with bradyzoites in the variety of tissues. It is well described that the parasite can persist within the intermediate host for a life span and can be found in all internal organs and muscles [67–69]. For instance, in pigs, viable *T. gondii* was recovered from porcine brain, heart, tongue, diaphragm, liver, and kidneys. Additionally, all edible commercial cuts of meat tested are also positive, representing thereby, a potential risk for consumers [4, 70]. It is a subject of discussion and ongoing research whether the host can clear the tissues during the chronic infection phase. In pigs, there is a scientific evidence that tissue cysts can gradually decrease in number and show a decline in viability, as tested by bioassay [66].

## 5. Risk factors associated with the porcine toxoplasmosis

Several factors can potentially modify the risk of *T. gondii* infection in pigs, such as the presence of cats on farms, rodent control, age of the animals, size and type of the herd, outdoor access, the carcass disposal, and feeding of unprocessed animal products such as goat whey to the pigs [41, 44, 49, 71].

The cat is responsible for the direct transmission of toxoplasmosis to farm animals such as pigs by entering the stables and shedding the oocysts in the animal facilities, or by contaminating the environment, and indirect spread of oocyts by animals entering the stables like dogs or birds. The free access to stables for people, without the application of strict hygienic measures (e.g., disinfecting foot bath or protective footwear and clothes for the exclusive use in the animal facilities) can also contribute to the dissemination of the oocysts within the herd or its transmission to the stables from the contaminated environment. The lack of these measures is especially important if domesticated or feral cats live in the close neighborhood of the animal facilities.

The second factor, namely the insufficient rodent control in the stables drives the persistence of the parasite on farm level in two ways: the rodents serve as a constant reservoir of the parasite for the cats, maintaining directly the infection risk within the herd; additionally, the rodents can directly be involved in the infection transmission by the predation or accidental ingestion of the mice by pigs [40, 56].

Age as a risk factor is strictly associated with a longer exposure and evidenced by an increased seroprevalence in older animals in comparison with piglets. As colostral antibodies disappear by 120 days of age, piglets and young raising pigs do not have any maternal immune protection, and are, therefore, exposed to the infection [71]. However, the humoral immunity alone is not sufficient in combating the parasite. Indeed, the antibodies facilitate the cytotoxicity by the innate immune cells toward the extracellular parasite, but the intracellular *T. gondii* can escape from that. The age-dependent increase in seroprevalence in pig farms have been described in numerous studies, showing a higher incidence in adult pigs (19.5%) than in young animals (10.9%) [28], or in breeding sows than in finishers (30.9% and 1.9%, respectively, in the Netherlands [72] and 24.2% and 9.7%, respectively, in Spain [28].

The age of the animals at slaughter has also an important implication for the transmission of the disease toward human consumers and the epidemiology of human toxoplasmosis. Indeed, the younger the animals, the more chance that the meat will be consumed fresh and unprocessed, while the meat derived from older animals such as sows, will undergo processing to different pork products, which is harmful for the parasite and thus, safer for the consumer in terms of parasitic load [49].

Two major factors contributing to porcine toxoplasmosis are the size of the herd and the management type of the herd with a reverse correlation between the size and the on-farm prevalence: small herds showed a higher rate of seropositive animals (4.1%) than medium (1.9%) or large (0.6%) herds [51]. The reason for that would be the higher exposure per animal in smaller farms due to the lower density of the pigs. Even more critical for the risk for toxoplasmosis is the management type of the farm. The recently observed decrease in seroprevalence of toxoplasmosis in the pig population in the developed countries might be due to the implementation of the modern management system in porcine herds, with a visible shift from housing of a smaller number of animals in less strictly confined establishments or outdoor, to large scale facilities with a high output and a fast turn-over, characterized by all-in-all-out or farrow-to-finish models [44, 48, 73]. The extensive pig production expressed by the increasing number and size of porcine herds is driven by the high consumption of porcine meat in the developed countries in Europe and in the USA. In Belgium for instance, the total yearly number of pigs comprise 6.5 million animals, housed in 5000 conventional farms, ranging between on average 700–1300 pigs, as estimated by the National Institute of the Calculations, Federal Public Service Economy, (Actualization of the Industrial Study on Pork, 2015). Consequently, nearly 12 million of animals are slaughtered each year, due to an excessive consumption rate per inhabitant (35 kg/year), in comparison with other countries.

Summarizing, in the modern large-scale herds, the risk of *T. gondii* infection and thus, the prevalence of seropositive animals can be substantially reduced by the employment of a strict confinement housing with restrictive biosecurity regulations [1, 44, 45, 48].

However, in the last years, a new tendency in animal husbandry deserves the attention, namely the animal-friendly herds, housing organic or free range animals, providing daily a permanent or a temporary outdoor access to the animals. The term 'organic' refers to the quality and safety of the porcine products, with constraints about the chemical compounds originating from the feed or drug treatment, while 'free range' stands for the life quality of the animals during the production round. Hence, organic pigs are mainly reared outdoor, receive an organic feed, are provided with an animal friendly living space, the piglets are weaned at the later age than 3–4 weeks as on the intensive farms, and undergo a restrictive use of the antibiotics. The free range pigs differ from the regular pigs by the outdoor access and straw bedding, but are fed with a standard porcine feed and may receive drug treatment, if necessary, without losing a label as in case of the organic pigs [43]. In both types of farming, pigs are continuously exposed to the parasite by contact with contaminated soil or ground water, and can easily transmit the infection further in the food chain [43, 44, 74].

As indicated above, an appropriate rodent control is of significant importance for the reduction of the risk for porcine toxoplasmosis; in addition to the latter, a proper carcass disposal seems to be equally essential, since both measures are intended to avoid the ingestion of formerly infected tissues [44, 56]. The cases of cannibalism by the accidental access to preliminary dead animals, especially when animal tissues are buried or composted are considerably common [41, 44, 49, 71]. Similarly, providing drink water of unknown quality to the pigs, possibly contaminated with the oocysts and feeding of raw animal products such as goat whey is also a potential risk, if made from unprocessed milk containing tachyzoites from a recently infected animal undergoing the dissemination phase [42, 75].

Finally, the prevalence of porcine toxoplasmosis may be influenced by the climate and geographical factors, for example, in altitude, temperature, and humidity, since they have a direct impact on the survival of *T. gondii* oocysts in the environment. As established previously, the oocysts remain infectious for a long period of time in a humid and cold environment, as long as they are not dried out or frozen. Hence, the prevalence of toxoplasmosis in pigs is higher in the mountains (32.1%) than in semi desert areas in Mexico (14%) [28], or in the coastal and northern regions of the USA (2.9–3.2%) than in the south continental part of the country [76].

## Acknowledgements

Belgian Federal Public Service of Health, Food Chain Safety and Environment through the contract RF 13/6274 for its support

## Author details

Malgorzata Jennes* and Eric Cox

*Address all correspondence to: malgorzata.jennes@ugent.be

Laboratory for Immunology, Faculty of Veterinary Medicine, Ghent University, Belgium

## References

[1] Tenter, A.M., Heckeroth, A.R. and Weiss, L.M. (2000). *Toxoplasma gondii*: From animals to humans. Int J Parasitol 30, 1217–1258.

[2] Robert-Gangneux, F. and Dardé, M.L.. (2012). Epidemiology of and diagnostic strategies for toxoplasmosis. Clin Microbiol Rev 25 (2): 264–296.

[3] Cook, A.J.C., Gilbert, R.E., Buffolano, W., Zufferey, J., Petersen, E., Jenum, P.A., Foulon, W., and Semprini, A.E. (2000). Sources of toxoplasma infection in pregnant women: European multicentre case-control study. BMJ 321 (July): 142–147.

[4] Opsteegh, M., Schares, G. and van der Giessen, J., on behalf of the consortium (2016). Relationship between seroprevalence in the main livestock species and presence of Toxoplasma gondii in meat (GP/EFSA/BIOHAZ/2013/01). An extensive literature review. Final report. In: EFSA Supporting Publication 2016, Parma, Italy: EN-996, 294 p.

[5] Fehlhaber, K., Hintersdorf, P., Kruger, G. (2002). [Study on the prevalence of *Toxoplasma gondii* in pigs of different management systems and in minced meat]. Fleischwirtschaft 83, 97–99.

[6] Venturini, M.C., Bacigalupe, D., Venturini, L., Rambeaud, M., Basso, W., Unzaga, J.M. and Perfumo, C.J. (2004). Seroprevalence of *Toxoplasma gondii* in sows from slaughter-houses and in pigs from an indoor and an outdoor farm in Argentina. Vet Parasitol 124: 161–165.

[7] de Sousa, R.Á., Lemos, J.F., Farias, L.A., Lopes, C.D. and dos Santos, K.R. (2014). Seroprevalence and risk factors for *Toxoplasma gondii* infection in pigs in southern Piauí. Braz J Vet Parasitol 23:98–100.

[8] Cademartori, B.G., Santos, L.M.J.F., Oliveira, F.C., Quevedlo, P., Oliveira, P.A., Ramos, T.S., Rocha, A.S.R., Ruas, J.L. and Farias, N.A.R. (2014). Isolation and pathogenicity of *Toxoplasma gondii* in naturally infected (rustic farm) pigs in southern Brazil. Vet Parasitol. 203:207–211.

[9] Luciano, D.M., Menezes, R.C., Ferreira, L.C., Nicolau, J.L., das Neves, L.B., Luciano, R.M., Dahroug, M.A., and Amendoeira, M.R. (2011 Oct–Dec). Occurrence of anti-*Toxoplasma gondii* antibodies in cattle and pigs slaughtered, State of Rio de Janeiro. Rev Bras Parasitol. 20(4):351–353.

[10] Piassa, F.R., de Araú jo, J.B., da Rosa, R.C., Mattei, R.J., da Silva, R.C., Langoni, H., and da Silva, A.V. (2010). Prevalence and risk factors for *Toxoplasma gondii* infection in certified and non-certified pig breeding farms in the Toledo microregion, PR, Brazil. Rev Bras Parasitol Vet 19:152–156.

[11] Poljak, Z., Dewey, C.E., Friendship, R.M., Martin, S.W., Christensen, J., Ojkic, D., Wu, J., and Chow, E. (2008). Pig and herd level prevalence of *Toxoplasma gondii* in Ontario finisher pigs in 2001, 2003, and 2004. Can J Vet Res. 72:303-310. Pulawy 52:545–549.

[12] Munoz-Zanzi, C., R. Tamayo, J. Balboa, and D. Hill (2012). Detection of oocyst-associated toxoplasmosis in swine from southern Chile. Zoonoses Public Health 59:389–392.

[13] Chang, Q. C., Qiu, J.H., Wang, C.R., and Zhu, X.Q. (2013). Seroprevalence of *Toxoplasma gondii* infection in fattening pigs in northeast China. J Parasitol 99:544–545.

[14] Du, F., Zhang, Q., Yu, Q., Hu, M., Zhou, Y., and Zhao, J. (2012). Soil contamination of *Toxoplasma gondii* oocysts in pig farms in central China. Vet Parasitol 187:53–56.

[15] Wu, D., Lv, R., Sun, X., Shu, F., Zhou, Z., Nie, K., Duan, G., and Zou, F. (2012). Seroprevalence of *Toxoplasma gondii* antibodies from slaughter pigs in Chongqing, China Trop Anim Health Prod 44:685–687.

[16] Tao, Q., Wang, Z., Feng, H., Fang, R., Nie, H., Hu, M., Zhou, Y. and Zhao, J. (2011). Seroprevalence and risk factors for *Toxoplasma gondii* infection on pig farms in central China. J Parasitol 97:262–264.

[17] Yu, H.J., Zhang, Z., Liu, Z., Qu, D.F., Zhang, D.F., Zhang, H.L., Zhou, Q.J., and Du, A.F. (2011). Seroprevalence of *Toxoplasma gondii* infection in pigs, in Zhejiang Province, China J Parasitol 97:748–749.

[18] Huang, C.Q., Lin, Y.Y., Dai, A.L., Li, X.H., Yang, X.Y., Yuan, Z.G., and Zhu, X.Q. (2010). Seroprevalence of *Toxoplasma gondii* infection in breeding sows in western Fujian Province, China Trop Anim Health Prod 42:115–118.

[19] Bártová, E., and Sedlák, K. (2011). Seroprevalence of *Toxoplasma gondii* and *Neospora caninum* in slaughtered pigs in the Czech Republic. Parasitology 138:1369–1371.

[20] Roqueplo, C., Halos, L., Cabre, O., and Davoust, B. (2011). *Toxoplasma gondii* in wild and domestic animals from New Caledonia. Parasite 18:345–348.

[21] de Buhr, K., Ludewig, M., and Fehlhaber, K. (2008). *Toxoplasma gondii*—seroprevalence: Current results in German swine herds. Arch Lebensmittelhyg. 59:5–8.

[22] Damriyasa, I.M., Bauer, C., Edelhofer, R., Failing, K., Lind, P., Petersen, E., Schares, G., Tenter, A.M., Volmer, R., and Zahner, H. (2004). Cross-sectional survey in pig breeding farms in Hesse, Germany: Seroprevalence and risk factors of infections with *Toxoplasma gondii*, Sarcocystis spp. and *Neospora caninum* in sows. Vet Parasitol 126:271–286.

[23] Halová, D., Mulcahy, G., Rafter, P., Turcekova, L., Grant, T., and de Waal, T. (2013). *Toxoplasma gondii* in Ireland: Seroprevalence and novel molecular detection method in sheep, pigs, deer and chickens. Zoonoses Public Health 60:168–173.

[24] Veronesi, F., Ranucci, D., Branciari, R., Miraglia, D., Mammoli, R., and Fioretti, D.P. (2011). Seroprevalence and risk factors for *Toxoplasma gondii* infection on finishing swine reared in the Umbria region, central Italy. Zoonoses Public Health 58:178–184.

[25] Villari, S., Vesco, G., Petersen, E., Crispo, A., and Buffolano, W. (2009). Risk factors for toxoplasmosis in pigs bred in Sicily, southern Italy. Vet Parasitol 161:18.

[26] Deksne, G., and Kirjusina, M. (2013). Seroprevalence of *Toxoplasma gondii* in domestic pigs (Sus scrofa domestica) and wild boars (Sus scrofa) in Latvia. J Parasitol 99:44–47.

[27] Chandrawathani, P., Nurulaini, R., Zanin, C.M., Premaalatha, B., Adnan, M., Jamnah, O., Khor, S.K., Khadijah, S., Lai, S.Z., Shaik, M.A.B., Seah, T.C., and Zatil, S.A. (2008). Seroprevalence of *Toxoplasma gondii* antibodies in pigs, goats, cattle, dogs and cats in peninsular Malaysia. Trop Biomed. 25:257–258.

[28] Alvarado-Esquivel, C., Estrada-Malacó, n M.A., Reyes-Hernández, S.O., Pérez-Ramírez, J.A., Trujillo-López, J.I., Villena, I. and Dubey, J.P. (2012). High prevalence

of *Toxoplasma gondii* antibodies in domestic pigs in Oaxaca State, Mexico. J Parasitol 98:1248–1250.

[29] Devleesschauwer, B., Pruvot, M., Joshi, D.D., De Craeye, S., Jennes, M., Ale, A., Welinski, A., Lama, S., Aryal, A., Victor, B., Duchateau, L., Speybroeck, N., Vercruysse, J., Dorny, P. (2013 Dec). Seroprevalence of zoonotic parasites in pigs slaughtered in the Kathmandu Valley of Nepal. Vector Borne Zoonotic Dis. 13(12):872–876. doi: 10.1089/vbz.2013.1313.

[30] Correa, R., Cedeño, I., de Escobar, C., and Fuentes, I. (2008). Increased urban seroprevalence of *Toxoplasma gondii* infecting swine in Panama. Vet Parasitol. 153:9–11.

[31] Saavedra, G.M., and Ortega, Y.R. (2004). Seroprevalence of *Toxoplasma gondii* in swine from slaughterhouses in Lima, Peru, and Georgia, U.S.A. J Parasitol 90:902–904.

[32] Sroka, J., Cencek, T., Ziomko, I., Karamon, J., and Zwolinski, J. (September 2008). Preliminary assessment of ELISA, MAT, and LAT for detecting Toxoplasma gondii antibodies in pigs. Bull Vet Inst. in Pulawy, 52(4): 545–549.

[33] Lopes, A.P., Dubey, J.P., Neto, F., Rodrigues, A., Martins, T., Rodrigues, M., and Cardoso, L. (2013). Seroprevalence of *Toxoplasma gondii* infection in cattle, sheep, goats and pigs from the north of Portugal for human consumption. Vet Parasitol. 193:266–269, 44

[34] Pastiu, A.I., Gyorke, A., Blaga, R., Mircean, V., Rosenthal, B.M., and Cozma, V. (2013). In Romania, exposure to *Toxoplasma gondii* occurs twice as often in swine raised for familial consumption as in hunted wild boar, but occurs rarely if ever among fattening pigs raised in confinement. Parasitol Res. 112:2403–2407.

[35] Klun, I., Vujanić, M., Yera, H., Nikolić, A., Ivović, V., Bobić, B., Bradonjić, S., Dupouy-Camet, J. and Djurković-Djaković, O. (2011). *Toxoplasma gondii* infection in slaughter pigs in Serbia: Seroprevalence and demonstration of parasites in blood. Vet Res 42:17–22.

[36] Turcekova, L., Antolova, D., Reiterova, K., and Spisak, F. (2013). Occurrence and genetic characterization of *Toxoplasma gondii* in naturally infected pigs. Acta Parasitol. 58:361–366.

[37] Garcia, J.L., Gennari, S.M., Navarro, I.T., Machado, R.Z., Sinhorini, I.L., Freire, R.L., Marana, E.R., Tsutsui, V., Contente, A.P., Begale, L.P. (2005). Partial protection against tissue cysts formation in pigs vaccinated with crude rhoptry proteins of *Toxoplasma gondii*. Vet Parasitol 129(3/4):209–217.

[38] Berger-Schoch, A.E., Bernet D., Doherr, M.G., Gottstein, B., and Frey, C.F. (2011). *Toxoplasma gondii* in Switzerland: A serosurvey based on meat juice analysis of slaughtered pigs, wild boar, sheep and cattle. Zoonoses Public Health 58:472–478.

[39] Tsai, Y.J., Chung, W.C., Fei, A.C.Y., Kaphle, K., Peng, S. and Wu, Y.L. (2007). Seroprevalence of *Toxoplasma gondii* in pigs from slaughterhouses in Taiwan. J Parasitol 93:1540–1541.

[40] Kijlstra, A. and Jongert, E. (October 2008). Control of the risk of human toxoplasmosis transmitted by meat. Int J Parasitol. 1359–1370.

[41] van der Giessen, J., Fonville, M., Bouwknegt, M., Langelaar, M., and Vollema, A. (2007). Seroprevalence of *Trichinella spiralis* and *Toxoplasma gondii* in pigs from different housing systems in The Netherlands. Vet Parasitol 148:371–374.

[42] Meerburg, B.G., van Riel, J.W., Cornelissen, J.B., Kijlstra, A., and Mul, M.F. (2006). Cats and goat whey associated with *Toxoplasma gondii* infection in pigs. Vector Borne Zoonotic Dis 6:266–274.

[43] Kijlstra, A., Eissen, O.A., Cornelissen, J., Munniksma, K., Eijck, I., and Kortbeek, T. (2004). *Toxoplasma gondii* infection in animal friendly pig production systems. Invest Ophthalmol Vis Sci 45: 3165–3169.

[44] Hill, D.E., Haley, C., Wagner, B., Gamble, H.R., and Dubey, J.P. (2010). Seroprevalence of and risk factors for *Toxoplasma gondii* in the US swine herd using sera collected during the National Animal Health Monitoring Survey (Swine 2006). Zoonoses Public Health 57:53–59.

[45] Gebreyes, W.A., Bahnson, P.B., Funk, J.A., McKean, J., and Patchanee, P. (2008). Seroprevalence of Trichinella, Toxoplasma, and Salmonella in antimicrobial-free and conventional swine production systems. Foodborne Pathog Dis. 5:199–203.

[46] Dubey, J.P., Hill, D.E., Sundar, N., Velmurugan, G.V., Bandini, L.A., Kwok, O.C.H., Pierce, V., Kelly, K., Dulin, M., Thulliez, P., Iwueke, C., and Su, C. (2008). Endemic toxoplasmosis in pigs on a farm in Maryland: Isolation and genetic characterization of *Toxoplasma gondii*. J Parasitol 94:36–41.

[47] Huong, L.T.T., and Dubey, J.P. (2007). Seroprevalence of *Toxoplasma gondii* in pigs from Vietnam. J Parasitol 93:951–952.

[48] Guo, M., Dubey, J.P., Hill, D., Buchanan, R.L., Gamble, H., Jones, J.L., Pradhan, A.K. (2015). Prevalence and risk factors for *Toxoplasma gondii* infection in meat animals and meat products destined for human consumption. J Food Prot 78, 457–476.

[49] Dubey, J.P. (2009 Oct 14). Toxoplasmosis in pigs – The last 20 years. Vet Parasitol 164(2-4):89-103. doi: 10.1016/j.vetpar.2009.05.018. Review.

[50] European Food Safety Authority, European Centre for Disease Prevention and Control 2012. The European Union summary report on trends and sources of zoonoses, zoonotic agents and food-borne outbreaks in 2010; EFSA Journal; 10(3):2597. [442 pp.] doi:10.2903/j.efsa.2012.2597

[51] Hill D.E., Chirukandoth, S., Dubey J.P., Lunney, J.K., Gamble, H.R. (2006 Oct 10). Comparison of detection methods for *Toxoplasma gondii* in naturally and experimentally infected swine. Vet Parasitol. 141(1-2):9–17.

[52] Jones J.L., and Dubey, J.P. (2012 Sep). Foodborne toxoplasmosis Clin Infect Dis. 55(6): 845–851. doi: 10.1093/cid/cis508. Review.

[53] Sibley, L.D., LeBlanc, A.J., Pfefferkorn, E.R., Boothroyd, J.C. (1992 Dec). Generation of a restriction fragment length polymorphism linkage map for *Toxoplasma gondii*. Genetics. 132(4):1003–1015.

[54] Howe, D.K., Sibley, L.D. (1997 Oct). Development of molecular genetics for *Neospora caninum*: A complementary system to *Toxoplasma gondii*. Methods. 13(2):123–133.

[55] Innes, E.A. (2010 Feb). A brief history and overview of *Toxoplasma gondii*. Zoonoses Public Health. 57(1):1–7. doi: 10.1111/j.1863-2378.2009.01276.x. Review.

[56] Lehmann, T., Graham, D.H., Dahl, E., Sreekumar, C., Launer, F., Corn, J.L., Gamble, H.R., Dubey, J.P. (2003 Jul). Transmission dynamics of *Toxoplasma gondii* on a pig farm. Infect Genet Evol. 3(2):135–141.

[57] de Sousa, S., Ajzenberg, D., Canada, N., Freire, L., da Costa, J.M., Dardé, M.L., Thulliez, P., Dubey, J.P. (2006 Jan 30). Biologic and molecular characterization of *Toxoplasma gondii* isolates from pigs from Portugal. Vet Parasitol. 135(2):133-136. Epub 2005 Sep 26.

[58] Belfort-Neto, R., Nussenblatt, V., Rizzo, L., Muccioli, C., Silveira, C., Nussenblatt, R., Khan, A., Sibley, L.D., Belfort, R. Jr. (Mar 2007). High prevalence of unusual genotypes of *Toxoplasma gondii* infection in pork meat samples from Erechim, Southern Brazil. An Acad Bras Cienc. 79 1 Rio de Janeiro. http://dx.doi.org/10.1590/S0001-37652007000100013.

[59] Dubey, J.P. (1986). A review of toxoplasmosis in pigs. Vet Parasitol 19: 181–223.

[60] Lind, P., Haugegaard, J., Wingstrand, A., Henriksen, S.A. (1997). The time course of the specific antibody response by various ELISAs in pigs experimentally infected with *Toxoplasma gondii*. Vet Parasitol 71, 1–15.

[61] Dawson, H.D., Beshah, E., Nishi, S., Solano-Aguilar, G., Morimoto, M., Zhao, A., Madden, K.B., Ledbetter, T.K., Dubey, J.P., Shea-Donohue, T., Lunney, J.K., Urban, J.F. Jr. (2005). Localized multigene expression patterns support an evolving Th1/ Th2-like paradigm in response to infections with Toxoplasma gondii and Ascaris suum. Infect Immun 2005 Feb;73(2):1116–28.

[62] Jongert, E., Melkebeek, V., De Craeye, S., Dewit, J., Verhelst, D., Cox, E. (2008a). An enhanced GRA1-GRA7 cocktail DNA vaccine primes anti-Toxoplasma immune responses in pigs. Vaccine 26, 1025–1031.

[63] Solano Aguilar, G.I., Beshah, E., Vengroski, K.G., Zarlenga, D., Jauregui, L., Cosio, M., Douglass, L.W., Dubey, J.P., Lunney, J.K. (2001 Feb). Cytokine and lymphocyte profiles in miniature swine after oral infection with *Toxoplasma gondii* oocysts. Int J Parasitol. 31(2):187–195. Erratum in: Int J Parasitol 2001 Jun;31(8):852.

[64] Dawson, H.D., Royaee, A.R., Nishi, S., Kuhar, D., Schnitzlein, W.M., Zuckermann, F., Urban, J. Jr., Lunney, J.K.. (2004 Jul). Identification of key immune mediators regulating T helper 1 responses in swine. Vet Immunol Immunopathol. 100(1-2):105–111.

[65] Verhelst, D., De Craeye, S., Jennes, M., Dorny, P., Goddeeris, B., Cox, E. (2015). Interferon-gamma expression and infectivity of Toxoplasma infected tissues in experimentally infected sheep in comparison with pigs. Vet Parasitol 207 (2015) 7–16.

[66] Verhelst, D., De Craeye, S., Melkebeek, V., Goddeeris, B., Cox, E., Jongert, E. (2011 Jun 30). IFN-γ expression and infectivity of Toxoplasma infected tissues are associated with

an antibody response against GRA7 in experimentally infected pigs. Vet Parasitol. 179 (1-3):14–21.

[67] Dubey, J.P., Lindsay, D.S., Speer, C.A. (1998 Apr). Structures of *Toxoplasma gondii* tachyzoites, bradyzoites, and sporozoites and biology and development of tissue cysts. Clin Microbiol Rev. 11(2):267–299. Review.

[68] Black, M.W., and Boothroyd, J.C. (2000). Lytic cycle of *Toxoplasma gondii*. Microbiology and Molecular Biology Reviews, 64, 3, pp. 607–623.

[69] Montoya, J.G., Liesenfeld, O. (2004 Jun 12). Toxoplasmosis. Lancet. 363(9425):1965–1976.

[70] Dubey, J.P. (1988). Long-term persistence of *Toxoplasma gondii* in tissues of pigs inoculated with *T. gondii* oocysts and effect of freezing on viability of tissue cysts in pork. Am J Vet Res. 1988 Jun;49(6):910–913.

[71] García-Bocanegra, I., Simon-Grifé, M., Dubey, J.P., Casal, J., Martín, G.E., Cabezó n, O., Perea, A., and Almería, S. (2010). Seroprevalence and risk factors associated with *Toxolasma gondii* in domestic pigs from Spain. Parasitol Int. 59:421–426.

[72] van Knapen, F., Kremers, A.F., Franchimont, J.H., Narucka, U. (1995 Sep). Prevalence of antibodies to *Toxoplasma gondii* in cattle and swine in The Netherlands: Towards an integrated control of livestock production. Vet Q. 17(3):87–91.

[73] Davies, P.R., Morrow, W.E., Deen, J., Gamble, H.R., Patton, S. (1998 Jul 17). Seroprevalence of *Toxoplasma gondii* and *Trichinella spiralis* in finishing swine raised in different production systems in North Carolina, USA. Prev Vet Med. 36(1):67–76.

[74] Dubey J.P., Hill, D.E., Rozeboom, D.W., Rajendran, C., Choudhary, S., Ferreira, L.R., Kwok, O.C., Su, C. 2012 Aug 13 High prevalence and genotypes of *Toxoplasma gondii* isolated from organic pigs in northern USA. Vet Parasitol. 188(1-2):14–18. doi: 10.1016/j.vetpar.2012.03.008.

[75] Boughattas, S. (2015 Oct 14). Toxoplasma infection and milk consumption: Meta-analysis of assumptions and evidences. Crit Rev Food Sci Nutr. 0.

[76] Hill, D.E., and Dubey, J.P. (2013). *Toxoplasma gondii* prevalence in farm animals in the United States. Int J Parasitol. 43(2):107–113. doi: 10.1016/j.ijpara.2012.09.012. Review.

# Permissions

All chapters in this book were first published in TOXOPLASMOSIS, by InTech Open; hereby published with permission under the Creative Commons Attribution License or equivalent. Every chapter published in this book has been scrutinized by our experts. Their significance has been extensively debated. The topics covered herein carry significant findings which will fuel the growth of the discipline. They may even be implemented as practical applications or may be referred to as a beginning point for another development.

The contributors of this book come from diverse backgrounds, making this book a truly international effort. This book will bring forth new frontiers with its revolutionizing research information and detailed analysis of the nascent developments around the world.

We would like to thank all the contributing authors for lending their expertise to make the book truly unique. They have played a crucial role in the development of this book. Without their invaluable contributions this book wouldn't have been possible. They have made vital efforts to compile up to date information on the varied aspects of this subject to make this book a valuable addition to the collection of many professionals and students.

This book was conceptualized with the vision of imparting up-to-date information and advanced data in this field. To ensure the same, a matchless editorial board was set up. Every individual on the board went through rigorous rounds of assessment to prove their worth. After which they invested a large part of their time researching and compiling the most relevant data for our readers.

The editorial board has been involved in producing this book since its inception. They have spent rigorous hours researching and exploring the diverse topics which have resulted in the successful publishing of this book. They have passed on their knowledge of decades through this book. To expedite this challenging task, the publisher supported the team at every step. A small team of assistant editors was also appointed to further simplify the editing procedure and attain best results for the readers.

Apart from the editorial board, the designing team has also invested a significant amount of their time in understanding the subject and creating the most relevant covers. They scrutinized every image to scout for the most suitable representation of the subject and create an appropriate cover for the book.

The publishing team has been an ardent support to the editorial, designing and production team. Their endless efforts to recruit the best for this project, has resulted in the accomplishment of this book. They are a veteran in the field of academics and their pool of knowledge is as vast as their experience in printing. Their expertise and guidance has proved useful at every step. Their uncompromising quality standards have made this book an exceptional effort. Their encouragement from time to time has been an inspiration for everyone.

The publisher and the editorial board hope that this book will prove to be a valuable piece of knowledge for researchers, students, practitioners and scholars across the globe.

# List of Contributors

**Antonio Sorlozano-Puerto**
Department of Microbiology, School of Medicine, University of Granada and Biosanitary Research Institute ibs, Granada, Spain

**Jose Gutierrez-Fernandez**
Area of Microbiology, Granada University Hospital Complex, Spain

**María de la Luz Galván Ramírez**
Department of Physiology, University Center of Health Sciences, University of Guadalajara, Guadalajara, Jalisco, Mexico

**Laura Verónica Sánchez Orozco**
Department of Molecular Biology, University Center of Health Sciences, University of Guadalajara, Guadalajara, Jalisco, Mexico

**Cynthia Guadalupe Temores Ramírez**
Department of Cellular and Molecular Biology, University Center of Biological and Agricultural Sciences, University of Guadalajara, Guadalajara, Jalisco, Mexico

**Alessandra F. Gomes and Helene S. Barbosa**
Laboratory of Structural Biology, Oswaldo Cruz Institute, Oswaldo Cruz Foundation, Rio de Janeiro, RJ, Brazil

**Sprakel-Leyke Silja and Presber Wolfgang**
Institute of Microbiology and Hygiene, University of Medicine Berlin (Charité), Berlin, Germany

**Paulke Bernd-Reiner**
Fraunhofer Institute for Applied Polymer Research, Potsdam-Golm, Germany

**Sandra K. Halonen**
Dept. of Microbiology and Immunology, Montana State University, Bozeman, MT, USA

**Oymak Sibel**
Department of Public Health, Faculty of Medicine, Çanakkale Onsekiz Mart University, Canakkale, Turkey

**Hız Meliha Merve**
Department of Medical Biology, Faculty of Medicine, Çanakkale Onsekiz Mart University, Canakkale, Turkey

**Kılıç Sevilay**
Department of Dermatology, Faculty of Medicine, Çanakkale Onsekiz Mart University, Canakkale, Turkey

**Büyük Başak**
Department of Histology and Embriology, Faculty of Medicine, Çanakkale Onsekiz Mart University, Canakkale, Turkey

**Halil İbrahim Taş**
Department of Psychiatry, Faculty of Medicine, Çanakkale Onsekiz Mart University, Canakkale, Turkey

**Ülken Tunga Babaoğlu**
Department of Public Health, Faculty of Medicine, Ahi Evran University, Kırsehir, Turkey

**Chung-Da Yang**
Graduate Institute of Animal Vaccine Technology, College of Veterinary Medicine, National Pingtung University of Science and Technology, Pingtung, Taiwan

**Mariana Acquarone**
Laboratory Frontiers in Neurosciences, Institute of Biomedical Sciences, Federal University of Rio de Janeiro, RJ, Brazil

**Marialice da F. Ferreira-da-Silva**
Institute for Medical Microbiology, Immunology and Hygiene, CECAD, University of Cologne, Cologne, Germany

**Erick V. Guimarães and Helene S. Barbosa**
Laboratory of Structural Biology, Oswaldo Cruz Institute, Oswaldo Cruz Foundation, Rio de Janeiro, RJ, Brazil

**G. F. Dzib Paredes and M. Jiménez-Coello**
Institutional Postgraduate Agricultural Science and Resource Management, CCBA/ UADY, Mérida, Yucatán, México

**A. Ortega-Pacheco and J. A. Rosado-Aguilar**
Department of Animal Health and Preventive Medicine, CCBA/UADY, Merida, Yucatan, Mexico

**K. Y. Acosta-Viana and E. Guzmán -Marín**
Laboratory of Cell Biology, CIR, Dr. Hideyo Noguchi, CA Biomedicine of Infectious and Parasitic Diseases, Autonomous University of Yucatan, Mérida, Yucatán, México

**Aléx Martins Nasaré and Roberto Carlos Tedesco**
Federal University of São Paulo, São Paulo, Brazil

**Alvaro Ferreira Júnior, Jandra P. Santos, Paula B. Bassi, Joely F.F. Bittar and Eustáquio R. Bittar**
Veterinary Medicine School, University of Uberaba, Minas Gerais, Brazil

**Zeehaida Mohamed**
Department of Medical Microbiology & Parasitology, School of Medical Sciences, Universiti Sains Malaysia, Kubang Kerian, Kelantan, Malaysia

**Khalid Hajissa**
Department of Zoology, Faculty of Science and Technology, Omdurman Islamic University, Omdurman, Sudan

**Malgorzata Jennes and Eric Cox**
Laboratory for Immunology, Faculty of Veterinary Medicine, Ghent University, Belgium

# Index

www.ingramcontent.com/pod-product-compliance
Lightning Source LLC
LaVergne TN
LVHW080638210926
848485LV00003B/291